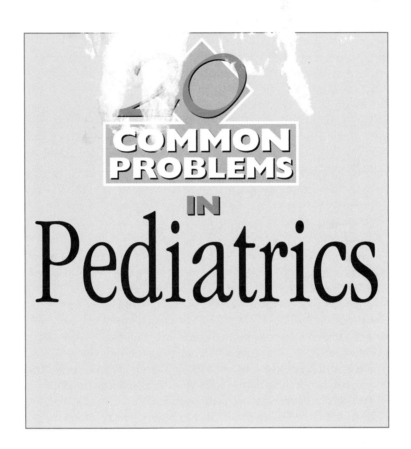

20 COMMON PROBLEMS IN Pediatrics

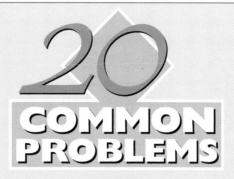

20 COMMON PROBLEMS IN Pediatrics

EDITOR

ABRAHAM B. BERGMAN, M.D.

Director of Pediatrics
Harborview Medical Center, and
Professor of Pediatrics
University of Washington School of Medicine
Seattle, Washington

McGraw-Hill

Medical Publishing Division

New York   St. Louis   San Francisco   Auckland   Bogotá   Caracas   Lisbon   London   Madrid
Mexico City   Milan   Montreal   New Delhi   San Juan   Singapore   Sydney   Tokyo   Toronto

McGraw-Hill

A Division of The McGraw·Hill Companies

618.92

1234567890 DOCDOC 09876543210

ISBN 0-07-134901-4

This book was set in Garamond by Better Graphics, Inc.
The editors were Barbara Holton, Susan Noujaim and Andrea Seils.
The production supervisor was Phil Galea.
The index was prepared by Deborah Tourtlotte.

R R Donnelley and Sons, Inc. was printer and binder.

This book is printed on acid-free paper.

€ 46.00

052052

Library of Congress Cataloging-in-Publication Data

20 common problems in pediatrics / editor, Abraham B. Bergman.
  p. ; cm.
 Includes bibliographical references and index.
 ISBN 0-07-134901-4
  1. Pediatrics. I. Title: Twenty common problems in pediatrics. II. Bergman, Abraham
B., 1932-
 [DNLM: 1. Pediatrics. WS 200 Z999 2001]
 RJ47 .A15 2001
 618.92--dc21
                    00-020236

To Suzanne Fiala,
my wife, lover, friend, medical colleague,
and irreplaceable bookend.

Contents

List of Contributors

Ronald G. Barr, MDCM, FRCP(C)
Professor of Pediatrics and Psychiatry
McGill University Faculty of Medicine

Abraham B. Bergman, MD
Professor of Pediatrics
University of Washington
    School of Medicine
Seattle, Washington

Thomas J. Bowen, MD, FRCPC
Clinical Professor of Pediatrics and Medicine
University of Calgary
Calgary, Alberta, Canada

Peter K. Domoto, DDS, MPH
Chairman, Department of Pediatric Dentistry
University of Washington School of Dentistry
Seattle, Washington

Kenneth W. Feldman, MD
Clinical Professor of Pediatrics
University of Washington School of Medicine
Seattle, Washington

William Feldman, MD, FRCPC
Professor Emeritus of Pediatrics, University of Toronto
Toronto, Ontario, Canada

John M. Freeman, MD
Lederer Professor of Pediatric Epilepsy and
Professor of Neurology and Pediatrics
Johns Hopkins Medical Institutions
Baltimore, Maryland

Frances Page Glascoe, PhD
Associate Professor of Pediatrics
Vanderbilt University
Nashville, Tennessee

Alan L. Goldbloom, MD, FRCPC
Associate Professor of Pediatrics
University of Toronto
Toronto, Ontario, Canada

Saul Greenberg, MD, FRCPC
Associate Professor of Pediatrics
University of Toronto
Toronto, Ontario, Canada

Camille Haisley-Royster, MD
Resident in Medicine (Dermatology)
Duke University
Durham, North Carolina

Julie Lessard, MD, FRCP (C)
Fellow in Developmental Pediatrics
McGill University-Montreal Children's Hospital
    Research Institute
Montreal, Quebec, Canada

Alexander K. C. Leung,
MBBS, FRCP (UK & Irel), FRCPCH, FRCPC, FAAP, FRSH,
FHKAM, FHKCPaed
Clinical Associate Professor of Pediatrics
University of Calgary
Calgary, Alberta, Canada

Ronald L. Lindsay, MD
Clinical Assistant Professor of Pediatrics
Department of Pediatrics
The Ohio State University
Columbus, Ohio

Edward M. McMahon, Jr., MD
Clinical Associate Professor of Pediatrics
University of Washington School of Medicine
Seattle, Washington

Neil S. Prose, MD
Professor of Medicine (Dermatology) and Pediatrics
Duke University
Durham, North Carolina

Michael I. Reiff, MD
Assistant Professor of Pediatrics
University of Minnesota
Minneapolis, Minnesota

Frederick P. Rivara, MD, MPH
George Adkins Professor of Pediatrics
University of Washington School of Medicine
Seattle, Washington

Lance E. Rodewald, MD
Associate Director for Science,
  National Immunization Program
Centers for Disease Control and Prevention
Atlanta, Georgia

Jeanne M. Santoli, MD, MPH
Medical Epidemiologist
National Immunization Program
Centers for Disease Control and Prevention
Atlanta, Georgia

Richard H. Schwartz, MD
Clinical Professor of Pediatrics
University of Virginia
Charlottesville, VA

Sam R. Sharar, MD
Associate Professor of Anesthesiology
University of Washington School of Medicine
Seattle, Washington

F. Estelle R. Simons, MD, FRCPC
Bruce Chown Professor of Pediatrics & Child Health
University of Manitoba
Winnipeg, Manitoba, Canada

James A. Taylor, MD
Associate Professor of Pediatrics
University of Washington School of Medicine
Seattle, Washington

Monica S. Vavilala, MD
Acting Assistant Professor of Anesthesiology
  and Pediatrics
University of Washington School of Medicine
Seattle, Washington

Jeffrey A. Wright, MD
Associate Professor of Pediatrics
University of Washington School of Medicine
Seattle, Washington

Preface

An editor's dilemma: What twenty subjects should be covered in a book on common pediatric problems and which authors should be asked to author them? Should the chapters cover the most frequent presenting symptoms or the most frequent conditions diagnosed by primary care clinicians? And what data should be used to determine which symptoms and/or conditions are most frequently seen? These are some of the questions I pondered after agreeing to edit this book.

As in most things, there are data on the subject, but are the data helpful? The National Center for Health Statistics carries out periodic systematic surveys of ambulatory health care visit encounters by children from a nationwide network of office-based physicians who are not federally employed (National Ambulatory Medical Care Survey) and from hospital outpatient departments and emergency departments (National Hospital Ambulatory Medical Care Survey). Their most recently published data collected in 1993–1995 showed that 75 percent of ambulatory visits occurred in physicians' offices, 8 percent in hospital outpatient departments, and 14 percent in hospital emergency departments. The following account for almost 40 percent of visits: well-child care, 15 percent; middle ear infection, 12 percent; and injuries, 10 percent. Not surprisingly, there was considerable variation in these figures among children on the basis of age, sex, and race.[1]

This information, however valuable as a statistical overview, was not helpful in identifying subjects of interest to individual clinicians. I decided to eschew any pretense of scientific objectivity and instead to exercise my own judgment, using a single criterion: What common symptoms or disorders do *I* have difficulty sorting out when they present to *me?* If I feel the need for guidance in managing a particular problem, then perhaps readers of this book might feel the same way. I thus ceased to worry whether the subjects in this book constituted the 20 symptoms or disorders *most* commonly seen by primary care clinicians. Instead I vouch that none of the subjects covered in this book are rare, and that, in whatever setting, all primary care clinicians who care for infants, children, or adolescents—be they pediatricians, family physicians, nurse practitioners, physicians assistants, or other clinicians—should have a basic understanding of the subject material.

The book is organized into sections on health supervision, acute problems, chronic problems, and development and behavioral problems. The chapters are not uniform in length. For example the chapter on attention deficit hyperactivity disorder (ADHD) is twice as long as several of the other chapters. Again, my personal bias influenced the decision not to edit the chapter down to a smaller one. My traditional pediatric training did not prepare me to diagnose and manage the increasing volume of children who present with ADHD. I thus welcome all the help I can get in dealing with this challenging problem. I also need more help with managing children with elimination disorders, school failure, and developmental problems than I do for children with fever, otitis, and urinary tract infections.

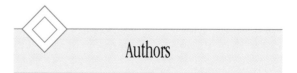

Authors

All of the authors have academic affiliations and are involved in teaching. But more importantly for the purposes of this book, all of them are engaged in active clinical practice. As recognized authorities in their respective fields, I asked the authors to be emphatic in their opinions; the chapters are not meant to be scholarly review articles. Thus Edward (Ted) McMahon, one of the preeminent pediatric practitioners in Seattle, starts off his chapter on fever with a Peggy Lee lyric, and says, "with the exception of the special case of infants under the age of three months, parental perception is all that is necessary for the diagnosis of fever. We do ourselves and our patients a disservice by succumbing to the peculiar predilection of Western medicine to want to measure everything. This leads to fussing and hair-splitting over axillary vs. rectal, mercury vs. digital, and ascribes undue importance to the absolute level of fever."

A reader might have difficulty believing that John Freeman is a distinguished tenured professor of pediatrics and neurology at Johns Hopkins University when coming across the following statement in his down-to-earth chapter on seizures: "There is no laboratory test or radiologic examination which will diagnose or rule out a seizure. The 'full' workup of a seizure does *not* require that every conceivable possible cause of the seizure be ruled out." Or the statement: "The *only* two consequences of a first febrile seizure are: another febrile seizure (chance 30%) and an anxious parent (chance close to 100%)."

Seven of the chapters are written by colleagues at the University of Washington. I hope this does not appear too provincial. I was familiar with their expertise and knew that the contributions of these authors would be of the highest quality. In an international touch, six of the chapters are authored by Canadians. I solicited the authors of three of the chapters, disorders of sleep, recurrent pain, and behavioral problems, after seeing their contributions in a marvelous book for parents prepared by members of the Division of General Pediatrics at the Hospital for Sick Children in Toronto.[2] In a turnabout, I asked Drs. Feldman, Goldbloom, and Greenberg to transpose their words for parents to an audience of physician readers.

There are important common pediatric problems not covered in this book, such as orthopedic, vision, and hearing impairments. But no book can be all-inclusive. Medical education must be a continuing process; there is no finite amount of knowledge to learn. I just hope that some children and their families are helped by the information contained in this book.

Big thank-yous go to the contributors who worked hard to produce chapters that are practical and helpful; to Dr. Barry Weiss, the editor of McGraw-Hill's 20 Common Problems Series, who carefully reviewed every sentence of every manuscript for accuracy and readability; Susan Noujaim, McGraw-Hill developmental editor, for her competence and affability; and my long-time colleague, Yvonne Koshi, for her ever-present capability in preparing the manuscript.

Abraham B. Bergman
Seattle, Washington

REFERENCES

1. Freid VM, Makuc DM, Rooks RN: Ambulatory health care visits by children: principal diagnosis and place of visit. National Center for Health Statistics. *Vital Health Stat* 13:137, 1998.
2. Feldman W (ed): *The 3 AM Handbook: The Most Commonly Asked Questions about Your Child's Health.* Toronto, Ontario, Key Porter Books, 1997.

Part

1

Health
Supervision

Ronald G. Barr
Julie Lessard

Excessive Crying

Toward the end of the nineteenth century, the editors of the *British Medical Journal (BMJ)* cited a contemporary opinion that "the human infant . . . is an interesting object of scientific research, and even a cross baby should be contemplated calmly by the philosophic mind." They went on to recommend that "Few persons have better opportunities of adding to the store of knowledge on these points than medical men."[1] One of the main reasons for this opportunity that medical men (and women) have is the problem often referred to as "excessive crying," "persistent crying," "paroxysmal fussing," or "colic."

Indeed, excessive crying might be considered one of the commonest of the common problems with which pediatric clinicians are faced. Estimates of incidence vary from 4 percent to almost 50 percent, depending on how it is defined. In their classic 1954 study,[2] Wessel and colleagues reported that 49 percent of their sample constituted "fussy" babies, and that half of these (26 percent of the whole sample) were considered "seriously fussy" because their paroxysms of fussing or crying "continued to recur for more than three weeks, or became so severe that the pediatrician felt that medication was indicated." Of course, whether parents *complain* of crying (or that crying is "excessive") is another question. This will depend on a number of factors, including whether the infant is a first-born, cultural attitudes toward crying, and access to medical services considered to be sympathetic to such complaints.

As it turns out, the *BMJ* recommendation was prescient, since the "cross baby" has become the subject of increasing interest and scientific investigation both to medical investigators and to others interested in growth and development of the human infant. Furthermore, these investigations, although far from having "solved" the problem, have changed our understanding of early excessive crying significantly. In particular, there are three important changes that provide a basis for a more rational approach to *complaints* of excessive crying.

The first is the concept that excessive crying or "colic" represents the upper end of the spectrum of crying behavior that is typical of normally developing infants, rather than a distinct crying pattern indicative of underlying organic pathology in the infant or psychopathology in the caregiver.

Second, individual differences in crying are likely to reflect differences in the way the central nervous system works rather than differences in the way the gastrointestinal system works.

Third, if parents and their infants can make it through the period of increased crying without it seriously affecting the way they think about each other or their infant, the prognosis is likely to be good.

In this chapter, we focus on some of the evidence that supports these three shifts in our understanding of crying, and then, in light of these findings, propose a strategy for a clinical approach to crying complaints.

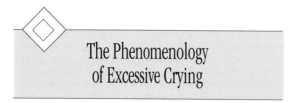

The Phenomenology of Excessive Crying

From most textbooks, the classic descriptions of the clinical presentation of early excessive, persistent crying focus on characteristics of the symptoms or signs that tend to cluster together in what is usually thought of as the "colic syn-

drome."[3] Of course, crying is the core symptom of the syndrome, but all infants cry. Thus the clinical descriptions attempt to identify whether there is a set of features that identifies a clinically distinct entity of colic from the crying of an otherwise normal infant.

Age Dependency

The first defining dimension is that the crying has *age-dependent* and *diurnal* characteristics. The age-dependent feature is that the increased crying of colic typically begins at about 2 weeks after birth, reaching a peak sometime in the second month, and then declines to baseline levels by about the fourth month of age. The diurnal feature is that the crying tends to cluster during the late afternoon and evening hours. In fact, these are two sides of the same phenomenon, since the age-related increase and decrease are mostly accounted for by changes in amounts of crying that tend to cluster late in the day.

Associated Behavioral Characteristics

The second defining dimension is that the crying tends to be accompanied by a number of *behavioral* characteristics, two of which are almost always present and others of which are more variably present. The two common features are that the crying occurs in prolonged bouts (sometimes called "colic" bouts), and these are resistant to all kinds of soothing attempts, even including feeding. During such bouts, infants may also clench their fists, flex their legs over the abdomen, arch their backs, have an active and grimacing face giving the impression that the infant is in pain ("pain facies"), and be flushed. Contributing to the idea that this is a gastrointestinal problem, the infant's abdomen may be hard and distended, and the crying bout may include regurgitation and the passing of gas per rectum.

Paroxysms

The third defining dimension is that the crying bouts are typically described as *paroxysmal*, an unfortunately vague term that tries to capture the facts that the onset of the crying bouts can be sudden, they tend to begin and to end without warning, and they are not easily related to other events in the environment (they appear to be spontaneous).

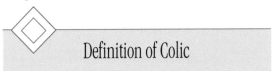

Definition of Colic

Because the above characteristics are qualitative descriptions and most infants do this some of the time, it is often difficult to determine when an infant should be considered to have colic. By far the most widely used definition is that proposed by Wessel and colleagues, which has come to be known as the "rule of threes."[2] They proposed that an infant can be considered to have colic if it cries for more than 3 h a day for more than 3 days a week for more than 3 weeks. This proposal has been very helpful for at least four reasons. First, it focuses on *duration* of crying, a characteristic that is more easily quantifiable. Second, it captures an important additional feature; namely, that the increased crying is very variable even within infants. The excessive crying does not happen every day like clockwork but may be present some days and not others. This lack of predictability adds to the frustration of trying to understand why it is happening. Third, it is becoming increasingly clear that most of the other defining features of the crying of colic syndrome occur in rough proportion to the overall duration of crying that infants do.[4] Thus, for example, the number of crying bouts that are unsoothable is greater in infants whose overall duration of crying and fussing is greater. Consequently, overall duration of crying is a fairly good index of the presence of the other, less easily quantifiable phenonomena. Finally, it is helpful because the clinical report can be confirmed by the use of a parental diary for a few days (Fig. 1-1). These diaries give a reasonably accurate (valid) measure of crying duration, including time of occurrence during the day, that is helpful for the clinician. Furthermore, they may also have a therapeutic benefit, in that parents discover that their infants do not actually cry all the time, even though it may seem like it on some days.

However, this definition also has a number of limitations when it is applied in the clinical setting. The first is that the amounts of crying used in the definition are arbitrary. There is no obvious reason why an infant who cries for just under 180 min per day for 3 days per week does not have colic syndrome, while another infant who cries just over 180 min per day does have the syndrome. There are not two populations of infants that are different, but rather one population of infants, some of whom cry more and some of whom cry less. In addition, the third "three" (crying at this level for 3 weeks) is not very helpful clinically. Few parents or clinicians are willing to wait for 3 weeks to see if the infant meets criteria for colic. As a result, the third criterion is usually dropped in both clinical and research settings (and then referred to as modified Wessel's criteria). Furthermore, the quantitative criteria do not take account of parental effort in calming the infant. If the mother is "working overtime" soothing and calming her infant, the infant may well cry less than the cutoff level (and therefore not be classified as having colic), whereas the infant of a mother who lets her infant "cry out" will meet the definition. The definition does not take account of the *quality* of the crying. To date, the evidence of whether there is an acoustically different colic cry is mixed, but it is clear that parents can detect differences in the quality of cries, and these differences contribute to whether or not the infant is brought to the physician as a complaint.[5]

Figure 1-1

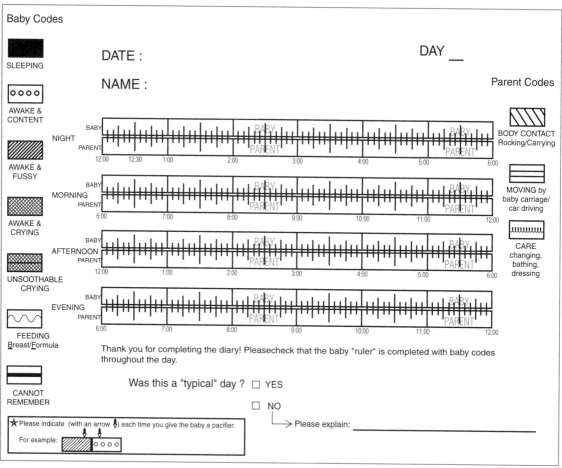

A sample of the *Baby's Day Diary* that can be used by parents to document the amount and timing of the fussing, crying, and unsoothable crying that occurs during 24 h. The "time rulers" allow parents to easily fill in the their baby's state with symbols. Most parents do this every 2 or 3 h, usually in association with a regularly recurring care event, such as feeding. The bottom half of the ruler can be used for parenting behaviors, such as time spent carrying the infant.

However, perhaps the most important reason why this kind of definition is so limited is what has been termed "the crying paradox," which can be stated as follows: the very same crying behavior (or amounts of crying) may function to bring about good or bad consequences to the infant *depending on the context.* An extreme illustration of this phenomenon is that infants that were irritable and cried more were more likely to survive a famine than infants that cried less.[6] Infants who cry more also receive more attention, mutual gaze, patting, caressing, moving, and rocking stimulation from their caregivers. One way to think of this is to understand that crying acts not simply as a symptom or a sign that something may be wrong or abnormal but also as a signal to which the caregiving environment may (or may not) respond. The important clinical decision is whether the crying functions to bring about good or bad consequences for the infant (and its caregivers) rather than determining whether a certain amount of crying is normal or abnormal.[7]

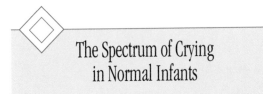

The Spectrum of Crying in Normal Infants

The textbook descriptions and most definitions imply that the phenomenology of excessive crying is defining of a distinct clinical syndrome indicating that something is wrong or abnormal in the infant, the caregiver, or the infant-caregiver interaction. However, more recent work has indicated that it is both more accurate and more helpful to understand early excessive crying as the upper end of the spectrum of crying in normally developing infants. There are two types of evidence that contribute to this shift in our understanding: (1) evidence that most or all of the phenomena thought to be defining of colic are also present in infants without colic except that they are less in amount, duration or intensity and (2) evidence that organic diseases and/or caregiver psychopathology contribute to only a small proportion (probably 5 to 10 percent) of cases of excessive crying.

Crying in Normal States

We can illustrate that these characteristics of crying are present in normal infants by considering the three dimensions cited in textbook descriptions. With regard to the age-dependent curve, it is now clear that this is a characteristic crying pattern in almost all infants and in almost all cultures studied to date, despite radical differences in caregiving styles. Figure 1-2 presents crying and fussing data for a sample of normal

Figure 1-2

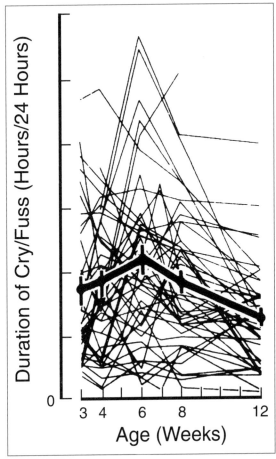

Cry/fuss duration by week of age of 50 infants, with superimposed mean and S.E.M. values for the whole group. (Data are from the Hunziker and Barr control group. Hunziker UA, Barr RG. Increased carrying reduces infant crying: a randomized controlled trial. *Pediatrics* 77:641–648, 1986. Figure reproduced by permission from Barr RG: The normal crying curve: what do we really know? *Dev Med Child Neurol* 32:356–362, 1990.)

infants. Note that the thick line, clearly showing an n-shaped curve, represents the mean crying for the group of infants. Note also how variable the crying is for individual infants, with some infants crying much more and some much less. Some infants have their peak earlier and some later.

A recent study suggests that the peak may be earlier in infants that are formula fed compared to those that are breast-fed.[8] Furthermore, the curve pattern is not as distinct or smooth for individual infants as for the group of infants together, so that it may not be so easy to recognize the pattern in a single infant. Some 30 to 40 percent of the infants at the upper end of the spectrum would meet (modified) Wessel's criteria for colic, while other infants would not.

This pattern of crying is remarkably robust. It has been found in almost all samples of infants in western cultures. However, its importance as a normal developmental phenomenon has also been supported by finding similar patterns in other cultures where caregiving is radically different, as among the !Kung San hunter-gatherers of Botswana[9] and communities in Manali, India.[10] In addition, the crying curve is similar in premature infants, occurring at about 6 weeks *corrected* age rather than 6 weeks after birth.[11] Consequently, far from being definitive of a distinct clinical syndrome, this pattern of crying (as per the n-shaped curve) is more likely to be a behavioral manifestation of normal developmental processes.

Similar results are being found for all the other "definitive" characteristics of colic crying. For example, infants with colic are more likely to show a pain facies when they cry, but most of the time infants without colic do too.[5] Infants with colic do cry after a feed if left alone, but at only a slightly higher rate than infants without colic.[5] Infants without colic are more likely to have bouts of crying that are unsoothable, but only proportionately to the overall amount of crying that they do.[4] In short, the crying characteristics of infants with colic is *continuous* with that of normal infants rather than distinct.

Crying in Pathologic States

The second type of evidence indicates that pathologic entities (either in the infant or in the parents) account for only a small percentage of infants with colic syndrome. The ideal study to determine this percentage has not been done, but most current estimates suggest that less than 5 percent will be due to recognizable organic diseases.[12–15] This may seem surprising, since clinical descriptions of colic are usually accompanied by long lists of organic causes. This is because almost any disease condition can present with crying in infants. However, if the diagnosis of colic is limited to infants who have crying complaints without fever, that occur during the first 3 months, and that are chronic (as opposed to acute), then the percentage due to organic disease is much lower. (For helpful reviews of acute crying presenting in the emergency department, see Poole[16] and Trocinski and Pearigen.[17])

Although the evidence is less well established, a similar pattern is emerging in regard to caregiver pathologies; that is, most cases of colic cannot be accounted for by preexisting maternal personality characteristics, postpartum depression, or inappropriate or nonoptimal caregiving. This is not to say that these conditions are not risk factors that may exacerbate the increased crying typical of this age and put the infant at greater risk. They are also risk factors for maternal distress and mother-infant interactions after colic has resolved ("persistent caregiver-infant distress syndrome"[18,19]). However, they are insufficient explanations of the *cause(s)* of colic. A number of observations support this. Because of inexperience, first-time mothers may bring their crying infants to the physician as a concern, but there is no difference in crying amounts between first- and later-born infants.[20] In addition, third-trimester emotional lability in mothers is no different with regard to infants that subsequently meet criteria for colic.[21] Importantly, mothers with persistently crying infants are as interactively sensitive, show similar affection, and hold and soothe their infants more as compared with other mothers.[4]

Consequently, most cases of infant colic are unlikely to be accounted for by clinical pathology either in the infant or in the mother, and most cases are due to the increase in crying that is typical of normally developing infants, especially those at the upper end of the crying spectrum. Differences in caregiving (such as amounts of contact, frequency and type of feeding) are likely to modify the duration and possibly the pattern of crying, but they may or may not be sufficiently efficacious to allay caregiver concerns about the crying. Nevertheless, understanding that the increase and decrease in crying is typical of normal development, rather than a clinically distinct pattern of crying implicating abnormality, is an important starting point in understanding and evaluating early complaints of excessive crying.

Identifying Infants with Organic Disease

Even though most cases can be accounted for by normal developmental processes, this does not reduce the important challenge to the clinician of identifying those infants in which organic disease "presents as" a colic-like syndrome. Although the number of diseases that may present in this way is much less than usually assumed (once acute illnesses and illnesses with fever are removed), they nevertheless remain important. One reason why identifying such infants is so difficult is that the coexistent disease may simply exacerbate the pattern of increased crying that would be present even in the absence of disease. In a recent review,[15] Gormally and Barr systematically searched for those entities for which there was evidence that a colic-like syndrome could be a presenting symptom. Their list will continue to evolve as more and better-described clinical presentations are added to the clinical literature. In Table 1-1, we have updated their list, adding qualitative descriptors concerning the strength of the evidence for each as well as how likely it is that they will account for colic cases in a primary care setting.

Of course, such lists always have the benefit of "hindsight," since they are derived from reports of clinical experience, including follow-up of the cases. The clinician, however, must

Table 1-1

Organic Diseases Implicated in Colic Syndrome

ORGANIC ENTITIES PRESENTING WITH "COLIC-LIKE" SYNDROME	STRENGTH OF EVIDENCE IMPLICATING THIS ENTITY	ESTIMATED PREVALENCE (IN PRIMARY CARE SETTINGS)
Cow's milk protein intolerance	Strong	<5%
Isolated fructose intolerance	Strong	Rare
Maternal drug effects [esp. fluoxetine hydrochoride (Prozac)]	Strong	Unknown, changing
Anomalous left coronary artery from the pulmonary artery	Strong	Very rare
Infantile migraine	Moderate	Rare
Reflux esophagitis	Moderate	Rare
Shaken baby syndrome	Moderate	Difficult to distinguish cause and effect
Congenital glaucoma	Weak, but suggestive	Rare
CNS abnormalities, esp. Chiari type I malformation	Weak, but suggestive	Rare
Urinary tract infection	Weak	Probably rare
Lactose intolerance	Very weak	Probably not etiologic

make decisions prospectively in the absence of complete information, including the clinical course. Gormally and Barr suggest that there are at least four clinical clues that increase the possibility that organic causes might be implicated. First, infants whose crying is described as "high-pitched," who *regularly* arch their backs during crying bouts (most infants will do that occasionally if the crying is very forceful), and whose crying does not manifest a diurnal pattern (after-noon-evening clustering) may be more at risk for an organic etiology. Second, the principle may hold that colic syndrome is not due to organic disease in the absence of additional signs and symptoms, although the evidence is not systematic enough as yet that this can be said with complete confidence. However, it is extremely rare that excessive crying alone was the only clue to organic disease in all descriptions to date. Other symptoms by history (increased regurgitations, diarrhea, vomiting, respiratory distress) or by examination (bruises, retinal hemorrhages, etc.) were almost always reported. Third, a late onset of increased crying in the third month or following a switch from breast to formula may implicate cow's milk protein intolerance. Such symptoms may but rarely do begin in the first 2 or 3 weeks of life. Finally, it was common for the unusual and excessive crying of infants *with organic disease* to persist beyond 4 months. This clue is not helpful at the beginning of the complaint but clearly justifies the importance of regular monitoring of the complaint until the crying resolves.

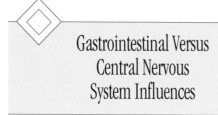

Gastrointestinal Versus Central Nervous System Influences

For understandable reasons, early excessive crying has been presumed to be primarily a condi-tion related to the gastrointestinal tract. In part, this is a reflection of the name *colic*. It is thought to imply reference to the colon or, more generally, the abdomen regardless of etiology. Second, many of the accompanying symptoms are thought to implicate the gastrointestinal system—notably including crying that persists after a feed, the expulsion of gas at either end, the tenseness of the abdomen, and drawing legs up over the abdomen. Third, there are many anec-dotal accounts of "cures" after an infant has been switched from one formula to another or sometimes from breast feeding to formula feeding, seeming to confirm that there is some nutrient that is not well tolerated by the gastrointestinal tract of the infants with colic. In fact, there is reasonable evidence that cow's milk protein intolerance can present as colic-like syndrome, or that cow's milk protein can exacerbate colic-like crying in some infants. However, many of the anecdotal "cures" due to formula changes are due to coincident reduction in crying at about the time the formula change occurs rather than because the causal stimulus was removed by the formula change. It is also clear that cow's milk protein intolerance accounts for only a small proportion (less than 5 percent) of infants with colic.[3,12,15] A fourth reason that colic is considered gastrointestinal is the presence of gas. In fact, infants do produce more colonic gas during the first 3 months of life due to incomplete absorption of lactose.[22] But the evidence to date that gas is etiologic or that treatment for gas is efficacious is extremely weak.[3,15]

Role of the Nervous System

Although there is more to learn about the gastrointestinal tract and early excessive crying, there are a number of reasons to consider excessive crying a reflection of central nervous system differences rather than gastrointestinal ones. The first is that all of the behavioral symptoms presumed to indicate gastrointestinal differences could be effects of the crying rather than causes. To take but one example, the increased gas expulsion at either end may be due to air swallowing or the Valsalva maneuver associated with crying. More importantly, however, more careful studies of the crying symptoms suggest that what is different in the crying of infants with colic is not that they cry *more often* but rather that they cry *longer* once they start.[5] In other words, the issue is not what causes the crying in the first place but what regulates the crying once it starts. This fits with the common observation that these infants are unsoothable.

Indeed, there are now a few studies that have documented experimentally that the difficulty in soothing (or regulating) crying is typical of infants with colic. In one, infants who met Wessel's criteria for colic cried longer, cried more intensely, and were less soothable in response to a mock physical exam than infants without colic.[23] Since it was so situation-specific, it seems unlikely that this crying was due to gastrointestinal problems. There were two other interesting findings. First, the crying that occurred during the physical exam correlated very well with the amount of crying that occurred at home. This suggests that the experimental crying in the laboratory was probably indicating something important about the crying in the home. If so, then the differences in ability to regulate crying (independent of gastrointestinal or other stimuli) may be important in both settings. Second, although the infants with colic cried more, they did not show more physiologic distress, as indexed by cardiovascular or salivary cortisol measures. Nor did they secrete more cortisol at home. Consequently, the differences seemed to be quite specific to regulating their *crying*. Evidence for differences in crying regulation was also found in a second study comparing calming responses to sucrose taste. The response to sucrose taste is of particular interest, since this appears to access a central opioid-dependent distress reduction system. Newborn infants who are in a crying state are dramatically

calmed by just two drops of sucrose solution. Sucrose taste also works to calm crying infants at 6 weeks of age (when crying is at its peak) but not nearly as well as with newborns. This diminished responsiveness would be expected if this central opioid-dependent regulatory system were relevant to the prolonged crying at this age. In addition, when the response to sucrose of already crying 6-week-old infants *with colic* was compared to the response of those without, the sucrose taste was even less effective.[24] Again, this diminished response to sucrose taste would be expected in infants with colic if this system were implicated in the differential abilities of infants to stop crying once it had started. Although still not conclusive, this is the most specific evidence yet that the behavioral differences in infants with colic may reflect central nervous system rather than gastrointestinal differences.

Indicators of a Good Prognosis

The third shift in our understanding of early excessive crying is that, if caregivers can make it through the colicky period, the prognosis for the infant is likely to be good. We still do not have enough appropriate longitudinal studies, and those that we do have are not consistent in their definitions of early excessive crying, the outcome measures they use, or the rigor of their methodologies. Despite this, there is a consistent finding to date that, on all objective measures of the infants—including growth, health (including allergies), behavior (including sleep), and temperament—they are not distinguishable from their peers who had colic.[25] On the other hand, these infants are *perceived* differently. Their parents are more likely to see them as more temperamentally difficult and as more vulnerable to illness up to 3 years later. Consequently, there is an important role to play in diminishing this outcome in the parents of infants with early excessive crying.

However, there are three important caveats to this positive prognostic picture. The first is that, even if the infants turn out all right, there is the potential for some negative effects on the caregiver (usually the mother), including an increased risk to report depressive symptoms, a challenge to her self-esteem,[4,26] and more difficulties in family interactions.[27–29] The second caveat is that most of these studies were carried out in relatively low-risk samples of families. As a result, it may be that colic can be a significant perturbation in the context of a high-risk family, even if this condition is a normative developmental phenomenon. This seems to be the experience in specialized clinics, in which excessively crying infants in high-risk families sometimes develop a "persistent caregiver-infant distress syndrome" that includes a breakdown in normal caregiving responses and continues well after colic usually resolves.[18,19] The third caveat is that these follow-up studies do not capture the very low incidence but high-severity outcomes that include infant abuse and even death. Such cases are eloquent testimony to the power of crying to bring about very serious negative consequences for the infant.

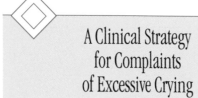

A Clinical Strategy for Complaints of Excessive Crying

In light of the above, it remains a significant challenge to deal with the complaint of excessive crying in the early months of life. The challenge is heightened because increased crying is a normal developmental phenomenon, and the crying that is characteristic of infants with colic

is continuous with, rather than distinct from, this normal behavioral development. Since infants with organic disease can present with 'colic-like syndrome' and the likelihood of pathology is rare, it is more difficult to identify and distinguish those with or without a disease process contributing to the crying. Finally, because even normal crying can elicit negative consequences both for the infant and its caregivers, there is an important role in prevention of these consequences even if the crying cannot be affected.

To accommodate these realities, the clinical approach needs to consider all crying complaints seriously, whether or not they are due to an organic disorder in the infant or psychopathology in the caregivers. As a way of doing this, it is most helpful to have a clinical strategy to approach *crying complaints* rather than "colic." Using Gormally and Barr's "clinical pie" approach (Figure 1-3),[15] one can think of all crying complaints in terms of the phenomenologic presentation of the crying behavior. Infants within the circle represent those whose crying is a concern for their caregivers, regardless of how much they cry. Those outside of the circle may cry as much, but they are not brought to the clinician as a concern. The sizes of the slices represent a rough approximation of the size of the groups. Of course, this will depend on the setting. For example, in tertiary care consultative settings, the "organic" slice is more likely to be bigger than it is in primary care settings.

In this approach, infants with "normal concern" crying are those whose crying and physical exam is not exceptional in any way. The caregivers simply were unaware that this increased crying would occur and were anxious about its possible meaning. Infants with "non-Wessel's crying" are also not unusual nor is their crying excessive (i.e., it does not meet Wessel's criteria for quantity—see opening discussion), but the parents may be concerned about the *quality* of crying. We still know very little about such infants, but they represent a significant proportion of early complaints.[5] Infants with

Figure 1-3

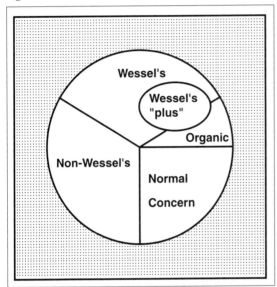

Gormally and Barr's "clinical pie" for crying complaints. The stippled background represents all crying infants, and the circle represents those that present to the clinician with a complaint about crying. The pie slices represent different presentations of the complaint based on phenomenology rather than etiology. In only one slice (organic) is etiology suggested; it is represented as accounting for about 5 percent of cases. (Reproduced by permission from Gormally S, Barr RG: Of clinical pies and clinical clues: proposal for a clinical approach to complaints of early crying and colic. *Ambul Child Health* 3:137–153, 1997.)

"Wessel's crying" *do* meet the traditional textbook criteria for increased amounts of crying but do not have additional cues on history and physical examination. Most of what has been described previously in terms of patterns, quantity, quality, unsoothability, and prognosis refers to these infants because they have been studied in most depth. "Wessel's plus" infants are those that meet Wessel's criteria but, in addition, have other cues that raise concern, have failed trials of therapy, and/or have additional risk factors (such as a fragile family). These are also the infants in whom additional signs of distress (clenched fists; legs flexed; arched back; flushed face; tense, distended abdomen; regurgitation with crying; and a pain facies when crying) are most likely to be seen. The clinical course of these infants sometimes evolves to manifesting organic disease but often does not (which is why they are represented as a circle on the border of the pie slices). It is this subgroup (especially if diarrhea and/or vomiting is an additional symptom) in whom a *trial* of cow's milk protein elimination (either from the mother's diet if breast-feeding or from the infant's diet through formula change) is indicated. Finally, the "organic" slice is the only slice representing infants in whom an organic etiology is identified by history (other noncrying clues), physical examination (positive findings), and follow-up (total less than 5 percent: see Table 1-1 for most likely causes).

Evaluative Phase

The *evaluative* phase of the clinical approach consists of careful description of the phenomenology of the crying, assessment of the consequences for the infant (e.g., has the caregiver stopped expressing affection for the infant?) and for the caregiver (e.g., are there symptoms of depression or lack of self-confidence?), and a search for clinical clues of organicity other than the crying itself. If all of these are negative, then the most important evaluative procedure is monitoring the infant until the expected resolution of the crying occurs. Monitoring is indicated in *all* infants whose parents complain of crying because of the small but important possibility that organic disease tends to be associated with excessive crying that persists beyond the first 4 months. It cannot be explained away as colic after that.

Management Phase

The *management* phase is graded in the sense that the number and intensity of strategies used to help the infant and the mother increase depending on the extent to which the above questions are answered in the affirmative. Beginning with the case of an infant in whom evidence for organic disease is uncovered, specific therapy directed at the pathophysiology of the condition is indicated. For the remainder, therapy can be directed (1) at reducing the crying in the infant, (2) at reducing the psychological "pressure" on the caregivers, and (3), in the difficult "Wessel's plus" infants (especially those with accompanying diarrhea or vomiting), at a therapeutic trial of the elimination of cow's milk protein.

Medications

In regard to reducing crying, it must be understood and acknowledged that crying *may* be temporarily reduced by various interventions (that is, *while* the interventions are being used), but it is not likely to be "fixed" or "cured" or to "go away" until the infant matures sufficiently that the infant's own regulatory controls on crying behavior become more efficient. At the current time, there is no medication with proven efficacy that is available to be used with infants with colic. The only medication with appropriate clinical trials of effectiveness is dicyclomine hydrochloride, and colic has been removed as an indication for its use because of possible problematic side effects. Preparations to eliminate problems with gas have not been shown to be effective in large, appropriately designed studies.

Education and Stress Reduction

Leaving the infant to "cry out" so that it "learns to control its crying" is neither a useful nor an effective strategy. Being responsive to the infant does not "spoil" the infant. A good functional outcome for the infant is that more contact, interaction, and soothing, occurs, not less, even

if this increased contact does not sufficiently reduce the crying. There are many devices available (e.g., bed shakers, heart sounds) that essentially provide "analogue" stimulation to that which would be provided by more contact with a caregiver. In general, however, temporary soothing is most often provided by anything that provides relatively constant background motion or sound. Many devices around the house can be recruited for this purpose (e.g., the sounds of a fish-tank aerator). However, putting the infant on a washer or drier is to be avoided because of the danger of skull fractures from falling off due to the vibrations.

By far and away the most important component of the management phase is directed at reducing the psychological pressure on the caregivers. Roughly speaking, more of these strategies will be required as one progresses from "normal concern" crying complaints to (moving clockwise around the pie) Wessel's-plus colic infants. They are:

1. Acknowledge the reality of the concern, regardless of amount of crying.
2. Provide information about the pattern of increased and decreased crying, its continuity with the behavior of infants with less crying, its universality as a behavioral phenomenon of normally developing infants, and its lack of association with organic disease (in the absence of other symptoms and signs). Often, simply informing parents about the normal crying curve (Figure 1-2) will be sufficient, especially in first-time mothers who have not heard about it.
3. Determine where the pressure on the primary caregiver is coming from (her significant other, parents-in-law, friends or internalized cultural beliefs that having an infant with colic is a sign of a "bad" mother). It is helpful if all of the primary caregiver's significant support persons are "on the same page" with regard to how the crying is perceived and handled.

4. Ask caregivers to keep a diary (as in Fig. 1-1). This provides you with more objective information about the pattern of the crying and also makes it more evident to parents that the infant does other things than cry, even though it might not seem like it at times.

5. Provide "boundary" suggestions for what is *not* an appropriate response, no matter how problematic the crying. It is important to raise the issue that such crying can make parents feel very negatively toward their infant. However, should it seem too much to handle, it is important to stress that, no matter how badly they feel, physically shaking the infant is never an appropriate response. Removing oneself from the infant's crying and having someone to call when it seems "too much" are important alternative coping strategies.

6. Ask the parents to weigh the infant and include the weights in the diary. If the *trend* (as opposed to the day-to-day variations) in weight is rising, this provides important information for the clinician and the parent that organic disease is less likely.

7. Provide parent support through regular contact and encouragement to call in the event of new symptoms or signs.

8. Arrange for regular "respite" periods for the primary caregiver. This is best provided by the spouse or other partner, if available, especially for crying periods during the night. However, other family members and baby sitters are also useful. The primary caregiver may resist having help, believing the infant needs her more.

9. In severe cases, and especially if the increased crying is occurring in the context of a fragile and otherwise challenged family, referral to specialized clinics or services is indicated and important. The increased crying may unmask caregivers and families with significant issues that need clinical attention as well as be helpful as a useful "reason" for the family to seek help.

Conclusions

Despite increasing interest, the problem of excessive crying (or colic) in infancy continues to be a rather mysterious and difficult clinical challenge for both parents and clinicians. As the *BMJ* recommendation to contemplate and study the "cross baby" has increasingly been acted upon, more systematic observations and studies have begun to provide a more complete, empirically based understanding of the phenomenology and some of the determinants of early increased crying.

Clinical studies (both case reports and clinical trials) have contributed two findings. On the one hand, they have confirmed that a number of organic diseases can present with "colic-like crying syndromes" and, on the other hand, they have shown that these organic diseases only account for a small proportion of infants that present with colic syndrome.

Developmental studies have contributed two main findings important for the clinical approach to crying problems. They have shown that the early increasing and decreasing pattern of crying is a normal pattern of behavior and that virtually all of the behaviors thought to be characteristic of a distinct clinical crying syndrome are continuous with the crying of normal infants but exaggerated in infants that cry more. Consequently, it is probably more helpful to think of colic as something normally developing infants "do" rather than as a condition that infants "have."[7]

However, this continuity of "excessive" crying behavior with the behavior of normally developing infants increases the difficulty of identifying those infants in whom there is organic disease or of identifying those caregivers in whom the increased crying stresses the psychological fragility of the infant's caregiver or family. Further, this normal pattern of early increased crying sets up the possibility of a "double hit" for unsuspecting parents. A relatively calm infant may not come to clinical attention even if the parents are fragile or stressed, nor will a relatively highly crying infant in whom the caregivers are confident of their skills. However, some combinations of the increased crying and lack of confidence, varying uniquely from family to family, will manifest themselves as complaints about excessive crying in the early postnatal months.

This developing understanding of early increased crying has some clear implications for the clinical approach outlined above. There is much good news that provides guidelines for parents and clinicians as to what this crying means. This includes the findings that the likelihood of disease as a cause of the crying is low, and that most of our usual techniques available in a primary care setting for detecting disease (careful history, physical examination, and monitoring for additional cues in addition to the crying) work. This permits careful clinicians to have confidence that they can contribute to the important responsibility of detecting organic disease, allowing the parents to focus their attention and care on the infant's distress. The other important finding is that the outcomes appear good for the infant, contingent upon successfully coping with the challenge of the increased crying typical of this period.

Our understanding of early increased crying implies three clear "don'ts" in the clinical setting. First, *don't ignore the complaint and the parents concern or downplay its importance.* Increased anxiety in the face of crying that is unsoothable and increases even in the face of the best caregiving is appropriate and should not be dismissed. Indeed, although less well studied, it might be a worse prognostic indicator if parents *don't* manifest concern than if they do. It is better to use the increased crying as an *opportunity* to focus the natural anxiety that it elicits by encouraging parents to increase their closeness, responsiveness, availability, and sharing of care for their infant. Successfully negotiating this

early caregiving challenge can increase the confidence of caregivers to the benefit of their infants and themselves, just as unsuccessfully handling it can diminish their confidence.

Second, *don't fail to monitor the crying.* Persistence of increased crying is common in infants with organic diseases and an important clue to the need for further investigation. There are differences in the amounts of crying that older infants do too (especially those with "difficult temperaments"), so increased crying does not necessarily imply organic determinants. But it remains an important clue. The problem of increased crying is not resolved with the initial evaluation but only when the crying (and the concern it generates) is resolved.

Third, *don't focus solely on the infant.* The more likely negative consequences of this early challenge are the effect(s) on the infant's caregivers. Preventing lack of confidence in parenting skills or depressive symptoms in the parents constitutes a therapeutic success.

References

1. One hundred years ago: the instincts and habits of babies. *BMJ* 309:8957, 1994 (reprinted from *BMJ* 2:1264, 1894).
2. Wessel MA, Cobb JC, Jackson EB, et al: Paroxysmal fussing in infancy, sometimes called "colic." *Pediatrics* 14:421–434, 1954.
3. Barr RG: Colic, in Walker WA, Durie PR, Hamilton JR, et al (eds): *Pediatric Gastrointestinal Disease: Pathophysiology, Diagnosis, and Management.* 2nd ed. St. Louis, Mosby, 1996, pp 241–250.
4. St James-Roberts I, Conroy S, Wilsher K: Links between maternal care and persistent infant crying in the early months. *Child Care Health Dev* 24:353–376, 1998.
5. Barr RG, Rotman A, Yaremko J, et al: The crying of infants with colic: a controlled empirical description. *Pediatrics* 90:14–21, 1992.
6. DeVries MW: Temperament and infant mortality among the Masai of East Africa. *Am J Psychiatry* 141:1189–1194, 1984.

7. Barr RG: Normality: a clinically useless concept; the case of infant crying and colic. *J Dev Behav Pediatr* 14:264–270, 1993.

8. Lucas A, St.James-Roberts I: Crying, fussing and colic behaviour in breast-and bottle-fed infants. *Early Hum Dev* 53:9–18, 1998.

9. Barr RG, Bakeman R, Konner M, Adamson L: Crying in !Kung infants: a test of the cultural specificity hypothesis. *Dev Med Child Neurol* 33:601–610, 1991.

10. St.James-Roberts I, Bowyer J, Varghese S, Sawdon J: Infant crying patterns in Manali and London. *Child Care Health Dev* 20:323–337, 1994.

11. Barr RG, Chen S, Hopkins B, Westra T: Crying patterns in preterm infants. *Dev Med Child Neurol* 38:345–355, 1996.

12. Miller AR, Barr RG: Infantile colic: is it a gut issue? *Pediatr Clin North Am* 38:1407–1423, 1991.

13. Treem WR: Infant colic: a pediatric gastroenterologist's perspective. *Pediatr Clin North Am* 41:1121–1138, 1994.

14. Sauls HS, Redfern DE (eds): *Colic and Excessive Crying.* Columbus, OH, Ross Products Division, Abbott Laboratories, 1997

15. Gormally SM, Barr RG: Of clinical pies and clinical clues: proposal for a clinical approach to complaints of early crying and colic. *Ambul Child Health* 3:137–153, 1997.

16. Poole SR: The infant with acute, unexplained, excessive crying. *Pediatrics* 88:450–455, 1991.

17. Trocinski DR, Pearigen PD: The crying infant. *Emerg Clin North Am* 16:895–910, 1998.

18. Papousek M, von Hofacker N: Persistent crying in early infancy: a non-trivial condition of risk for the developing mother-infant relationship. *Child Care Health Dev* 24:395–424, 1998.

19. Barr RG: Crying in the first year of life: good news in the midst of distress. *Child Care Health Dev* 24:425–439, 1998.

20. St James-Roberts I, Halil T: Infant crying patterns in the first year: normal community and clinical findings. *J Child Psychol Psychiatry* 32:951–968, 1991.

21. Miller AR, Barr RG, Eaton WO: Crying and motor behavior of six-week-old infants and postpartum maternal mood. *Pediatrics* 92:551–558, 1993.

22. Barr RG, Hanley J, Patterson DK, Wooldridge JA: Breath hydrogen excretion of normal newborn infants in response to usual feeding patterns: evidence for "functional lactase insufficience" beyond the first month of life. *J Pediatr* 104:527–533, 1984.

23. White BP, Gunnar MR, Larson MC, et al: Physiological reactivity and daily rhythms in infants with and without colic. *Child Dev.* In press.

24. Barr RG, Young SN, Wright JH, et al: Differential calming response to sucrose taste in crying infants with and without colic. *Pediatrics* 103:1–9, 1999.

25. Lehtonen L, Gormally SM, Barr RG: Clinical pies and prognostic clues to outcome in infants with colic syndrome, in Barr RG, Hopkins B, Green J, (eds): *Crying as a Sign, a Symptom and a Signal: Clinical, Emotional and Developmental Aspects of Infant and Toddler Crying.* London: McKeith Press. In press.

26. Stifter CA, Bono MA: The effect of infant colic on maternal self-perceptions and mother-infant attachment. *Child Care Health Dev* 24:339–351, 1998.

27. Rautava P, Lehtonen L, Helenius H, Silanpaa M: Infantile colic: child and family three years later. *Pediatrics* 96:43–47, 1995.

28. Raiha H, Lehtonen L, Korhonen T, Korvenranta H: Family life one year after infantile colic. *Arch Pediatr Adolesc Med* 150:1032–1036, 1996.

29. Raiha H, Lehtonen L, Korhonen T, Korvenranta H: Family functioning three years after infantile colic. *J Dev Behav Pediatr* 18:290–294, 1997.

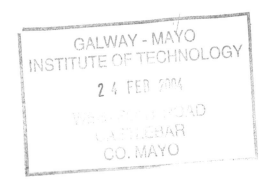

William Feldman

Disorders of Sleep

The most prevalent sleep problems of infancy and childhood are difficulty falling asleep, difficulty staying asleep, night terrors, nightmares, and sleepwalking. Rocking and head-banging by sleepy infants may also be seen. As a general rule children suffer no harm from sleep disorders; their parents most assuredly do. The sleep needs of children vary. The parents of children who require a lot of sleep are blessed; the parents of children who require little sleep feel cursed. Cultural factors and parental upbringing determine what they consider to be abnormal. Cosleeping, (the practice of allowing children to sleep in their parents' bed), for example, is normal in some cultures, even though it enhances dependence.

In this chapter, a clinical description of these problems is provided, as are current ideas about their causes and mechanisms and the best available evidence regarding their management.

Difficulty Falling and Staying Asleep

Difficulty Falling Asleep

This problem is usually first seen in the preschool period and is the most common sleep problem in school-age children, occurring in around 25 percent.[1] Although the relative roles of genetics and environment as causes of this problem are unknown, some children seem to be poor sleepers from infancy regardless of the approaches used by their parents, whereas in other cases the behavior is clearly learned.

Children with this problem will use a number of techniques to get out of staying in their beds; they will claim to be frightened of monsters, to be hungry or thirsty, or to have to go the bathroom. Many of these children had frequent nighttime awakenings as infants; i.e., they would be put into their cribs asleep but would frequently awaken during the night.

Although there are no good studies on causation, an approach that can be used in discussing this problem with parents is that there are some children who are temperamentally poor sleepers and who learn that their sleep problem can bring them a lot of extra attention. This attention is frequently positive, in the form of snacks, hugs, and extra time spent watching television with parents.

Difficulty Staying Asleep

Frequent nighttime awakenings are also common, most often seen in children between 6 months and 4 years of age. The milder forms (waking up around three times a week) are about three times as common as the severest forms (waking up at least twice per night). Many of these children also have daytime behavior problems, especially temper tantrums. A variety of causes have been proposed, from a difficult temperament[2] to maternal depression and stress within the family.[3] The family's handling of nighttime awakenings has also been associated with this problem, in that nighttime feeding after 6 months of age and taking the child into the parents' bed are considered to be risk factors.[3,4]

A popular theory of causation for the problem of frequent awakenings is the presence of "nonadaptive sleep associations." Sleep associations are described as the usual bedtime environment at the time the child falls asleep.[5] What defines these sleep associations as "nonadaptive" is the fact that they are bedtime conditions that the infant or child cannot reproduce himself or herself—for example, falling asleep while being rocked, held in a parent's arms, or while feeding. The theory is that most infants wake up periodically, as do older children, but if they initially fell asleep alone in their cribs or beds, they

fall asleep easily again. If they fell asleep in their parents' arms or while feeding, these "nonadaptive associations" are also required if the child wakes up during the night.

The usual nonadaptive sleep associations include the child falling asleep while breast- or bottle-feeding, falling asleep with a pacifier which the child cannot replace if he or she awakens in the night with the pacifier having fallen out, and falling asleep in the parents' bed or parents' arms and then being put into his or her own bed already asleep.

There are some studies that support nonadaptive sleep associations; that is, children put to bed already asleep (i.e., with nonadaptive sleep associations) have more nighttime awakenings than children put to bed awake.

Management

Because the management of children who have difficulty falling asleep is similar to that of children who have trouble staying asleep, approaches to dealing with these problems are discussed together. The most widely studied approaches to solving these problems involve behavioral management principles. The use of medications is also discussed briefly. It should be understood that many parents cannot or will not take the necessary behavioral steps because of their own limitations or needs. In addition, it is rare that two parents will concur completely in a behavioral management program. Men tend to be "tougher" and women "softer." It is important to bring theses issues out into the open so that such "natural" disagreements do not cascade into more serious marital conflict.

Behavioral Approaches

Several approaches to dealing with these problems involve identification and elimination of nonadaptive sleep associations (Table 2-1).

Table 2-1

Dealing with Sleep Problems

1. Help the parents identify nonadaptive sleep associations.
2. Impress upon the parents the importance of teaching the child to fall asleep alone and under conditions that they can control.
3. Identify and stop using those parental behaviors that reinforce the child not falling asleep or awakening (e.g., cuddling, feeding, bringing the child to the parents' bed, or allowing the child to come out of bed to play or watch television).
4. Keep the morning awakening time regular, so that the child cannot catch up the next morning on the sleep that was missed at night.
5. Reward good sleep behavior.

In addition to the steps outlined in Table 2-1, there should be a structured bedtime routine.[6] The routine should take about 15 minutes and should not change from night to night. For the infant, the feeding and diaper changes having been completed, the child should be put into his or her crib awake. The parent should then leave the room, but can come back from time to time to reassure the crying child. The parent should stay in the room for no longer than 1 min and should wait for progressively longer periods before going in again. Each night the length of time before the parent goes in to reassure the infant can be a bit longer.

For the child in a crib who has little difficulty falling asleep but who is a frequent nighttime awakener, the same approach can be used: reassure for no longer than 1 min in the child's room and wait progressively longer periods before reassuring again. (Tables 2-2 and 2-3)

GETTING THE OLDER CHILD TO FALL ASLEEP ALONE

It is more difficult to address these sleep problems in older children, who sleep in beds, than in infants who sleep in a cribs because the child who sleeps in his or her own bed can easily get out of bed and follow the parent out of the room. One approach that is commonly used

is the "chair-sitting" technique.[7] The first step, having put the child into bed awake after the structured bedtime routine, is for the parent to sit in a chair close to the child. Each night, the chair is moved further from the child's bed until it is out of the room. The parent's role is simply to sit there—not to speak with the child. Most children do well with this routine and will fall asleep without crying. When this happens with a child at least 3 years old, the child should

Table 2-2

Preventing Night Awakenings

The key to preventing night awakenings is teaching a child to fall asleep alone at an early age. Even a baby 10 or 12 weeks old can be put into a crib or cradle awake. To avoid creating positive reinforcement for waking,

- Keep night-time encounters short and boring.
- Do not do unnecessary diaper changes at night.
- Try to drop night-time feedings after 6 months of age.
- Follow a consistent bedtime routine at the same time every evening.

SOURCE: From Fehlings,[6] by permission.

Table 2-3

Handout for Parents

How do I get my child to fall asleep alone if I can't bear to ignore the crying?
You can retrain your child by simply waiting a little longer each day before going in. This works best in a child under age 2 who is still sleeping in a crib. (Do not use this method if your child is old enough to fall out of the crib.) Go through your normal bedtime routine and then put the child in the crib awake. Leave the room, but come back from time to time to reassure the child until he or she falls asleep—but stay only a minute or two each time, and do not pick the child up. Wait a little longer after each visit, and increase the intervals from night to night. For example:

	First Visit	Second Visit	Third Visit	Further Visits
Day 1	2 min	4 min	6 min	6 min
Day 2	4 min	6 min	8 min	8 min
Day 3	6 min	8 min	10 min	10 min
Day 4	8 min	10 min	12 min	12 min

Most children are quite upset during the first few nights of this change, but soon they learn to fall asleep alone. The same technique can be used to decrease your response when the child wakes up during the night.

SOURCE: From Fehlings,[6] by permission.

receive praise and a sticker the next morning. This approach teaches the child adaptive sleep associations.

For the few children who do not respond to the chair-sitting technique and who continue to cry even though the parent is sitting nearby, the parent should leave the room and hold the door shut for 1 min and then return to the chair. If the child continues to cry, the parent should again leave the room holding the door shut for 2 min, increasing the door-holding phase until the child stays in bed without crying.

The chair-sitting approach could also be tried for the child sleeping in a bed who has frequent nighttime awakenings.

DECREASING AND ELIMINATING NIGHTTIME FEEDINGS

Many parents continue to feed their infants during the night even though most healthy infants can sleep through the night without feeding by 4 to 6 months of age. This maladaptive sleep association reinforces nighttime awakening, and removing this factor should be the first approach taken. Stopping nighttime feeds in the poor sleeper over 6 months of age should be done gradually. For the bottle-fed infant, 1 oz of formula less should be put in the bottle each night. Adding water to the bottle should be discouraged because the parent then has to remove the water-feeding maladaptive sleep association. For breast-fed infants the feeding time can be decreased by 1 or 2 min each night and the interval between feedings lengthened by 1/2 h each night.

How good is the evidence in support of behavioral strategies for infants and children who either cannot fall asleep or who wake up frequently?

In one study, an approach called *systematic ignoring* (in which the parents were advised to check on the child and then leave the room) was found to be more effective than the parents' usual approach: comforting, feeding, etc. In this well-done randomized controlled trial there was a high dropout rate of families randomized to the systematic ignoring group.[8] In discussing this study with parents it may be wise to ask in advance whether they feel they would be able to tolerate the infant's crying. If not, another approach—such as consoling for no more than 1 min and gradually increasing the periods before going in again—should be tried.

The structured bedtime routine has also been studied in a randomized controlled trial.[9] In this study, the structured bedtime routine with several activities (tooth-brushing, washing, story) and with praise after completion of each activity was compared with graduated extinction (ignoring the crying child for progressively longer periods, with intermittent comforting for fewer than 15 s), and with a no-treatment control group. Both treatment groups improved significantly when compared to the controls.

The advice to teach infants to sleep through the night without feeding has also been studied in a randomized controlled trial.[10] In this study, breast-fed infants were fed before midnight and then the time between feedings was gradually lengthened. In the control group, mothers were advised to continue their usual regimen. In this study, 100 percent of the treatment group slept through the night, compared with only 23 percent of the controls. Both groups gained weight appropriately.

Medication

Most physicians are reluctant to use medication for healthy children who have problems falling asleep or staying asleep. However, medications such as choral hydrate and melatonin are used for children with developmental disorders whose sleep problems do not respond to behavior modification programs. Other drugs such as barbiturates, benzodiazepines, and antihista-

mines can sedate and induce sleep in these children at bedtime, but because of other side effects, they are rarely used.

Chloral hydrate, if it is to be used at all, should be used for the short-term only.[11] It is usually given in a dose of 10 mg/kg/dose about 1/2 h before bed-time. The dose may have to be increased up to 25 mg/kg/dose and should not be used for more than 4 weeks, at which time the dose should be gradually dropped to zero over about five nights. This advice is based on clinical experience alone; unfortunately there have been no randomized controlled trials of choral hydrate for childhood sleep disorders.

Melatonin has been studied, but the results are conflicting and there have been no long-term studies regarding the benefits and risks for its use in childhood sleep problems. It should probably still be considered an experimental drug.

In summary, behavioral interventions have been well studied and should be used for otherwise healthy children who have trouble falling asleep or staying asleep. Medications need rarely be used for these children. The use of hypnotic or sedative drugs should be considered a second-line treatment for developmentally disabled children who have failed a concerted behavioral approach.

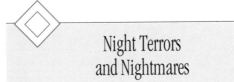

Night Terrors and Nightmares

Night terrors are very frightening for the parents of the affected child, but do not seem to disturb the child very much. They are biological, not psychological in origin, and happen when the affected children pass from non–rapid-eye-movement (non-REM) to REM sleep.[12] Night terrors are said to occur in approximately 6 percent of children.[13] There may be several episodes a week, followed by a period of up to a few months before a single episode or a cluster of night terrors recurs.

Night terrors usually begin after 18 months of age. In the typical case the child suddenly sits up in bed screaming, staring straight ahead with a blank gaze, breathing in an irregular pattern, possibly sweating. The child can usually not be consoled and does not recognize his or her parent. After a period of 30 s to 10 min (it may seem like 10 h to the terrified parent!) the child settles back to sleep and the next morning has no memory of the night terror.

The most important component of the treatment of night terrors is a careful explanation to the parents that this is not a nightmare and is probably a genetic sleep disorder. There are frequently other family members who had either night terrors, sleepwalking, or sleep-talking. The parents can be reassured that most children with night terrors outgrow the problem by adolescence. Once the parents understand the nature of this condition, they should be informed that there is no specific treatment other than being sure that the child does not injure himself or herself during the episode should there be some thrashing about. There is no point in either awakening the child during the episode or discussing it with the child or in the child's presence the next morning.

Other components of therapy, such as behavioral management or the use of medications such as benzodiazepines or tricyclic antidepressants, have not been well studied and are not needed in most cases. If medications are considered essential because the episodes occur nightly and the family is having problems coping, they should be used only for a short time—no more than 1 or 2 weeks.[13]

Nightmares are distinctly different from night terrors. Whereas night terrors occur in the first third of sleep, when the child goes from non-REM to REM sleep, nightmares happen in the last third of the night, when the child is in REM sleep. Nightmares usually start at a somewhat later age than night terrors, often between 3 and 6 years of age. They are much more prevalent than night terrors, occurring in up to 50 percent of children.[14] They can easily be distinguished clinically from night terrors on the basis of a careful history from the parents. The child will awaken crying, is agitated when the parents come in to his or her room, but is awake and easily comforted. The child with a nightmare can remember the dream and what it was that frightened him or her. The affected child may be too frightened to go back to sleep easily.

Just as the histories of the two sleep problems given by the parents are very different, so too is the management. In the case of nightmares, the parents should console their children by reassuring them that parents are there to protect them, that it was only a dream, and that nothing bad will happen to them. If a stressful event happened that day or if the child saw a frightening movie or TV show before going to bed, the possible cause-and-effect relationship can be discussed the next day and attempts made to decrease the frightening experiences.

Sleepwalking and/or Sleep-Talking

At least one episode of sleepwalking or sleep-talking has been reported in up to 30 percent of children, but these are rare in adults. Like night terrors, sleepwalking and/or sleep-talking occur when the child goes from non-REM to REM sleep during the first third of the night. It is also most likely an inherited sleep disorder. The child may both walk and talk during sleep, wandering aimlessly and talking incoherently. Some children walk sometimes and talk at other times while remaining in bed. Some children begin sleepwalking and/or sleep-talking when they have outgrown night terrors. It is most prevalent between ages 10 and 12 years.

These conditions are not caused by psychological or emotional problems. The most important part of the treatment is the explanation to the parents and child about what is known regarding the etiology and natural history: the parents are not to blame, the child is not emotionally disturbed, and it gets better with age.

The only other component of treatment is to have the parents ensure a safe environment. Some parents may sleep through an episode. What often helps is to place a bell on the child's door; this should be set up to ring when the door is opened. Behavior management, scheduled night awakenings, and late-afternoon naps have not been studied in controlled trials and should be considered experimental. Medications have also not been studied adequately, and since this is rarely a serious problem, the risks of using drugs outweigh the potential benefits.

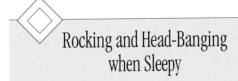

Rocking and Head-Banging when Sleepy

These are seen in normal children fairly commonly, usually in the second 6 months of life and rarely up to age 4 or 5 years. It is more common in boys. These infants rock in the crawling position; head-banging may occur in that position or in the sitting-up position. They occur usually at night when the child is drowsy but may occur during the day at nap time.

The cause of these phenomena is unknown; what is known is that these young children have no more emotional or psychological problems than their nonrocking and non-head-banging peers. Since it is the experience of all physicians who have cared for these children that it generally always disappears when ignored, no treatments have been developed or studied in controlled trials.

The key to successful management is to reassure the parents that their child is normal, that he or she will not be harmed, and that the child will outgrow the problem by age 4 or 5 years or perhaps sooner.

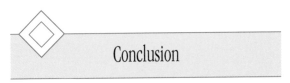

Conclusion

In summary, problems falling and staying asleep have been shown to respond to appropriate interventions. To determine the initial severity and progress, parents should keep a sleep diary. (Table 2-4) Night terrors and sleepwalking/talking are likely inherited sleep disorders that merely require attention to the child's safety. Nightmares are common and should be pursued for etiology only if they are frequent and persistent. Finally, head-banging and rocking in normal children are also fairly common, improve with age, and are harmless. Further attention should be paid only to children who continue to rock their beds or bang their heads past 5 years of age.

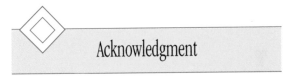

Acknowledgment

The author is grateful to Dr. Darcy Fehlings for her excellent contributions to the literature on sleep disorders in childhood.

References

1. Bramble D: Rapid-acting treatment for a common sleep problem. *Dev Med Child Neurolo* 39:543–547, 1997.
2. Richman N: A community survey of characteristics of 1–2 year-olds with sleep disruptions. *J Am Acad Child Psychiatry* 20:281–291, 1981.
3. Lozoff B, Wolf AW, Davis NS: Sleep problems seen in pediatric practice. *Pediatrics* 75:477–483, 1985.

4. Sandler LW, Stechier G, Burns P, et al: Early mother-infant interaction and 24-hour patterns of activity and sleep. *J Am Acad Child Psychiatry* 9:103–123, 1970.

5. Ferber R: *Solve Your Child's' Sleep Problems*. New York, Simon & Schuster, 1985.

6. Fehlings D: Sleeping patterns and problems, in Feldman W (ed): *The 3 am Handbook*. New York, Facts on File, 1998.

7. Richman N, Douglas J, Hunt M, et al: Behavioral methods in the treatment of sleep disorders: a pilot study. *J Child Psychol Psychiatry* 26:581–590, 1985.

8. Richert VI, Johnson CM: Reducing nocturnal awakenings and crying episodes in infants and young children: a comparison between scheduled awakenings and systematic ignoring. *Pediatrics* 81:203–212, 1988.

9. Adams LA, Richert VI: Reducing bedtime tantrums: comparison between positive routines and graduated extinction. *Pediatrics* 84:756–761, 1989.

10. Pinella T, Birch LL: Help me make it through the night: behavioral entrainment of breast-fed infant's sleep patterns. *Pediatrics* 91:434–444, 1993.

11. American Academy of Pediatrics: Use of choral hydrate for sedation in children. *Pediatrics* 92:471–473, 1993.

12. Lask B: Sleep disorders. *J Am Acad Child and Adolesc Psychiatry* 36:1161, 1997.

13. Blum N, Carey W: Sleep problems among infants and young children. *Pediatr Rev* 17:87–92, 1996.

14. Anders T, Eiben L: Pediatric sleep disorders: a review of the past 10 years. *J Am Acad Child Adolesc Psychiatry* 36:9–12, 1997.

Table 2-4

Sleep Diary for Parents

Please keep a record of your child's sleep patterns both day and night.

x – child put to bed

✔ – asleep

	NIGHT					A.M.							MORNING					P.M.					
	8	9	10	11	12	1	2	3	4	5	6	7	8	9	10	11	12	1	2	3	4	5	6	7
Week #____																								
Sunday																								
Monday																								
Tuesday																								
Wednesday																								
Thursday																								
Friday																								
Saturday																								
Week #____																								
Sunday																								
Monday																								
Tuesday																								
Wednesday																								
Thursday																								
Friday																								
Saturday																								
Week #____																								
Sunday																								
Monday																								
Tuesday																								
Wednesday																								
Thursday																								
Friday																								
Saturday																								

SOURCE: From Fehlings,[6] by permission.

Lance E. Rodewald
Jeanne M. Santoli

Immunizations

The provision of immunizations to U.S. preschool children has shifted significantly from health department clinics to primary care providers—predominantly community practitioners. During the late 1980s, approximately 50 percent of vaccinations were administered by health departments, but in 1997 only 14 to 20 percent of children received vaccinations in health departments. This shift was largely caused by vaccination financing programs and policies intended to reintegrate vaccinations into private-sector primary care practice and reduce missed opportunities to vaccinate. Vaccinating children in their medical home is consistent with the desires of pediatricians and family physicians as well as parents, but the shift has consequences for primary care providers because of the responsibility and accountability that accompany the job of providing immunizations. The increasing complexity of the immunization schedule and technical demands of vaccination make the job much more challenging than in the past.

Public health officials rely on clinicians to implement childhood immunization recommendations for the appropriate administration of vaccines to all patients not having valid contraindications. However, public health officials treat *populations*, while clinicians treat *individuals*. Although the primary goal of protecting children from vaccine-preventable diseases is shared by both public health officials and clinicians, certain of the considerations, decision making, and strategies to achieve this goal may differ between the two groups of professionals. The relationship between public health and private practice should be synergistic: together, they accomplish much more than could be accomplished separately.

This chapter explores some areas where differences in strategies and methods may become apparent to the clinician, with the goal of articulating public health practices that can be helpful to practitioners. It discusses the current status of childhood vaccination, implementation of new vaccines, vaccine safety and parental objection to vaccination, vaccination recommendation decision making, and evidence-based office strategies to raise and sustain high coverage levels among a panels of patients. Our intention is not to review all vaccine recommendations but rather to discuss issues involved in carrying them out.

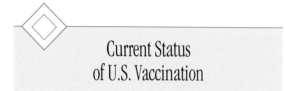

Current Status of U.S. Vaccination

Routine childhood vaccination is one of the major public health success stories in this century. Due to routine vaccinations administered throughout this century, it is estimated that almost half a billion cases of vaccine-preventable disease and 3 million premature deaths were prevented in the United States alone.[1] Further evidence of the effectiveness and importance of vaccination can be seen in the incidence rates of the traditional vaccine preventable diseases: diphtheria, tetanus, pertussis, measles, mumps, rubella, invasive Haemophilus influenzae type B disease, and paralytic polio. All of these diseases are currently at record low levels—each has seen a reduction in reported disease rates of over 97 percent compared with their peak, prevaccine incidences.[2] To achieve this reduction in

disease incidence, vaccination levels for the corresponding diseases had to be raised to the highest levels ever—greater than 90 percent population-level coverage for the most critical doses of the vaccines. Together, primary care practitioners and public health providers achieved this feat during a time of increasing complexity in the vaccination schedule, while the immunization delivery system underwent large-scale changes. At the same time, the burden of vaccination was shifted in large part away from health departments and toward primary care providers.

However, the successes of routine vaccination are somewhat illusory for two reasons. First and most important, yesterday's success means little for the babies of today. As the director of the National Immunization Program of the Centers for Disease Control and Prevention (CDC) Walt Orenstein, M.D., is fond of saying, there are 11,000 babies born each day with a vaccination status of zero who must receive 15 to 19 doses of vaccine by the time they reach 18 months of age. The goal of building an immunization delivery system that ensures timely vaccination, day in and day out, regardless of political interest or vaccine-preventable disease epidemics, is still a work in progress. Two critical inadequacies of the current immunization delivery system are (1) insurance plans that do not cover the costs of recommended vaccines and their administration and (2) the lack of an information infrastructure adequate to monitor coverage and help providers identify children in need of vaccination. To be sure, important elements of the delivery system have been built. An obvious example is the Vaccines for Children (VFC) program, which entitles eligible children to receive public-purchased vaccine in their medical home for primary care. But vaccine financing alone is insufficient to assure the vaccination of all children.

Second, the weak implementation of new vaccines and new recommendations has led to a situation in which preventable morbidity and mortality are widespread but not generally appreciated by the public. In contrast to traditional vaccine-preventable diseases such as measles and diphtheria, many patients and parents view diseases that have recently become vaccine-preventable as less important, and they are more willing to forgo immunization for themselves and their children. Even physicians have questioned the need for some vaccines, such as varicella and hepatitis B. However, consider the following examples: Each annual cohort of adolescents that "escapes" vaccination and becomes more difficult to reach as young adults will suffer over 160,000 cases of hepatitis B infection, leading to about 1400 hepatitis B–related deaths. Yet the hepatitis B coverage level remains at a stubborn plateau of about 85 percent.

More children die each year from varicella than died of measles during the peak year of the measles resurgence of 1989 to 1991, yet the coverage level of this vaccine is less than 50 percent. The heavy emphasis on the more traditional vaccine-preventable diseases has compromised prevention opportunities related to new populations and new vaccines.

Thus, the current status of the immunization delivery system is a mixture of good news, bad news, and significant challenges. Although there are unparalleled successes with the traditional vaccine-preventable diseases, there is need for improvement and for consolidation of the gains. Otherwise, the present inadequacies in our delivery system might set a pattern for future failures with the coming plethora of new vaccines.

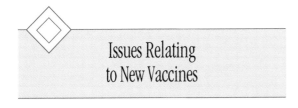

Issues Relating to New Vaccines

The ability of clinicians to protect their patients from vaccine-preventable diseases is becoming much more powerful and safe due to the fruits of biotechnology. This power and safety are accompanied by increasing invasiveness, complexity, cost, decision making, and communication challenges. In addition, new vaccines continue to be developed and new recommendations are being targeted to establish routine vaccination of adolescents. (*Table 3-1*)

Invasiveness

Twenty years ago 5 injections were recommended for children through 18 months of age: today at least 15 and as many as 19 injections are recommended by 18 months of age: more will follow soon. One important consequence of this growing number of recommended immunizations is the need for simultaneous injections. While everyone concerned desires to reduce the number of injections, parents appear willing to tolerate four simultaneous injections for babies. Empiric evidence can be found when looking at the recent change from oral poliovirus vaccination to a sequential schedule, which occurred at about the same time DTaP replaced DTP and uncoupled the popular DTP-Hib combination. The number of injections doubled from two to four injections at the 2- and 4-month visits. Monitoring studies showed that parents and providers tolerated the extra injections, and that there was no decrease in coverage or increase in missed opportunities.[3] However no one knows the theoretical upper bound for the number of injections tolerated at well-child visits, nor does anyone want to find out. Many clinicians suspect that we may be close to that limit.

Although combination vaccines that will reduce the number of injections are under development, it is unclear when the absolute number of injections will decrease to a level more comfortable for providers, parents, and (most importantly) patients. Solutions to multiple, simultaneous injections are only palliative until new combination vaccines become available in the United States. Examples of injection-reducing combination vaccines, currently in

Table 3-1

Challenges to the Implementation of New Vaccines and New Recommendations

CHALLENGE	EXAMPLES
Increased invasiveness	11 to 15 injections by 18 months of age 4 injections at 2- and 4-month visit
Complexity of the immunization schedule	Three new vaccines in last 5 years Harmonization of schedule created age ranges instead of specific ages Sequenced change in poliovirus vaccination to IPV Minimum spacing between vaccinations is confusing
Office decision making about offering new vaccines	New vaccines may have different storage requirements Insurance coverage may lag recommendation for use, creating cost barrier Some new vaccines are for milder diseases than older vaccines
Communicating with parents about new vaccines and vaccine safety	Parent education requires valuable time in well-child visits Some new vaccines protect against severe disease, but child may acquire mild disease Some new vaccines protect against diseases not specifically recognized by parents New Vaccine Information Statements are needed Groups opposed to routine vaccination are more visible and vocal
Vaccinating adolescents	May require change in practice to incorporate routine vaccination Need to implement recall system for unvaccinated older adolescents Adolescents tend to be less well insured

development at the phase III trial level for the U.S. market, include DTaP/Hep B/Hib/IPV and Hib/Hep B/IPV, both of which will greatly reduce the number of injections. Some progress has been made to reduce the pain associated with injections—for example, using a vapocoolant spray applied immediately prior to injection. While waiting for combination vaccines to become available, it is important to keep in mind that there are no contraindications to the simultaneous administration of any of the vaccines in the harmonized schedule.

Complexity

The most visible example of complexity caused by new vaccines and new recommendations is the childhood immunization schedule, which has been harmonized among recommending bodies for pediatricians, family physicians, and the federal government since 1994. Because childhood immunization is such a fast-moving field, the schedule changes annually (but not more often). As a result of harmonization, specific ages have been replaced by age intervals, and additional footnotes have been added to indicate minor variations among the three recommending groups. An obvious change over the years is in the number of new vaccines and in the nuances of their technical recommendations. The desire to keep the immunization schedule to one page with footnotes has necessitated the use of rather small-size type for the footnotes (*Fig. 3-1.*).

Unfortunately, not all vaccination scheduling information can be placed on the harmonized schedule. Missing is information about the minimum spacing intervals that can be used to catch up a child who is behind in his or her immunizations. Problems arise in the clinical situation of determining if a child is eligible for vaccination and in the distantly related situation of determining eligibility for kindergarten entry (which has considerable variation in the laws of the various states). New vaccines add new rules to be incorporated into practice. Furthermore, for many vaccines, the nuances of when to revaccinate if a dose was given too early can be extremely challenging to determine. The Advisory Committee on Immunization Practices (ACIP) and the Red Book Committee are investigating new methods to make rules of revaccination clearer.

With new vaccines come new Vaccine Information Statements (VIS), which the law requires providers to distribute and discuss with parents prior to vaccination. New vaccination recommendations about old vaccines require providers to replace outdated statements with new ones. Keeping current of the VIS forms is no easy matter, because the statements vary in their "shelf life," and they do not currently contain an explicit expiration date. One solution being investigated is notifying all physicians each year of the current version of the VIS that they should be using.

Finally, a less visible aspect of the complexity caused by new vaccines is the increase in vaccine storage and handling specifications and the need for additional training for office staff. Prior to the recommendation for universal varicella vaccine administration, for example, the coldest temperature required to store the recommended vaccines was −14°C. Varicella vaccine requires a temperature unattainable by small, dormitory-style refrigerators to remain viable, and many practices have had to purchase new refrigerators in order to offer this vaccine to their patients.

Cost

New vaccines are more expensive than vaccines that have been available for a number of years because manufacturers have attempted to recover the considerable costs associated with vaccine development. A problem arises for the clinician when a new vaccine is recommended, because most practices have a combination of publicly insured children and privately insured children, and the timing of the availability of coverage for new vaccines is likely to vary among insurance types. This disparity easily creates a double standard of vaccination coverage in a practice, although hopefully it is a temporary double standard. Children eligible for Vaccines for Children (VFC) vaccine become entitled for vaccination as soon as the ACIP votes the vaccine into the VFC program and a contract is negotiated between the CDC and the manufacturer. Managed care organizations, however, may negotiate their capitation rates only once a year, in which case the new vaccine would not be covered until the next negotiation period. An additional barrier for privately insured patients is the need to create vaccine-specific CPT-4 codes that allow reimbursement for vaccines administered. On occasion, the ACIP has recognized these financing issues and allowed a phase-in period to allow time for private insurance companies to incorporate the vaccine into their benefit packages.

A further concern is the possibility that a number of private insurance companies or self-insured corporations will fail to cover the cost of vaccinations for families. With the growing cost of routine vaccination, this might cause a shift back to health departments for free vaccine,

Figure 3-1

Recommended Childhood Immunization Schedule
United States, January - December 2000

Vaccines[1] are listed under routinely recommended ages. Bars indicate range of recommended ages for immunization. Any dose not given at the recommended age should be given as a "catch-up" immunization at any subsequent visit when indicated and feasible. Ovals indicate vaccines to be given if previously recommended doses were missed or given earlier than the recommended minimum age.

Age ▶ Vaccine ▼	Birth	1 mo	2 mos	4 mos	6 mos	12 mos	15 mos	18 mos	24 mos	4-6 yrs	11-12 yrs	14-16 yrs
Hepatitis B[2]	Hep B	Hep B		Hep B							Hep B	
Diphtheria, Tetanus, Pertussis[3]			DTaP	DTaP	DTaP		DTaP[3]			DTaP	Td	
H. influenzae type b[4]			Hib	Hib	Hib	Hib						
Polio[5]			IPV	IPV		IPV[5]				IPV[5]		
Measles, Mumps Rubella[6]						MMR				MMR[6]	MMR[6]	
Varicella[7]						Var					Var[7]	
Hepatitis A[8]									Hep A-[8]in selected areas			

Approved by the Advisory Committee on Immunization Practices (ACIP), the American Academy of Pediatrics (AAP), and the American Academy of Family Physicians (AAFP).

The harmonized, routine childhood immunization schedule.

On October 22, 1999, the Advisory Committee on Immunization Practices (ACIP) recommended that Rotashield® (RRV-TV), the only U.S.-licensed rotavirus vaccine, no longer be used in the United States (MMWR, Volume 48, Number 43, Nov. 5, 1999). Parents should be reassured that their children who received rotavirus vaccine before July are not at increased risk for intussusception now.

[1]This schedule indicates the recommended ages for routine administration of currently licensed childhood vaccines as of 11/1/99. Additional vaccines may be licensed and recommended during the year. Licensed combination vaccines may be used whenever any components of the combination are indicated and its other components are not contraindicated. Providers should consult the manufacturers' package inserts for detailed recommendations.

[2]**Infants born to HBsAg-negative mothers** should receive the 1st dose of hepatitis B (Hep B) vaccine by age 2 months. The 2nd dose should be at least one month after the 1st dose.   The 3rd dose should be administered at least 4 months after the 1st dose and at least 2 months after the 2nd dose, but not before 6 months of age for infants.

Infants born to HBsAg-positive mothers should receive hepatitis B vaccine and 0.5 mL hepatitis B immune globulin (HBIG) within 12 hours of birth at separate sites. The 2nd dose is recommended at 1-2 months of age and the 3rd dose at 6 months of age.

Infants born to mothers whose HBsAg status is unknown should receive hepatitis B vaccine within 12 hours of birth. Maternal blood should be drawn at the time of delivery to determine the mother's HBsAg status; if the HBsAg test is positive, the infant should receive HBIG as soon as possible (no later than 1 week of age).

All children and adolescents (through 18 years of age) who have not been immunized against hepatitis B may begin the series during any visit. Special efforts should be made to immunize children who were born in or whose parents were born in areas of the world with moderate or high endemicity of hepatitis B virus infection.

[3]The 4th dose of DTaP (diphtheria and tetanus toxoids and acellular pertussis vaccine) may be administered as early as 12 months of age, provided 6 months have elapsed since the 3rd dose and the child is unlikely to return at age 15-18 months. Td (tetanus and diphtheria toxoids) is recommended at 11-12 years of age if at least 5 years have elapsed since the last dose of DTP, DTaP or DT. Subsequent routine Td boosters are recommended every 10 years.

[4]Three Haemophilus influenzae type b (Hib) conjugate vaccines are licensed for infant use. If PRP-OMP (PedvaxHIB® or ComVax® [Merck]) is administered at 2 and 4 months of age, a dose at 6 months is not required. Because clinical studies in infants have demonstrated that using some combination products may induce a lower immune response to the Hib vaccine component, DTaP/Hib combination products should not be used for primary immunization in infants at 2, 4 or 6 months of age, unless FDA-approved for these ages.

[5]To eliminate the risk of vaccine-associated paralytic polio (VAPP), an all-IPV schedule is now recommended for routine childhood polio vaccination in the United States. All children should receive four doses of IPV at 2 months, 4 months, 6-18 months, and 4-6 years. OPV (if available) may be used only for the following special circumstances:
1. Mass vaccination campaigns to control outbreaks of paralytic polio.
2. Unvaccinated children who will be traveling in <4 weeks to areas where polio is endemic or epidemic.
3. Children of parents who do not accept the recommended number of vaccine injections. These children may receive OPV only for the third or fourth dose or both; in this situation, health-care providers should administer OPV only after discussing the risk for VAPP with parents or caregivers.
4. During the transition to an all-IPV schedule, recommendations for the use of remaining OPV supplies in physicians' offices and clinics have been issued by the American Academy of Pediatrics (see Pediatrics, December 1999).

[6]The 2nd dose of measles, mumps, and rubella (MMR) vaccine is recommended routinely at 4-6 years of age but may be administered during any visit, provided at least 4 weeks have elapsed since receipt of the 1st dose and that both doses are administered beginning at or after 12 months of age. Those who have not previously received the second dose should complete the schedule by the 11-12 year old visit.

[7]Varicella (Var) vaccine is recommended at any visit on or after the first birthday for susceptible children, i.e. those who lack a reliable history of chickenpox (as judged by a health care provider) and who have not been immunized. Susceptible persons 13 years of age or older should receive 2 doses, given at least 4 weeks apart.

[8]Hepatitis A (Hep A) is shaded to indicate its recommended use in selected states and/or regions; consult your local public health authority. (Also see MMWR Oct. 01, 1999/48(RR12); 1-27).

effectively undoing the considerable gains made during the 1990s to reintegrate vaccination into the medical home for primary care. Although there are recommendations to purchasers of health care that all recommended vaccines and their administration should be covered in full, these are only recommendations, not binding mandates, and the concern of inadequate private insurance coverage for vaccination is very real.

Decision Making

It is difficult to overstate the importance of the clinician's recommendation to parents about vaccination. Parents trust their child's doctor and tend to follow his or her advice about health matters for their children. Parents look to providers for education on the need for vaccination and the importance of vaccines to their child's health. This education and advice plays a determining role in parental vaccination decisions. For example, a survey of pediatricians, conducted as part of market research conducted by Merck, Inc., showed that a provider recommendation against varicella vaccination was a strong deterrent to parental acceptance (30 percent vaccinated); a neutral recommendation resulted in fewer than half of parents accepting vaccination; and a strong recommendation for vaccination resulted in a high degree of parental acceptance (more than 85 percent).[4]

Not all vaccines are equally compelling to practitioners. By definition, new vaccines prevent infectious diseases that have been handled with varying degrees of success by curative medicine. Hib vaccine was immediately popular because it solved a vexing clinical problem, meningitis, which was amenable only to primary prevention. In contrast, varicella tends to be mild, and clinicians and parents have experience treating it. Few clinicians will see a varicella-associated death in their practice because such fatalities are rare in the United States.

Accepted by many providers as an unavoidable childhood affliction, varicella has not yet made the transition from a nuisance disease to a disease that should be avoided by vaccination. Yet when public health officials look at the nation as a whole, they see varicella vaccine as a cost-saving method to prevent the suffering associated with tens of thousands of hospitalizations, many office illness visits, and over 50 premature deaths per year.

Pathman and colleagues developed and investigated a sequential model about the decision-making process that physicians go through to determine whether to adopt new guidelines or recommendations. Called the Awareness to Adherence Model, it outlines a four-step process: first, physicians must become *aware* of a new recommendation; second, they must intellectually *agree* with it; third, they must decide to follow the recommendation *by adopting* it; and fourth, they successfully follow the recommendation by *adhering* to it.[5]

Ongoing dialogue with primary care providers will be an important element in the implementation of new vaccines. Supporting their decision making with strategies designed to simplify the administration and financing of vaccines is part of the necessary work of the CDC and partner organizations that promote vaccination. Whether the nation achieves its immunization objectives for new vaccines will be determined largely by whether clinicians are aware of, agree with. adopt, and are able to adhere to the new recommendations.

Communication Challenges

Educating parents about new vaccines will continue to be a challenge for clinicians because of the length of time needed and the new messages to communicate. Teaching parents the benefits and risks of each vaccine can be time-consuming. Vaccine Information Statements are helpful, but the large number of vaccines given in the primary series implies a lengthy discussion period with the parents. Moreover, new vaccines pose additional challenges for parental education. It is important not to overpromise the likely impact of a vaccine for an individual patient. For example, varicella vaccine is highly effective against severe disease and hospitalization, but does not prevent all infections. Rather, the impact of this vaccine is to prevent much of the disease, to make mild disease inapparent, and to make what would be severe disease much milder.

The new conjugate pneumococcal vaccine provides an additional communication challenge in that the disease it prevents is not specifically recognized by parents, the way that varicella is. Most parents can tell if their child has chickenpox, but conjugate pneumococcal vaccine will not prevent all or even most ear infections. From a parent's point of view, this vaccine is likely to be perceived as ineffective, since his or her children will still get ear infections. Parents must be told clearly and honestly which benefits to expect from the new vaccines in order to keep their expectations in line with likely benefits. These communication challenges are perhaps more difficult for primary care providers than for public health officials because the benefit to an individual is not as apparent as is the benefit to a population.

Future of New Vaccines

The end is not in sight for the challenge of implementing new vaccines, as biotechnology will continue to place more diseases into the "vaccine-preventable" category. Recently, the Institute of Medicine published a description of a decision tool to help determine which vaccines might have the greatest impact on quality-adjusted years of life for U.S. people.[6] Although the report is not an exhaustive list of vaccines to be developed, the list of vaccines categorized by the tool as favorable to most favorable is inter-

esting. Examples include *Helicobacter pylori* vaccine for infants, hepatitis C vaccine for infants, respiratory syncytial virus vaccine for infants, parainfluenza virus vaccine for infants, cytomegalovirus vaccine for adolescents, influenza virus vaccine for the general population, *Chlamydia* vaccine for adolescents, herpes simplex virus vaccine for adolescents, human papillomavirus vaccine for adolescents, *Neisseria gonorrhoeae* vaccine for adolescents, and group B streptococcus vaccine for adolescent females.

Adolescent Vaccination

A new initiative is being developed to establish routine vaccination of U.S. adolescents. The strategy for protecting adolescents is targeted at children aged 11 to 12 years and includes (1) establishing a routine preventive care visit to the primary care provider, (2) vaccinating those without previous varicella vaccination or history of disease against varicella, (3) administering a second dose of MMR to those who have received only a single dose, (4) administering hepatitis B vaccine to those not previously vaccinated, (5) providing a booster dose of tetanus and diphtheria toxoids, (6) providing other vaccines (influenza, pneumococcal polysaccharide, and hepatitis B vaccines) as indicated for certain high-risk adolescents, and (7) providing other preventive care measures as described in the *Guidelines for Adolescent Preventive Services.* The Institute of Medicine's list of potential new vaccines includes several targeted specifically toward adolescents, further underscoring the importance of institutionalizing adolescent vaccination strategies.

Timing is an important consideration for adolescent vaccination. In general, adolescents are easier to access than young adults, since there are several points of access for adolescents, including their clinician and the school system. Also, many adolescents (but not adults) are entitled to public-purchased vaccine through the

Vaccines for Children (VFC) program. Strategies for reaching all adolescents will probably revolve around who should provide and pay for the vaccinations. School-based clinics have potential to vaccinate large groups of children, and several states are conducting school vaccination clinics. Managed care organization and private providers have responsibility for vaccinating their patients. A number of states have adopted school entry regulations that require the initiation of hepatitis B vaccination before middle school entry, regardless of who provides the vaccinations. Ideally, adolescent vaccination will be incorporated into routine office-based practice, so that the 11- to 12-year-old visit can be used to deliver a number of important clinical preventive services, prevention messages, and new vaccines. Until this degree of program maturity is achieved, however, many adolescents are escaping protection against vaccine-preventable diseases, especially hepatitis B.

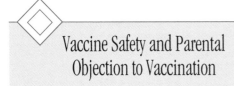

Vaccine Safety and Parental Objection to Vaccination

A core ingredient to the success of an immunization program is the assurance to parents, clinicians, and patients that the safest and most effective vaccines are recommended and used. Since immunization is recommended for all healthy children, it is held to a higher standard of safety than are curative services. Without widespread public support for routine vaccination, the protection of all children through vaccination is jeopardized. Examples where decreasing public support due to vaccine safety concerns led to epidemics of vaccine-preventable disease include the British, Japanese, and Swedish experiences with declining pertussis vaccination in the early 1980s. In these

situations, declining vaccination rates led to large epidemics of pertussis, with its concomitant morbidity and mortality.[7] The United States, in contrast, did not have significant decreases in coverage during this time, likely due to widespread support among practitioners and their professional organizations.

Although vaccines are rigorously tested for safety prior to licensure, the number of people exposed to the vaccine in the three phases of FDA testing is too small to detect adverse events occurring less frequently than approximately one in 10,000 vaccinations. Given the U.S. birth cohort size of 4 million, one can readily see the need for implementing postlicense surveillance to detect rare adverse events. This surveillance occurs via passive and active mechanisms. The passive surveillance method is the Vaccine Adverse Event Reporting System (VAERS), jointly administered by the FDA and the CDC. Active surveillance is conducted through the Vaccine Safety Datalink Project, administered by the CDC. Information about this project can be found at *http://www.cdc.gov/nip.*

Communication Challenges

A problem with the current situation is that the low levels of traditional vaccine-preventable diseases have created a major communication difficulty—the paucity of traditional vaccine-preventable diseases removes the public's stimulus for prevention. With so little traditional disease (e.g., a provisional total of 89 cases of measles in the entire United States in 1998!) to remind parents what their children are actively avoiding, it is understandable that many may question the need for high vaccination levels. Indeed, herd immunity, one of most helpful features of many vaccination programs, makes the communication challenge even more difficult because the many vaccinated protect the few unvaccinated. It requires little sophistication to see the advantage of relying on low levels of circulating pathogens rather than vaccination to protect an individual child. The chance of acquiring polio for the child who is not an international traveler is slim at best.

The combination of low vaccine-preventable disease levels and high immunization coverage levels makes vaccine adverse events (real or perceived) seem as more impressive than the damaged caused by traditional vaccine-preventable diseases. In addition, there is a natural human tendency to confuse association in time with causation. Moreover, primary prevention is a "silent" helper of children, because one cannot identify the actual individuals whose lives were saved by vaccination, even though it is well known that there are millions. Current vaccines are preventive rather than therapeutic, and primary prevention can be a thankless task as compared with curative medicine. Although no one knows which individuals' lives were saved by vaccination, individual practitioners know how their patients have benefited. Virtually all clinicians trained before the 1985 remember children in their practices who acquired and may have been damaged from invasive Hib disease. The implications of a febrile child were considerably more ominous when invasive Hib was prominent in the differential diagnosis. Helping parents understand the power of primary prevention will let them know they are making the best choice by vaccinating their children.

The media and the Internet provide a large amount of information to parents from groups opposed to routine vaccination. Regardless of the scientific validity of much of the available information, it may raise concerns about vaccination with some parents. Answering these concerns with accurate, unbiased information is important but time-consuming.

Philosophical and Religious Exemptions

Certain religions forbid vaccination, and almost all states recognize this by allowing religious exemption from school-entry vaccination laws. But some states also allow exemption from vaccination for philosophical reasons—i.e., the parents do not have a religious contraindication to vaccination but they are philosophically opposed. The decision by a parent to exempt his or her child from vaccination should not be taken lightly. Clinicians should help parents understand the critical importance of high vaccination coverage to protect not only the vaccinated children but also those children who cannot be vaccinated for medical or religious reasons. For example, failure to vaccinate healthy children jeopardizes children with cancer who cannot receive some vaccines due to the medical risk of a live virus vaccine or who cannot mount an adequate immune response to inactivated vaccines.

The actual decision making around exemption from school laws does not involve the child's doctor in most states because decisions for individual children are made by the schools (generally with quality assurance by the states' immunization programs). Some individuals may be taking "convenience" exemptions from vaccination, perhaps because they forgot their vaccination card during school registration or because they do not want to make an additional doctor visit to catch up on recommended vaccinations. Empiric evidence showing that states with a greater number of administrative barriers to taking an exemption have fewer students opting for exemption supports that concern.[8] Because of the relative ease of bypassing the primary care providers' desire to vaccinate all eligible patients, elimination of convenience exemptions may be the only solution. This means making sure that children about to enter school in the fall are completely up to date and have all of their immunization documentation before registration. Thus, the primary care provider can counsel parents about the importance of vaccination before the temptation to take a convenience exemption is allowed to arise at school registration.

Evidence-Based Office Strategies to Raise Coverage

It is within the power of the primary care provider to vaccinate virtually all of his or her patients for whom vaccination is recommended. A considerable body of research has been developed over that last two decades demonstrating methods for office-based physicians to raise and sustain vaccination coverage in their practices.[9] Before discussing two strategies for raising coverage that should be part of every immunization provider's practices (recall/reminder systems and practice-based coverage assessment), it will be helpful to discuss key barriers to vaccinating preschool children.

Barriers to Vaccination

Prior to the 1990s, parents were widely blamed for any failures to vaccinate their children—the rationale was that vaccines were freely available and that parents merely needed to take advantage of what was provided. Subsequent research has shown that parents are generally in favor of immunization, and, more to the point, parental attitudes toward vaccination are not significantly associated with vaccination status.[10] It was previously believed that the inability to identify an immunization provider was a major barrier to vaccination. This belief has also been shown to be incorrect. For example, parents of over 90 percent of undervaccinated children surveyed in the 1993 National Health Interview Survey were able to name their child's immunization provider.[11]

If parental attitudes and lack of immunization providers are not responsible for undervaccination, why are many children incompletely vaccinated? In addition to the barrier of poverty and its associated factors, there are five potentially changeable barriers that have been consistently described: (1) parents, although in general desirous of having their children vaccinated, do not know the vaccination status of their children, and they err on the side of believing that their child is up to date; (2) clinicians, although very desirous of vaccinating their patients, seldom operate information systems to identify patients in need of vaccination and to recall undervaccinated patients into the office; (3) practitioners seldom conduct self-assessments of the immunization coverage of their patients and in general believe the coverage to be higher than it actually is; (4) immunization records are sometimes scattered across multiple providers; and (5) providers frequently miss opportunities to vaccinate at non-well-child care visits.

These five barriers amount to an *information gap* that is causing children not to receive their vaccinations in a timely manner. Parents would like the doctor's office to let them know of any vaccination needs. But without a strategy that identifies immunization needs at office visits, recalls children who fall behind on the schedule, and reminds parents of upcoming appointments, there is little chance of filling the information gap. Furthermore, the increasing number of vaccinations and the shift of patients from health departments to private practices is exacerbating the problem of scattered records. It may become increasingly difficult to determine the vaccination needs of individual patients. The interventions described below (recall/reminder systems and practice-based coverage assessments) address this gap.

One additional barrier that may grow in importance as new vaccines become recommended for universal use in children needs to be mentioned. There is concern that significant numbers of practitioners may not recommend some new vaccines to their patients. At this point it is unclear how large a role this new provider barrier has played in the slow uptake of hepatitis B or varicella vaccines. Clearly, solutions other than those discussed below will need to be identified to overcome this potential barrier.

Table 3-2

Barriers to Timely Vaccination with Solutions to the Barriers

BARRIER	POTENTIAL REMEDY
Vaccination cost to parents	Join Vaccines for Children (VFC) program to help uninsured children. Encourage eligible children to join Child Health Insurance Plan or Medicaid. No remedy currently for children whose commercial insurance does not cover vaccinations.
Parents think their child is up to date when he or she may not be	Operate an office-based recall system to bring children in need of vaccination to the office
Most clinicians think their patients are better vaccinated than they are	Conduct an office-based assessment of coverage using self-assessment tool available at http://www.cdc.gov/nip. Work with VFC program to add coverage assessment at a VFC office visit.
Immunization records are scattered among different sites of care	Work with health department on communication arrangement for vaccinations given off site. Use recall system to identify children with incomplete records. Routinely ask for immunization records when new patient joins practice. Use one-page form in medical record to document all vaccinations. Join local immunization registry.
Vaccination opportunities are missed in the office setting	Use recall system to identify children in need of vaccination and flag their charts as a reminder at their next visit. Review practice policies for vaccination at all types of office visits.
Parents object to vaccination	Counsel parents about safety of current vaccinations and the need for full vaccination to protect children who cannot be successfully vaccinated.
Adolescents difficult to reach	Develop systematic reminder/recall system for adolescents. Initiate routine preventive visit for 11- to 12-year-olds that includes indicated vaccinations. Join VFC program to reduce vaccine costs to eligible adolescents.

Two ingredients are needed for successful office-based interventions. The first is an ability to identify or determine the patients for whom the practice is responsible, and the second is an ability to determine the immunization status of individual patients. The first issue is related to the concept of a "medical home" that provides a meaningful link of accountability between patient and provider. The second issue indicates the need to store and maintain up-to-date immunization histories in the medical record (or other available format such, as a community-based immunization registry).

Recall and Reminder Systems

The most consistently effective intervention to improve immunization coverage levels among a provider's patients is to operate a recall system to bring children who are getting behind in their immunizations into the office for vaccination. Over 60 studies have demonstrated their beneficial effect,[12] yet less than one-third of pediatricians use recall systems in their practice. A recall system does not need to be complicated or even computerized to be effective—simple card-file tickler systems work very well.

A simple method to set up a tickler file is to obtain a card file that has monthly dividers. Within each month, the patients are arranged alphabetically by name. The cards record the immunization history of the patient and are filed according to the date of the next vaccination appointment. New cards are created whenever a new patient (newborn infant or transfer) is added to the practice. As a patient is vaccinated, the vaccines administered are recorded on the card and the card is refiled into the month of the next vaccination appointment. At the end of the month, the remaining cards in the file identify the patients who should have been vaccinated during the month but who were not vaccinated. This forms the list of patients that need to be recalled into the practice for vaccination. After the routine vaccinations for the first 2 years of life are provided, the card is removed from the file. Recording the vaccination history on the cards is optional, but it does provide a double-check on the vaccination status.

A slightly higher-tech recall system uses a practice computer billing system. The billing system is modified to count the specific vaccinations given to each child turning 7 or 19 months of age. If the counts of the vaccinations are less than the office standard (e.g., 3 DTaP, 3 Hib, 2 hepatitis B, 3 rotavirus, and 2 IPV for a 7-month-

old), the chart is reviewed by office staff to determine whether the child is truly behind or whether there are missing billing data. Children truly behind are then recalled into the office. This particular technique was developed and used by a large urban group practice to vaccinate over 99 percent of all of the practice's 12- and 24-month-old children.[13] An additional benefit to the practice was the identification of gaps in the billing practices, which translated into lost revenue for services rendered.

As an adjunct to operating a recall system, charts of children who have missed vaccination appointments should be flagged to indicate that the children are overdue for vaccines and the vaccinations that are needed. This simple task will facilitate identification and vaccination of "past due" children when they come to the office for an acute care visit, thus reducing missed opportunities to vaccinate.

Cost is a consideration in determining the approach to setting up a recall system. Low-tech solutions obviously cost less in the short term, but taking advantage of computer technology by using the billing system might help optimize reimbursement for vaccinations administered.

Assessing Office-Based Coverage Levels

Most clinicians overestimate vaccination coverage levels among their patient population, frequently by a very large margin. Since a problem must be identified before there would be impetus to find a solution, overestimating one's practice coverage levels is a barrier to vaccination. A representative sample of California pediatricians and family physicians *estimated* their coverage to be 92 percent on average, while the *measured* coverage was a full 25 percentage points lower.[14] Thus, a key strategy to improve performance is to measure vaccination coverage and to provide feedback about coverage to the provider.

Two assessment tools are currently available for use in office practices. The most rigorous and well developed is the CDC's Clinic Assessment Software Application (CASA), which has become a standard for immunization performance measurement. In addition to calculating practice-based coverage levels, CASA also provides information about missed opportunities to vaccinate, children starting their vaccinations late; and children dropping out from the practice. It is available from CDC by downloading from *www.cdc.gov/nip* and is designed for use by trained personnel, usually from health department immunization programs. The second assessment tool is called Make Every Visit Count, and it is a provider self-assessment tool. It is easier to use than CASA, but the amount of information available from the assessment is less than that provided by CASA and the methodology has not been evaluated as rigorously. This tool kit is also available from the CDC's Internet home page.

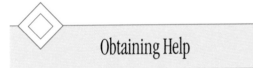

Obtaining Help

The CDC is available to help practitioners vaccinate their patients. CDC is the agency of the federal government that is accountable for implementing vaccination programs with federal and state governmental partners, and for coordinating with other organizations involved with routine childhood vaccination. It is a science-based agency that funds and conducts studies and disease surveillance, and synthesizes available evidence needed to implement a broad array of public health programs and policies.

Immunization resources provided by CDC are available at the National Immunization Program (NIP) home page, *www.cdc.gov/nip*, which provides one stop shopping for those interested in immunization.

In addition to these Internet materials, NIP conducts training courses on vaccination recommendations, new vaccines, and strategies to improve immunization practices. These courses are available in certain cities and by satellite hookup. Information about course topics and scheduling is published in the *Morbidity and Mortality Weekly Report.*

Another important resource to help primary care providers is the Vaccines for Children Program (VFC), which works actively with practitioners in every state. Most pediatricians and family physicians that vaccinate children are enrolled in VFC. Providers enrolled in VFC currently vaccinate over three-quarters of U.S. preschool children. Benefits to private providers include (1) the provision of vaccine at no charge to the provider, (2) enabling the practice to provide immunization services to many of their patients who would normally be referred to health departments for vaccination, and (3) education and quality improvement activities. The quality improvement activities included in the VFC program vary by state but generally include help with storage and handling of new vaccines and the use of the Vaccine Information Statements. Additionally, several states' VFC programs offer free vaccination coverage level assessments using CASA or a variation of CASA. (*Table 3-3*)

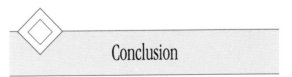

Conclusion

Childhood vaccination is the top-ranked service among all clinical preventive services for people of all ages.[15] Scientific advances will likely keep vaccination top-ranked and will increase the performance of immunization programs. But the price of increased performance is increased complexity, and the critical question is whether the U.S. immunization delivery system will be able and willing to handle the complexity that is needed to attain peak system performance. We are already falling short of today's potential, as indicated by the low coverage levels for varicella vaccine and adolescent hepatitis B vaccine.

Table 3-3

Sources of Helpful Information

ORGANIZATION AND INTERNET ADDRESS	SELECTED INFORMATION AVAILABLE
Centers for Disease Control and Prevention **www.cdc.gov/nip**	Current vaccination schedule Current Vaccine Information Statements (printable form) All Advisory Committee on Immunization Practices (ACIP) recommendations Textbook: "Epidemiology and Prevention of Vaccine-Preventable Diseases" "Six Common Misconceptions about Vaccination" Current and topical questions and answers about vaccine safety Guidelines for storage and handling of vaccines Office immunization coverage assessment tools Immunization registry information
Centers for Disease Control and Prevention **www.cdc.gov/travel**	Vaccination and other information for international travelers
Immunization Action Coalition **www.immunize.org**	Clinician educational material about vaccination Parent educational material about vaccination Links to many immunization sites
Health Resources and Services Agency **www.hrsa.dhhs.gov/bhpr/vicp**	Information on the National Childhood Vaccine Injury Table
Food and Drug Administration **www.fda.gov/cber**	Vaccine Adverse Events Reporting System

Primary care pediatricians, family physicians, and nurse practitioners have a most important role to play in ensuring the timely vaccination of children, and they also have a most valuable ingredient for successful implementation of vaccination programs: the trust of parents of their patients. The challenges faced by primary care practitioners are many, including navigating an increasingly complex immunization schedule, financing additional vaccines, and helping parents to understand why vaccines are important and worth the small but finite risks involved. Though these challenges might seem daunting, children's health care providers are in the enviable position of having to manage an ever-increasing arsenal of proven preventive tools.

References

1. Bernier R, Deuson R, Wharton M, et al: The epidemiological and economic impact of vaccines universally recommended for children in the United States in the 20th century. Presented before the 2nd World Conference of the International Health Economics Association, June 6, 1999.

2. Orenstein WA, Hinman AR, Rodewald LE: Public health considerations—United States, in Plotkin SA and Orenstein WA (eds): *Vaccines*, 3rd ed. Philadelphia, Saunders, 1999, p 1024.

3. Davis RL, Mell LK, Zavitkovsky A, et al: Impact of the sequential IPV/OPV schedule on vaccination coverage levels—United States, 1997. *MMWR* 47: 1017–1019, 1998.

4. Merck Vaccine Division. Business Research, October 1997.

5. Pathman DE, Konrad TR, Freed GL, et al: The awareness-to-adrenence model of the steps to clinical guideline compliance: the case of pediatric vaccine recommendations. *Med Care* 34: 873–889, 1996.

6. Stratton KR, Durch JS, Lawrence RS: *Vaccines for the 21st Century: A Tool for Decision Making.* Washington, DC, National Academy Press, 1999.

7. Gangarosa E, Galazka A, Wolfe C, et al: Impact of anti-vaccine movements on pertussis control: the untold story. *Lancet* 351:356–361, 1998.

8. Rota JS, Salmon DA, Chen RT, et al: Religious and philosophical exemptions to immunization requirements: additional steps to get an exemption correlate with fewer exemption claims. *Am J Prev Med* Submitted.

9. Udovic SL, Lieu TA: Evidence of office-based interventions to improve childhood immunization delivery. *Pediatr Ann* 27:355–365, 1998.

10. Strobino D, Keane V, Holt E, et al: Parental attitudes do not explain underimmunization. *Pediatrics* 98:1076–1083, 1996.

11. Tarande M, Dietz V, Lewin M, Zell E: Health care characteristics and their association with the vaccination status of children (abstr). *Arch Pediatr Adolesc Med* 150(4 supp):161, 1996.

12. Shefer A, Briss P, Rodewald L, et al: Improving immunization coverage rates: an evidence-based review of the literature. *Epidemiol Rev* 21(1): 96–142, 1999.

13. Tobin J: Immunization tracking and outreach in an office setting. Proceedings of the 31st National Immunization Conference. Detroit, 1997, pp 139–142.

14. Watt J, Kahane S, Smith N, et al: The difference between measured and estimated vaccination coverage among private physicians in California. Presented before the Pediatric Academic Societies Meeting, New Orleans, 1998.

15. Partnership for Prevention, reported in *Intern Med News*, July 15, 1998, p 34

Peter K. Domoto

Chapter 4

Dental Problems

Early Childhood Caries
Fluoride Supplements
Dental Infection
Eruption of Teeth
Nonnutritive Sucking
Common Oral Conditions
  Acquired
    Candidiasis
    Geographic Tongue
    Primary Herpetic Gingivostomatitis
    Aphthous Ulcers
    Discolored Teeth

  Developmental
    Mucocele
    Fusion/Gemination
  Congenital
    Natal Teeth
    Hemangioma
Dental Trauma
  Fracture
  Displacement
  Avulsion
Orthodontics
Conclusions

The aim of this chapter is to present a practical oral health guide for clinicians that provide primary care to children. Because the interval from conception to 3 years is the most dramatic period of growth and development for children, emphasis is given to the oral health of infants, toddlers, and preschool children. By age 3, children usually have all 20 primary teeth erupted and have begun to develop enamel on 28 permanent teeth.

The chapter discusses caries, dental infections, dental trauma, nonnutritive sucking, some common oral conditions, and orthodontics. Several publications are available for readers who desire a more comprehensive look at dentistry for the pediatrician.[1–3] In addition, the websites for the American Academy of Pediatrics and the American Academy of Pediatric Dentistry are useful resources for the primary care provider and the families whom they serve.[4–8]

Early Childhood Caries

In spite of dramatic reductions in caries, 50 percent of U.S. children have decay in their primary teeth.[9] Caries are an expression of a bacterial infection acquired during the first 2 years of life. Methods for the prevention of caries are effective, but the infants and toddlers who would benefit most from these methods often do not have access to them. Poverty, social and cultural isolation, and other factors are barriers to primary preventive services.

More than 90 percent of children under 5 years of age use medical services in the United States. With the success of universal access to immunizations, children in the United States are seen by medical providers early and often during the first 3 years of life. *In stark contrast to medical utilization, only about one in four children 5 years of age and younger use the services of a dentist.*[10] Primary care medical providers, therefore, are often in a better position than dentists to provide effective and timely caries-prevention services for their young patients and thus to reduce the incidence of early childhood caries (ECC). ECC was previously called *baby-bottle tooth decay, nursing caries,* and a number of other names.[3]

To address prevention of ECC, it is necessary to have a clear understanding of the etiology. *Caries is now recognized to be an infection that is transmissible, diet-dependent, and saliva-mediated. Streptococcus mutans,* the principal bacteria implicated in the initiation of the infection, is typically transmitted from the mother or caretaker during infancy. The bacteria require carbohydrate (largely sucrose) to produce an acid that attacks susceptible teeth and demineralize the enamel below its surface. The first clinical signs of this demineralization are chalky white areas on the surface of the enamel. In the infected child, these white spots are characteristically found on the maxillary incisors. These teeth are among the first to erupt, so white spots can be observed as early as 8 months of age. Figures 4-1 and 4-2 (see Color Plates 1 and 2) demonstrate the typical progression of decay: from white spots to devastated teeth with abscesses.

In addition, research indicates that there is a strong association of enamel hypoplasia with caries (Figs. 4-3 and 4-4, see Color Plates 3 and 4). Hypoplastic teeth of young children are at greater risk for ECC. The first primary molars erupt around 12 to 15 months of age and can also be observed to have white lesions and/or enamel hypoplasia.

Preventive measures are predicated on the three etiologic factors. Therefore measures that affect the pathogenic bacteria—e.g., antibacterial or bactericidal activity of topical fluoride, chlorhexidine, or povidone-iodine (Betadine)—are useful.[3] Such interventions can be used on infants and toddlers as well as to prevent transmission from caretakers to babies. In like manner, measures to prevent the loss of integrity of teeth (e.g., incorporation of systemic fluoride into enamel) will provide protection against decay attack. Finally, topical fluoride, both professionally applied and self-applied via dentifrice, supports remineralization of teeth that have begun to decay.

ECC affects children as young as 9 or 10 months. Feeding patterns in infants at risk for ECC are considered to be critical in the initiation of caries. Use of sugared drinks, including fruit juices, in a nursing bottle are highly implicated in the initiation of decay. Even milk and formula can be cariogenic in the susceptible infant. At-will breast-feeding during sleep also appears to be dangerous in the decay-susceptible youngster.

The following steps should be recommended for ECC prevention:

First, vigorous and effective oral hygiene measures by the mother to reduce her own oral bacterial infection during the prenatal and postnatal period.

Second, babies weighing 10 lb or more seldom require nutrition during sleep; therefore bottle propping in the crib and excessive nighttime bottle- or breast-feeding should be avoided. The child should be comforted with a pacifier or favorite toy or blanket instead of using the bottle or breast.

Third, a child's teeth should be cleaned daily as soon as they erupt. Parents should use a damp cloth or a toothbrush to clean the baby's teeth. A thin "smear" of a dentifrice-containing fluoride will help prevent decay.

Fluoride Supplements

Community water fluoridation is a safe and effective means to significantly reduce the risk of tooth decay in children and adults. When possible, it is best for the family to drink fluoridated water. Families who prefer to use bottled water should choose a brand that has fluoride added at a concentration of approximately 0.8 to 1.0 mg/L (ppm).

When fluoride concentrations in the water supply of a community fall below 0.6 ppm, dietary fluoride supplementation is necessary for children 6 months to 16 years of age. Continuous compliance with fluoride supplementation has been shown to produce caries reductions of

around 30 to 50 percent. Table 4-1 delineates the dosage schedule that was approved by the Council on Dental Therapeutics of the American Dental Association and the American Academy of Pediatric Dentistry in 1994.

Both the form and dosage of the fluoride must be tailored to the needs of the individual children in the family. The dosage of fluoride is 0.05 mg/kg body weight. It is currently recommended that supplementation not be initiated before 6 months of age. Excessive fluoride intake results in fluorosis, a staining of the permanent incisors, illustrated in Figure 4-5 (see Color Plate 5).

Dietary fluoride supplements are available in liquid, lozenges, tablets, chewable tablets, and preparations combined with vitamins. Infants and toddlers should receive liquid fluoride supplements when indicated on the basis of fluoride testing. When the appropriate dosage for an infant is determined, a liquid fluoride supplement with a calibrated dropper should be used, since a calibrated delivery system provides a reliable measure.

As soon as children are able to chew and swallow a tablet, they should be switched to a chewable tablet. The chewable form of fluoride is most advantageously given at bedtime after brushing. The tablet should be chewed or sucked and "swished" around the mouth prior to swallowing. "Chew, swish, and swallow" will produce both the systemic and topical benefits of fluoride.

Table 4-1

Dietary Fluoride Supplement Schedule

	FLUORIDE ION LEVEL IN DRINKING WATER (PPM)*		
AGE	<0.3 PPM	0.3–0.6 PPM	>0.6 PPM
Birth to 6 months	None	None	None
6 months to 3 years	0.25 mg/day*	None	None
3 to 6 years	0.50 mg/day	0.25 mg/day	None
6 to 16 years	1.0 mg/day	0.50 mg/day	None

Table 4-2

Questions Commonly Asked about Fluorides

> Q. Should pregnant women take fluoride supplements to benefit the developing teeth of their babies?
> A. Prenatal administration of dietary fluoride supplements cannot be recommended at this time.
>   Conclusive evidence is lacking to support the benefit to the fetus.
> Q. Should breast-fed infants receive fluoride supplementation?
> A. The fluoride concentration in breast milk is low. Since the earliest age that an infant might receive
>   supplementation is 6 months, there is initially no need for supplementation whether the baby is
>   exclusively breast-fed or not. If the infant is *exclusively* breast-fed after 6 months of age,
>   supplementation of 0.25 mg of fluoride should be prescribed even in a fluoridated community. When
>   the baby begins to ingest Seattle water, whether it be in foods or beverages, the supplementation
>   should be discontinued.
> Q. Should I prescribe vitamin-fluoride combinations for children?
> A. Since vitamins do not enhance or potentiate the effect of fluoride, the Council on Dental Therapeutics
>   of the ADA does not endorse any vitamin-fluoride preparation. However, if vitamins are needed, a
>   vitamin-fluoride combination would be more convenient and less expensive than two separate
>   preparations. A combination prescription should be coordinated with the child's health care provider
>   when vitamins are being taken. As with any prescription, the content and dosage should be reviewed
>   periodically for efficacy and appropriateness.

Dental Infection

Eruption of Teeth

If caries are left untreated, these tooth infections lead to pain and inflammation in bone and soft tissue. Tooth pain from inflammation of the tooth pulp tissue and abscess is common.

Antibiotic coverage is needed where there is frank cellulitis, swelling, and fever. This may appear as a gumboil in young children or a more diffuse soft tissue swelling in older children. An antibiotic such as amoxicillin, 40 mg/kg for 1 week, is appropriate. In the absence of clinical signs of swelling, antibiotics are of no benefit. In the case of marked swelling in the lower jaw and difficulty swallowing, a compromised airway should be suspected and the patient referred immediately. Consultation with the local dentist about management preferences is recommended.

Teething in infants and toddlers is a normal physiologic process and occurs as the tooth penetrates the gum. It is frequently associated with increased drooling and the desire to bite and chew on things and may be associated with mild pain. Despite popular opinion, there is no evidence that high fevers, diarrhea, or facial rashes are caused by teething. A wide variety of remedies for teething are available; some folk remedies caretakers use actually work. I recommend rubbing and cleaning the area where the teeth are erupting with a massaging brush or finger-cot massager and giving the baby something safe to bite on, such as a teething ring, a cool spoon, or a cold or frozen wet washcloth.

In primary dentition, the mandibular central incisors are the first to erupt, usually around

6 months of age. Eruption is typically symmetrical, and commonly mandibular teeth erupt before maxillary teeth. The timing of tooth eruption in both the primary and permanent dentition is highly variable. By 12 months, four primary incisors have usually erupted; by 15 months, all eight primary incisors may have erupted. The first primary molars erupt around 18 months, and the primary cuspids at around 24 months. All 20 primary teeth are usually erupted by 36 months of age. Consultation should be sought for the child who has not erupted any primary teeth by the second birthday. In the absence of other systemic or developmental diagnoses, premature or delayed eruption is of little concern in the young child and would not be an indication for further consultation.

Nonnutritive Sucking

Thumb and finger sucking is normal in babies and young children. Babies begin to suck on their fingers and thumbs in utero. Most children who suck digits, use a pacifier, or suck other objects give up these behaviors on their own between the ages of 2 and 4 years. Consultation with a pediatric dentist would be appropriate after age 5 if these nonnutritive sucking habits are intense and occur for long periods of time, because the upper front teeth may tip toward the lip or not come in properly if the habit persists. When the child is old enough to understand the possible results of a sucking habit, behavioral approaches can be used to reduce and/or eliminate the habit. With behavioral or mechanical approaches to the habit, it is essential initiate the intervention only after the child has agreed to "own the problem." In addition, determining the frequency and intensity of the habit is important in order to understand the nature of the problem and thus design an effective intervention. When the child agrees that some kind of "reminder" would be helpful, simple interventions like bitter ointments on the digit or mittens/socks over the hands for sleeptime thumbsuckers are very effective. If the habit is very refractory and is associated with a malocclusion, the dentist may place an appliance in the mouth to interrupt the sucking habit. Pacifier-, thumb-, and finger-sucking habits affect the teeth essentially the same way. However, a pacifier habit is often easier to correct.

Common Oral Conditions

Common oral conditions[5] in children fall into the following categories:

1. Acquired conditions
2. Developmental conditions
3. Congenital conditions

Acquired

CANDIDIASIS

Candidiasis is characterized clinically by raised, white, curdlike plaques that leave a raw, bleeding surface when scraped. Immunosuppressed children and immunoincompetent children who have been on antibiotic therapy (especially long-term therapy) are at risk of developing candidiasis.

The patient may be asymptomatic or may complain of a sore throat if the esophageal tissues are involved. In the newborn, secondary infection may occur and lesions may be found on any mucosal surface. Topical or systemic antifungal agents are the drugs of choice.

GEOGRAPHIC TONGUE

Geographic tongue is a benign condition of unknown etiology that is clinically characterized by multiple areas of desquamation of filiform papillae. The tongue appears "bald" in areas of varying size and shape. The condition may persist for weeks or months. These areas may change in size and location. The condition may resolve spontaneously, only to recur at a later date. No treatment is indicated or needed.

PRIMARY HERPETIC GINGIVOSTOMATITIS

Primary herpetic gingivostomatitis is caused by an initial infection with the herpes simplex virus type 1. It is characterized by painful, erythematous, and swollen gingival tissues and oral vesicles throughout the mouth. In addition, the youngster usually experiences fever, malaise, and lymphadenopathy. The vesicles rupture, leaving painful ulcers. Lip vesicles with subsequent ulcers and fissuring can also occur. This initial infection occurs most commonly from 6 months to 6 years. Lesions heal spontaneously in 1 to 2 weeks, with the acute phase lasting 7 to 10 days.

Palliative and supportive treatment is used. Antipyretics and analgesics are helpful in relieving discomfort, so that the child can drink—an important consideration in infants and toddlers, who may become dehydrated when they have painful infections. Palliative mouth rinses may also be helpful in controlling the oral discomfort. The following mouth rinses are useful in providing palliative care: alcohol-free Benadryl elixir (diphenydhydramine HCl) and Maalox (magnesia and alumina) in a 1:1 ratio (OTC); Benadryl/lidocaine/Maalox mouth rinse, mix 1.5 mL diphenhydramine injectable (50 mg/mL), 45 mL xylocaine viscous 2%, and 45 mL magnesium aluminum hydroxide solution; and Carafate (sucralfate) suspension 1 g/10 mL. Orabase may also be used as a protective barrier.

Information to the caregiver should include an explanation of the contagious aspects of this disease. Antibiotics are contraindicated unless secondary infection is present. Steroids are also contraindicated because suppression of the host response may allow dissemination of the herpesvirus.

APHTHOUS ULCERS

Recurrent aphthous ulcers, or canker sores, are the most common recurrent oral ulcers in the United States. These lesions present with a central area of necrosis and ulceration with an erythematous halo. The ulcers are less than a centimeter in diameter and occur on oral mucosa, including the tongue, soft palate, and oropharyngeal mucosa.

Although the etiology of aphthous stomatitis is unknown, viral, bacterial, autoimmune, allergic, and nutritional causes have been suspected. Treatment is palliative, and the minor lesion heals in 7 to 10 days without scarring. Topical steroids offer some hope for long-term management of recurrence. A medium-potency topical corticosteroid ointment suitable for management of aphthous ulcers is triamcinolone acetonide 0.025 percent to 0.1 percent (Kenalog in Orabase). Topical corticosteroids should not be used for longer than 7 to 10 days.

DISCOLORED TEETH

A darkened tooth may be the result of trauma to the tooth with resultant internal hemorrhage. Darkened primary teeth are of little concern in the absence of other clinical and radiographic evidence of pathology. In contrast, discolored permanent teeth (especially secondary to trauma) eventually result in nonvital, inflamed teeth that will require root canal therapy.

Intrinsic stain of the tooth enamel may be the result of excess fluoride or tetracycline ingestion during tooth formation. Fluorosis is associated with excessive fluoride ingestion during enamel formation. Common sources of excess fluoride are inappropriate fluoride supplement regimens and swallowing of fluoridated dentifrices in the child less than 3 years of age. Most fluorosis is mild and does not require treatment. However, when fluorosis is more severe and requires treatment, bleaching and/or covering the surface of the tooth with tooth-colored materials effective.

Use of tetracycline for periods exceeding 10 days and in children less than 8 years of age may result in yellow, brown, or gray discoloration.

Extrinsic stains of the enamel are caused by an accumulation of pigmented material on the surfaces of teeth. Foods, medications, or microorganisms may be the source of extrinsic stain. These extrinsic stains are primarily of esthetic concern. The dental provider will usually remove these stains by polishing the enamel surface.

Developmental

MUCOCELE

A mucocele develops when a salivary gland duct is injured or severed and the saliva leaks into the adjacent connective tissue. Granulation tissue forms and becomes the lining of a cyst-like structure. Unlike the case with a true cyst, the cystic space is not lined by epithelium. The most common location is the lower lip. The mucocele is bluish in color if it is located near the surface and normal in color if deeper in the tissues. Surgical excision is recommended.

FUSION/GEMINATION

Fusion is the union of two embryologically separate developing teeth; gemination is the incomplete division of a single tooth bud. Fusion/gemination appears as two joined crowns, usually in the incisor regions. (Fig. 4-6, see Color Plate 6). Radiographic examination usually determines whether it is fusion or gemination. Radiographs reveal that fused teeth have two pulp chambers and two canals, while the geminated tooth has one pulp chamber and canal. Referral for follow-up is indicated, since the vertical crease (the interface between the

two teeth) may be an entry for bacteria directly into the pulp.

Congenital

CONDITIONS SEEN IN THE NEWBORN

Three congenital conditions commonly observed at birth are Epstein's pearl, Bohn's nodule, and dental laminar cyst. Each of these conditions is benign and generally does not require treatment. Almost all of these conditions are sloughed and are resolved by 3 months. Epstein's pearl is a white, pearl-like lesion that is located along the midpalatal raphe. It is thought to represent epithelial remnants along the fusion line of the palatal halves. These cysts are visible in 80 percent of newborns.

Bohn's nodule is a lesion believed to be related to salivary gland remnants. It appears as a raised area located on the lateral portion of the alveolar ridge or between the midpalatal raphe and alveolar crest in the maxilla (Fig. 4-7, see Color Plate 7) Dental laminar cysts are remnants of the dental lamina (embryonic origin of tooth buds) (Fig. 4-8, see Color Plate 8). They are epithelial in origin and are located on the alveolar ridge in either the mandible or the maxilla.

NATAL TEETH

Natal teeth (present at birth) or neonatal teeth (erupting shortly after birth) are prematurely erupting teeth. In 85 percent of cases, natal or neonatal teeth are normal primary teeth and should be allowed to remain in place unless they are extremely loose and pose a risk of aspiration.

HEMANGIOMA

Hemangiomas occur with the first decade of life, typically within the first year. A female predilection is evident. The lesion may be localized or diffuse, red to blue in color, and flat or nodular. Hemangiomas are soft and blanch when compressed. Common sites of occurrence are the lips, tongue, and buccal mucosa. Hemorrhage from trauma is common.

Hemangiomas may undergo spontaneous involution, but if they persist and are cosmetically unacceptable, they may be successfully treated by surgical excision, the use of sclerosing agents, or cryotherapy.

Dental Trauma

Orofacial trauma is most common in the period from 6 months to 2 1/2 years. The most frequently injured teeth are the maxillary central incisors. When these teeth or other primary teeth are injured, an assessment by a dentist is indicated. Trauma is considered a dental emergency; therefore an assessment should be completed as soon as possible.

Fracture

Fractures in the primary and permanent dentition require evaluation, often including radiographs. Generally, the larger the fracture, the more extensive the required dental treatment. Small fractures of enamel may not require treatment or only need smoothing of the roughened surface; larger fractures may require protective restorations or root canal therapy.

Displacement

Trauma resulting in displacement of the teeth should be evaluated by a dentist, who will determine the nature and severity of the displacement and provide appropriate intervention. Intruded primary teeth (teeth displaced into the bony socket) are often left to reerupt sponta-

neously without intervention. For permanent teeth, as an emergency measure, a medical provider should reposition teeth that are displaced by trauma. Splinting of the repositioned teeth by an experienced dentist is often required later.

Avulsion

Avulsion refers to a traumatic injury in which a tooth is knocked completely out of its socket. Most avulsions occur in the maxillary anterior. First aid in traumatic dental injuries varies with the development of the child's dentition. Specifically, *in the avulsion of teeth, primary teeth are not reimplanted and permanent teeth are reimplanted.* A child 5 years of age or younger with an avulsed primary tooth should not have the tooth replaced in the socket. In contrast, an individual 6 years of age or older who has avulsed a permanent tooth should have that tooth reimplanted as soon as possible.

It is appropriate first aid to insert the tooth or teeth in the sockets, but it is important not to handle the root surface. The procedure is simple: Wash the tooth gently with clean water to remove debris and then insert the tooth into the socket. Some effort should be made to place the tooth or teeth in the correct position. However, time is of the essence. It is more important to return the teeth to the avulsion site quickly (ideally within an hour) than it is for the tooth to be correctly positioned. There is a direct relationship between the time out of the socket and the prognosis for the tooth. Even teeth that have to be removed and then later repositioned by a dentist have a better prognosis than teeth that have been out of the mouth for too long a period of time. If reinsertion is not possible, the tooth should be stored in milk and the patient brought to a care provider as soon as possible for reimplantation.

Most teeth that are reimplanted are nonvital and will eventually require root canal therapy.

Reimplanted teeth may undergo rapid patho-logic root resorption and/or ankylosis. This is the undesirable outcome of delay in reimplanta-tion. There is no consensus on antibiotic cover-age, but tetanus prophylaxis is an important consideration.

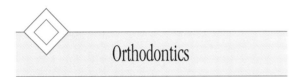

Orthodontics

Epidemiologic data indicate that the majority of adolescents could benefit from orthodontic ther-apy. However, "There are thus many variations from ideal occlusion that are both normal and compatible with good dental health and func-tion." Only 10 to 20 percent of children have severe or handicapping malocclusions.

Since orthodontic therapy can be the largest health-related expense for healthy children prior to adulthood, prevention and early intervention are desirable. As discussed earlier, pediatricians can play a key role both in prevention of caries and timely intervention for orthodontic prob-lems. Because decay is still the major cause of premature loss of baby teeth, and premature loss of teeth leads to space loss and subsequent crowding, prevention of caries is essential in minimizing the need for orthodontic treatment.

The child with a noticeable convex profile and protruding maxillary incisors is at risk for trauma to these incisors; early intervention should be sought to position these teeth in a safer relationship. In addition, athletic mouth guards should be used for all active children.

Fields described a simple method for pedia-tricians to recognize craniofacial growth prob-lems not associated with craniofacial anomalies and to determine if the child or adolescent requires referral for a skeletal problem.[2] The procedure is to view the child's face from the side and visualize the bridge of the nose, the base of the nose, and the point of the chin. By connecting these three points with line seg-ments, the facial profile can be described. A slightly convex profile is acceptable for most preschool and grade school children. An extreme convexity or concavity is cause for con-cern at any age. Referral for further evaluation would be appropriate for conditions where the craniofacial and/or dental relationships appear to be abnormal.

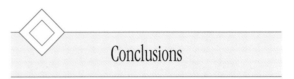

Conclusions

With the successful implementation of compre-hensive primary prevention programs for infants and toddlers, a dramatic decrease in the preva-lence and severity of caries in the primary denti-tion can be anticipated. Pediatricians and other primary care providers can play a significant role in reducing the incidence of early child-hood caries in the context of prenatal, well-child, and other primary care responsibilities, including anticipatory guidance.[11] Since the teeth of infants and toddlers are, for the most part, surprisingly uniform in color, shape, and texture, primary care providers should trust their assessments of teeth during infant and toddler examinations, as abnormalities are usually easily detected. Introduction and reinforcement of sound nutritional practices will enhance caries prevention in the young child. Daily brushing by the caretaker with a fluoridated dentifrice will also reduce bacterial levels and enhance remineralization. While this method is still in preliminary development, the application of flu-oride varnishes by primary care medical providers is a feasible approach to primary caries prevention. In light of the high utilization of medical services by preschool children and the low utilization of dental services, an expan-sion of effective preventive services in medical well-child care seems reasonable.

Table 4-3

Questions Commonly Asked by Caregivers about Infant Oral Health

Q. When should my child first see a dentist?

A. "First visit by first birthday" sums it up. Your child should visit a dentist when the first tooth comes in, usually between 6 and 12 months of age. Early examination and preventive care will protect your child's smile now and in the future.

Q. Why so early? What dental problems could a baby have?

A. Dental problems can begin early. A big concern is baby-bottle tooth decay (BBTD), which is preventable. BBTD can result from long periods of exposing baby teeth to liquids that contain sugar, including formula, milk, breast milk, and juice. A baby who has a habit of sleeping with a baby bottle filled with any sugary liquid or a breast in its mouth is at risk of getting BBTD. Frequent snacking on sweet or sticky foods can also cause decay.

   The earlier the first dental visit, the better the chance of preventing dental problems. Children with healthy teeth can chew food well, speak clearly, and share precious smiles. Start your child on a lifetime of good dental habits now!

Q. How can I prevent tooth decay from nursing or a bottle?

A. Taking your baby off of the breast when she or he falls asleep can prevent tooth decay. Hold your baby while bottle feeding. Always take a bottle filled with milk or juice away from the sleeping child. If your child requires a bottle at bedtime, provide a bottle filled with water. Instead of a bottle, try comforting your child with a pacifier or a favorite toy or blanket. Check with your health care provider to make sure your child is getting the right amount of fluoride. Brush your baby's teeth with a soft toothbrush daily.

Q. When should bottle-feeding be stopped?

A. Begin teaching your baby to use a cup by 7 months. It is a good idea to introduce juice in a cup. Your baby can be off the bottle by 12 months.

Q. Should I worry about thumb- or finger-sucking?

A. Thumb-sucking is perfectly normal for infants; most stop by age 2. Prolonged (beyond age 5 or 6 years) thumb-sucking can create crowded, crooked teeth or bite problems. Your dentist will be glad to suggest ways to address a prolonged thumb-sucking habit.

Q. When should I start cleaning my baby's teeth?

A. This is a good habit to start early! The teeth must be cleaned as they erupt. Use a damp washcloth or a toothbrush. If your dentist agrees, use a tiny dab of fluoride toothpaste. Tooth-brushing is definitely a parent job in the preschool years. Children are usually able to brush their teeth well by the time they are 8 years old. Be sure to check your child's teeth regularly for any chalky white or brown spots, which could indicate early decay.

Q. Any advice on teething?

A. Sore gums from teething often occur for a few days at a time between 6 months to age 3 years. Babies often get relief from a clean teething ring, cool spoon, cold wet washcloth, or toothbrush. Offering a chilled teething ring or rubbing a clean finger on the sore gum may also often help.

SOURCE: Adapted by permission from American Academy of Pediatric Dentistry.[4]

Primary care providers, both medical and dental, have determined that it is in the best interest of the children whom they serve to work in close collaboration. The biology of oral health is inextricably entwined with the developing child's general health. Teamwork, particularly in the pre- and postnatal periods, appears to have great promise for the health of children and the effectiveness of medicine and dentistry.

References

1. Creighton PR: Common pediatric dental problems. *Pediatr Clin North Am* 45:1579–1600, 1998.
2. Fields HM: Craniofacial growth from infancy through adulthood. *Pediatr Clin North Am* 38:1053–1088, 1991
3. Smith RJ: Normal and abnormal development of dental occlusion. *Pediatr Clin North Am* 38:1149–1172, 1991.
4. American Academy of Pediatric Dentistry. (http://www.aapd.org)
5. American Academy of Pediatric Dentistry: *Smiles for Tomorrow* slide presentation
6. American Academy of Pediatrics: *A Guide to Children's Dental Health.* (http://www.aap.org/family/dental.htm)
7. American Academy of Pediatrics: *Baby Bottle Tooth Decay-How to Prevent It.* (http://www.aap.org/family/toothdec.htm)
8. American Academy of Pediatrics: *Thumbs, Fingers, and Pacifiers.* (http://www.aap.org/family/thumbs.htm)
9. Edelstein BL, Douglas CW: Dispelling the myth that 50 percent of U.S. schoolchildren have never had a cavity. *Public Health Rep* 110(5):522–530, 1995.
10. Burt BA, Eklund SA: *Dentistry, Dental Practice, and the Community*, 5th ed. Philadelphia, Saunders, 1999, chap 2, Fig. 2-8, p 20.
11. *Bright Futures: Guidelines for Health Supervision of Infants, Children, and Adolescents.* (http://www.brightfutures.org)

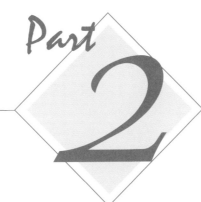

Part

2

Acute Problems

Edward M. McMahon, Jr.

Chapter

5

Fever

"Everybody's got the fever, that is somethin' you
  all know
Fever isn't such a new thing, fever started long
  ago . . .
You give me fever, fever when you hold me tight
Fever in the morning, fever all through the
  night . . ."

Peggy Lee: All Time Greatest Hits, *vol. 1. lyrics*
  by John Davenport and Eddie J. Cooley. Fort
  Knox Music, Inc., and Trio Music Co., Inc.
  Used by permission.

Fever, sad to say, is the most common problem in pediatrics. The nurses in our six-person pediatric office are unanimous that it is the topic they are called about most frequently. A recent 2-month sample of calls in our Seattle pediatric after-hours telephone triage service found "fever" to be the most frequent concern (3848 of 29,835 calls, or 12.8 percent). Fever is also a frequent subject in the medical literature. In my Medline search, I counted 80 review articles alone written since 1990, and much continues to be said.[1] I say sad because, except for infants, the less said about fever and the less attention paid to the degree of fever the better. The large number of telephone calls and office visits solely for fever reflects a culture of "fever phobia" that has developed over two or three generations in the United States.

This chapter does not deal with the pathophysiology of fever as a normal reaction to endogenous pyrogens. The interested reader is referred to an excellent article by Kluger.[2] Neither does it offer a systematic review of fever in children. Rather, it examines the response of parents and health care professionals to the presence of fever in their children or patients as a cultural phenomenon. That is because fever has been misinterpreted as a disease to be battled or controlled rather than as a symptom (a potentially health-enhancing symptom?) that should, ideally, result in more careful observation of the child for other more specific signs of illness.

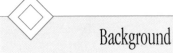

Background

The pattern and duration of fever have been important markers of disease since at least the time of Hippocrates, centuries before the development of thermometer technology. The numbers were simply unavailable for most of recorded history; hence, fever was a subjective sign, perhaps difficult to isolate from other aspects of illness. Even today, Cambodians newly settled in the United States have no word for the concept of fever as a number—rather, there are at least a dozen Cambodian terms describing fever in the context of an illness, such as malaria fever (*krun jang*) or fever with a cold or flu (*krun pradas sai*). The word that translates to "fever" (*krun*) has at least four different meanings in Cambodian, from "feeling ill" or "out of balance," to increased sensation of warmth in the body, to a reference to a specific illness.[3]

For centuries in the West, fever was felt to have a salutary effect, ridding the body of an excess of "humours" such as "phlegm." For a time, fever therapy was the accepted treatment for neurosyphilis. In the mid-eighteenth century, the English physician Thomas Sydenham is said to have declared, "Fever is nature's engine which she brings into the field to remove her enemy."[4]

However, after the invention of the thermometer, the French physiologist Claude Bernard, experimenting with artificial fevers in animals, demonstrated that animals died when their body temperatures were raised 5° to 6°C above normal, disrupting enzyme systems critical to maintenance of the *milieu intérieur*. Isolated cases of encephalopathy, seizures, and death due to hyperpyrexia (heat stroke) added credence to the theory that fever per se could be harmful. Apparently overlooked at the time was evidence suggesting that the highest and most "damaging" fevers were those occurring in individuals with either primary central nervous system (CNS) infections or preexisting conditions (trisomy 21, hydrocephalus, brain tumors) that might be expected to interfere with proper hypothalamic function.

Much of the above background information was published in 1980 by Barton Schmitt in a landmark paper entitled "Fever Phobia: Misconceptions of Parents about Fevers."[5] His survey of 81 parents attending an inner-city clinic revealed a high level of parental concern about the potential for severe neurologic damage following even moderate fevers, which was reflected in the parents' aggressive approach to early sponging and to early and frequent administration of antipyretics. In 1984 Kramer et al. extended these observations to middle- and upper-income parents, suggesting that "at least part of the reason for parental fever phobia is the message that pediatricians and other health care workers convey to parents."[4] In 1992 May and Bauchner surveyed 234 Massachusetts pediatricians about their beliefs and practices related to fever. They noted that the majority of responders recommended treating fevers between 101° and 102°F with antipyretics—yet 88 percent agreed with the statement that a sleeping child with fever should not be disturbed! These inconsistent recommendations, according to the authors, had the potential for parental confusion. They conclude, "Since parents learn from both our actions and our words, it is important that our actions be consistent with our beliefs."[6] Amen to that!

Diagnosis of Fever

"Not everything that matters can be measured, and not everything that can be measured, matters"

Attributed to Albert Einstein.

Almost invariably, the diagnosis of childhood fever begins with the parent's perception that the child "seems ill" or "feels warm." There are, of course, rare parents who routinely and regularly measure their child's temperature. To them I relate the story of a 7-year-old patient who, when asked if she had a temperature, replied crossly, "Of course I have a temperature! Even rocks have temperatures!"

With the exception of the special case of infants under the age of 3 months, parental perception is all that is necessary for the diagnosis of fever. We do ourselves and our patients a disservice by succumbing to the peculiar predilection of Western medicine to want to measure everything. This leads to fussing and hair-splitting over axillary vs. rectal, mercury vs. digital, and ascribes undue importance to the absolute level of fever.

A number of authors have attempted to correlate the degree of fever with the likelihood of serious and treatable illness.[7] These studies were all performed in the era before effective and nearly universal immunization against *Haemophilus influenzae* type b, and all are inescapably flawed in that the patients with fever were brought to medical attention (usually to emergency rooms) because they were ill. We have no real idea of the denominator—those children with moderate to high fevers, associated with mild or no illness, who were never brought to medical attention and who did just fine resolving their viral illness on their own.

All that being said, my arbitrary definition of fever is a rectal temperature, obtained with a mercury thermometer, of 100.5°F (38°C) or above. A child 3 months of age or older meeting the above definition should be observed for other signs and symptoms of illness (pain, shortness of breath, swelling or erythema, alteration in level of consciousness, duration of fever, or high level of parental concern). To the extent that the fever itself is contributing to the child's discomfort, anorexia, or irritability, attempts to lower the temperature with acetaminophen or ibuprofen are reasonable, as discussed further on.

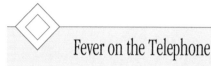

Fever on the Telephone

Experienced professionals understand that how a child looks is more important than the height of a fever in degrees. And yet they unintentionally reinforce fever phobia when parents call, as do the architects of the algorithms for after-hours telephone triage. More often than not, the first question asked is, "How high is the fever?" And worse, when the worried parent stammers out a number, the response is, "How did you measure it? Oral, rectal, or ear temperature?" What is a parent to conclude? That the absolute height of the fever is *critical* and that they are somehow remiss in not having measured it to two decimal places. We could do a great deal of good by reworking the algorithms to begin as follows: (1) How old is your child? (2) How long has he or she had the fever? and (3) How does he or she look to you?

The goal of telephone triage is not to make a diagnosis or even a presumptive diagnosis. It is simply to determine which patient with fever should be seen in the office. My criteria are these: (1) Any feverish child under 3 months of age should be seen. (2) Fever accompanied by significant localized pain (headache, chest, throat, or abdominal pain or dysuria) or dysfunction (persistent vomiting, bloody diarrhea, limping, or altered level of consciousness), calls for an office visit, as does (3) fever over 4 days' duration unexplained by other illness, such as upper respiratory infection or varicella. Finally, an office visit is appropriate (4) for the child who does not meet the above criteria but whose parents are very concerned.

Children with fever alone, not fulfilling the above criteria, may be safely observed at home.

(I emphasize *observed* because they may later develop symptoms that warrant examination.) The parents should be commended for calling for advice and assured that they are acting appropriately in providing comfort measures for their child's symptoms while the child's immune system copes with what should be a mild and self-limited viral illness. I make no attempt to assign some teleologic value to fever vis-à-vis enhancing the immune response. Although these theories are appealing,[2] it may be that fever merely represents some vestigial adaptive response of no more benefit than, say, the appendix or a twelfth rib.

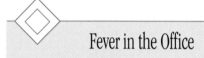

Fever in the Office

The primary care office setting is the optimal place to distinguish the very sick child from the mildly ill. Ideally, a telephone triage staff should bring in all of the seriously ill children, sprinkled throughout the melange of those with self-limited illness. My estimate of the ideal ratio is 1:20. Many surgeons, in contrast, feel that the proper ratio of appendicitis to appendectomy is 1:4. In children 3 months of age or older, a careful history, observation of the child (preferably by someone already acquainted), and a brief physical exam should identify those needing further evaluation (rapid strep test/throat culture, urinalysis and culture, chest x-ray, or complete blood count).

The younger and the more "ill-appearing" (i.e., "toxic") the child, the more useful the ancillary tests (increased positive predictive value). Nothing, however, will substitute for a caring attitude in informing the parents that (even if tests were not done), if the child's condition worsens, they should not hesitate to contact the office for a return appointment. This is the great advantage of an office or clinic setting

where family and physician have had the opportunity to develop a relationship of reciprocal trust.

Even in the absence of positive physical findings, my threshold for obtaining a urine specimen from febrile female infants and children is quite low. If the urinalysis is abnormal, I often begin empiric antibiotic treatment pending the results of a urine culture in those children who do not appear ill enough to warrant hospitalization. The debate continues over the usefulness of the "bag" urine specimen. When I suspect that a child has a viral illness, the finding of a normal bag urinalysis and a negative culture is reassuring. In the more ill-appearing child or in situations where the bag specimen is contaminated or inconclusive, a catheter-collected specimen can be obtained. I have found it impossible to convince parents that a bladder tap in the office setting has a favorable risk/benefit ratio.

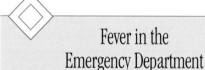

Fever in the Emergency Department

A febrile child who reaches the emergency department (ED) by whatever means should be presumed to be seriously ill until convincing data to the contrary are collected. This approach, although diametrically opposed to that which I have proposed for the primary care office, has much to recommend it. First, the large pool of febrile children has been distilled down, so that the proportion of seriously ill children is higher, increasing the prior probability of discovering serious illness. (For facilities that serve mostly as after-hours services for children who are not ill and are EDs in name only, the office-based approach is probably more appropriate.) Second, the ED offers less opportunity to establish a level of physician-parent trust. Lack of trust makes it more difficult to be reassuring in the absence of data provided by "tests." Third, for similar reasons, the reliability of follow-up is often in doubt. Fourth, risk of medicolegal liability attached to "missing" a serious, treatable illness is increased. An ED is expected not to miss anything.

So, after a careful history (which ought to include an inquiry about what the parent fears might be wrong) and physical exam, if a diagnosis is not apparent, further evaluation of the febrile child over 3 months of age should include a complete blood count (CBC) and differential, a "clean" (catheterized?) urinalysis and culture, and a chest x-ray if respiratory symptoms are present. The younger and more toxic-appearing the child, the more likely I am to request a blood culture be drawn along with the CBC. What about a lumbar puncture? There is no "one-size-fits-all" criterion. In the child over 3 months of age, I believe that the old adage, "If you have any suspicion of central nervous system infection, do a lumbar puncture" still applies. We are truly fortunate that almost universal immunization against *H. influenzae* type b has resulted in a higher proportion of taps that produce normal spinal fluid.

The decision about presumptive antibiotic treatment of the febrile toddler or child without a definite diagnosis is a difficult one. The 1993 guidelines proposed by Baraff and coworkers[8] for evaluation and treatment of the febrile toddler recommend that all children (whether or not "ill-appearing") 3 to 36 months of age with a fever above 39°C and no source should have a CBC performed; if the white blood cell count is greater than 15,000 the child should undergo a blood culture and empiric treatment with a parenteral antibiotic such as ceftriaxone. These guidelines also recommend catheterization for urinalysis and culture of all males under 6 months of age, and all females under age 2 years prior to antibiotic administration.[8]

These recommendations have recently been disputed by Kramer and Shapiro as methodologically flawed, excessively invasive, and inappro-

priate in an era of almost universal immunization against *H. influenzae* type b.[9] The recent surge of relative penicillin resistance in *Streptococcus pneumoniae* makes empiric antibiotic treatment even more problematic.

If the physical exam or lab results suggest the presence of a potentially serious bacterial infection, the options of (1) hospitalization, (2) parenteral antibiotics and outpatient observation, and (3) oral antibiotics and outpatient observation should be candidly discussed with the parents (with the assistance of an interpreter if necessary). Just as some passengers on a jetliner will be unable or unwilling to perform the tasks that might become necessary in an emergency, were they seated in an exit row, so not every family will be comfortable with reliably observing and assessing their ill child at home or able to do so. That is what hospitals are for.

For the majority of families, however, home observation is preferable if careful follow-up can be assured unless the child requires intravenous fluids or supplemental oxygen. My bias toward avoiding hospitalization if at all possible is based on the real risks of iatrogenic injury or serious errors in medication administration (which occur at rates approaching 10 percent of admissions, even in the "best" hospitals.)[10] Finally, no febrile child should leave the ED without definite arrangements for a source of outpatient follow-up care and a list of symptoms that would warrant a return to the ED.

Fever in the Very Young Infant

Fever in the infant below 3 months of age is a serious and often frustrating challenge to the clinical skills and judgment of the pediatric practitioner. During my first week in private practice, I was called to the ED to consult on a febrile 3-week-old girl who had been started on oral amoxicillin two days before by another physician based on a phone call about symptoms of an upper respiratory infection. She was poorly responsive, with a bulging fontanelle, and her spinal fluid quickly grew group B streptococci. She survived seizures, apnea, and brain abscesses but was left with a moderate developmental delay, deafness, and severe behavioral problems. No one wants to hear such a story. How can it be avoided?

In 1993, guidelines were published simultaneously in *Pediatrics* and the *Annals of Emergency Medicine*, with the disclaimer that "These Guidelines are those proposed by the authors and do not constitute Practice Guidelines of the American Academy of Pediatrics." These guidelines recommend a full "septic workup," hospitalization, and empiric parenteral antibiotic treatment for febrile infants less than 29 days old. The same complete workup is recommended for infants 1 to 3 months old, with the option of outpatient parenteral antibiotic treatment for those meeting "low risk" criteria[8] (Table 5-1).

Other authors have suggested other algorithms.[11] The recommendations for the care of febrile 1 to 2-month-olds that make the most sense to me are the "Philadelphia criteria" pro-

mulgated by Baker, Bell, and Avner.[12] These guidelines reliably separate the 60 percent of infants with fever (38.2°C or above) with risk factors for serious bacterial illness (SBI) from the remainder with self-limited viral illness by using an infant observation score composed of six items (quality of cry, reaction to parent stimulation, state variation, color, hydration, and response to social overtures)[13] combined with a complete laboratory evaluation (blood, urine, and cerebrospinal fluid) of all febrile infants. Treatment is reserved for those who appear ill or have abnormal laboratory findings.

Thus, hospitalization and unnecessary antibiotics are avoided in approximately 40 percent of those infants 29 to 59 days of age who would otherwise have undergone the standard "rule-out" (sepsis)—2 to 3 days of hospitalization and parenteral antibiotics until all bacterial cultures were negative. The negative predictive value following this protocol[12] was 100 percent in approximately 600 infants over a 5-year period. Thus, the chance of sending home a seriously ill infant was no greater than 1 in 600. Most parents, and I hope most physicians, would be comfortable with this degree of risk.

There is little disagreement about the evaluation of febrile infants less than 1 month of age—bacterial cultures and hospitalization for

Table 5-1

Low-Risk Criteria for Febrile Infants

CLINICAL CRITERIA	LABORATORY CRITERIA
Previously healthy	WBC count 5K to 15K, < 1.5K bands/mm^3
Nontoxic clinical appearance	Normal urinalysis (<5 WBC/hpf) or negative gram-stained smear
No focal bacterial infection on examination (except otitis media)	
When diarrhea present	< 5 WBC/hpf in stool

SOURCE: Modified by permission from Baraff LJ, Bass JW, Fleisher GR, et al: Practice guidelines for the management of infants and children 0 to 36 months of age with fever without source. *Pediatrics* 92:1, 1993.

observation and parenteral antibiotics until the cultures are negative for 48 to 72 h.

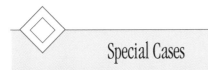

Special Cases

Febrile Seizures

There is rarely a more shocking event for parents to witness than their child's first febrile seizure. A more effective reinforcer of fever phobia would be hard to imagine, given the reported incidence of febrile seizures of 4 percent in children under 5 years of age. Fortunately, there is no evidence of long-term negative effects on brain function due to such seizures, and recurrence risk is well under 50 percent. Attempts to prevent recurrent febrile seizures through the use of ibuprofen or acetaminophen at the first suspicion of fever have not been shown to be effective.[14] Alternative strategies, such as reduction of exposure to viral illnesses (i.e., no day care) and the use of rectal benzodiazepine preparations, make sense for those children with recurrent or atypical febrile seizures, or for those with very anxious parents. Prophylactic treatment with anticonvulsants, especially phenobarbital, is no longer recommended.

Factitious Fever

I have not identified a case of factitious fever in 24 years of outpatient pediatric practice. A recent review of "Munchausen syndrome by proxy" in the psychiatric literature does not even mention factitious fever.[15] Although factitious fever has no place in a discussion of common pediatric problems, keep in mind that in prolonged unexplained fever, as with any other story that does not play out according to the script of common illness with which the clini-

cian has become familiar, consultation with a subspecialist should be considered early.

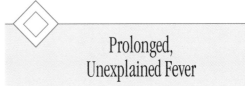

Prolonged, Unexplained Fever

"I mean Negative Capability, that is when a man is capable of being in uncertainties, Mysteries, doubts, without any irritable reaching after fact & reason. . ."

John Keats[16]

Appropriate, stepwise evaluation of the child with prolonged, unexplained fever is a real test of the clinician's diagnostic skills and of his or her relationship with a concerned family. The child I refer to is one with documented fever for over a week, without focal or organ-specific findings on physical exam, and with negative or nonspecific screening laboratory findings [complete blood count (CBC) with differential, urinalysis and culture, sedimentation rate +/or C-reactive protein (CRP) level].

Where to go next? This topic has been well-reviewed by Gartner[17] and by Miller et al.,[18] and the answer is back to another careful history, and another careful physical exam. If the child is asymptomatic except for fever, without recent travel or unusual animal exposure, and the parents are comfortable, then observation for another week or so is reasonable, followed by another set of screening laboratory studies. Most viral illnesses will have declared their identity by this time or will have resolved. If documented fever persists, further laboratory evaluations and imaging studies listed in Tables 5-2 and 5-3 can be considered.

As a practical matter, I recommend cultivating a collegial relationship with a pediatric rheumatologist who is amenable to telephone consultation. Rheumatologists see plenty of unusual

Table 5-2

Laboratory and Skin Tests to Consider in Evaluating the Child with Prolonged Fevers

TEST	REASON
CBC, differential, platelet count	Leukocytosis suggests infection, rheumatic disease Screen for leukemia Screen for thrombocytopenia, thrombocytosis
ESR / CRP	Persisting elevation suggests unresolved process requiring further evaluation
Liver function tests	Screen for hepatitis
Urinalysis	Abnormalities may suggest cystitis, pyelonephritis, or inflammatory nephritis
Blood cultures	Exclude bacteremia, SBE
Lyme titers	Exclude Lyme disease (in areas endemic for Lyme disease or patients who have traveled to such areas)
Antistreptococcal enzyme titers	Exclude recent steptococcal infection
Antinuclear antibody	Screen for lupus
Stool cultures (including O&P, *Clostridium difficile*)	If history includes diarrhea
PPD, *Candida* skin tests	Exclude exposure to tuberculosis

KEY: CBC, complete blood count; ESR, erythrocyte sedimentation rate; CRP, C-reactive protein; SBE, subacute bacterial endocarditis; O&P, ova & parasites; PPD, purified protein derivative.
SOURCE: Modified by permission from Miller ML, Szer I, Yogev R, et al: Fever of unknown origin. *Pediatr Clin North Am* 42:999, 1995.

Table 5-3

Imaging Tests to Consider in Evaluating the Child with Prolonged Fevers

IMAGING MODALITY	REASON
Chest radiograph	Exclude infiltrate, cardiomegaly, pleural fluid
Radiographs of specific bones	When other findings raise possibility of osteomyelitis or tumor
Electrocardiogram, echocardiogram	Exclude abnormalities suggestive of pericarditis in patient with possible systemic juvenile rheumatoid arthritis (JRA)
Bone scan	Screen for osteomyelitis, JRA
Gallium scan, abdominal ultrasound	Screen for intraabdominal abscesses or tumors
Magnetic resonance imaging	
Of spine	Exclude tumor, abscess, diskitis
Of abdomen (with contrast)	Exclude abscess

SOURCE: Modified by permission from Miller ML, Szer I, Yogev R, et al: Fever of unknown origin. *Pediatr Clin North Am* 42:999, 1995.

diseases presenting in common ways (and unusual presentations of common, harmless diseases) and can often provide reassurance against ordering every serology test on the laboratory requisition. Ordering only those tests that might rule in or out a clinical suspicion has a number of benefits: (1) conservation of healthcare resource dollars (sometimes I find it helpful to imagine that the parents are paying for everything out of pocket), (2) reduction of the likelihood of false-positive lab results (by definition, 5 percent, or one test in twenty, can be expected to be spuriously abnormal), and (3) less discomfort for the child.

There are advantages to identifying serious illnesses with potentially bad outcomes avoidable by early treatment (i.e., Kawasaki's disease); therefore, for the child with prolonged unexplained fever who appears ill or is in significant pain, hospitalization for observation and coordination of subspecialty consultation (infectious disease, rheumatology, hematology-oncology) should be considered early.

Treatment of Fever

It would be inconsistent to portray fever as a harmless (and possibly helpful) symptom of illness and then to concentrate too heavily on its treatment. Most parents, however, even if talked down from their height of fever phobia, wish to make their children more comfortable during illness and to try to get a decent night's sleep. Parents of children who have experienced a febrile seizure are anxious to prevent a recurrence, although evidence that early or prophylactic treatment with antipyretics will accomplish this is lacking.[14]

For children and infants over 3 months of age who "feel warm" and seem mildly ill, I recommend acetaminophen at a dose of 15 mg/kg no more often than every 4 h, or, put another way, 5 doses in 24 h. A satisfactory alternative is ibuprofen at a dose of 10 mg/kg no more often than every 6 h. Infants under 3 months of age who seem febrile should be brought in for evaluation if their rectal temperature exceeds 38°C (100.5°F) or if they appear ill.

Evidence is lacking for the efficacy of "stacking" or alternating acetaminophen and ibuprofen during the same illness. Such recommendations serve only to reinforce fever phobia.[19] Aspirin has no place in the management of fever in the child or young adolescent because of the association of influenza, aspirin, and Reye's syndrome. Those few children with documented fever above 105°F (40.5°C) should probably be examined rather than treated over the phone unless they are otherwise asymptomatic.

References

1. McCarthy PL: Fever. *Pediatr Rev* 19:401, 1998.
2. Kluger MJ: Fever revisited. *Pediatrics* 90:846, 1992.
3. Graham E, Chitnarong J: Ethnographic study among Seattle Cambodians: fever. November 1997. (http://healthlinks.washington.edu/clinical/ethnomed/ethno_fever/html)
4. Kramer MS, Naimark L, Leduc DG: Parental fever phobia and its correlates. *Pediatrics* 75:1110, 1985.
5. Schmitt BD: Fever phobia. *Am J Dis Child* 134:176, 1980.
6. May A, Bauchner H: Fever phobia: the pediatrician's contribution. *Pediatrics* 90:851, 1992.
7. Baraff LJ, Lee SI: Fever without source: management of children 3 to 36 months of age. *Pediatr Infect Dis J* 11:146, 1992.
8. Baraff LJ, Bass JW, Fleisher GR, et al: Practice guidelines for the management of infants and children 0 to 36 months of age with fever without source. *Pediatrics* 92:1, 1993.
9. Kramer MS, Shapiro ED: Management of the young febrile child: a commentary on recent practice guidelines. *Pediatrics* 100:128, 1997.

10. DeAngelis C, Joffe A, Wilson M, et al: Iatrogenic risks and financial costs of hospitalizing febrile infants. *Am J Dis Child* 137:1146, 1983.

11. Baskin MN, O'Rourke EJ, Fleisher GR: Outpatient treatment of febrile infants 28 to 89 days of age with intramuscular administration of ceftriaxone. *J Pediatr* 120:22, 1992.

12. Baker MD, Bell LM, Avner JR: Outpatient management without antibiotics of fever in selected infants. *N Engl J Med* 329:1437, 1993.

13. McCarthy PL, Sharpe MR, Spiesel SZ, et al: Observation scales to identify serious illness in febrile children. *Pediatrics* 70:802, 1982.

14. van Stuijvenberg M et al: Randomized, controlled trial of ibuprofen to prevent febrile seizure recurrences. *Pediatrics* November 1998. (e51@www.pediatrics.org)

15. Forsyth BWC: Munchausen syndrome by proxy, in Lewis M (ed): *Child and Adolescent Psychiatry: A Comprehensive Textbook*, 2nd ed. Williams & Wilkins, 1996, p 1048.

16. Keats J, in Oliver, M (ed): *A Poetry Handbook*. New York, Harcourt Brace, 1994, p 80.

17. Gartner JC: Fever of unknown origin. *Adv Pediatr Infect Dis* 7:1, 1992.

18. Miller ML, Szer I, Yogev R, et al: Fever of unknown origin. *Pediatr Clin North Am* 42:999, 1995.

19. Mayoral CE, Marino RV, Rosenfeld W, Greensher J: Alternating Antipyretics: Is It an Alternative? *Pediatrics* 195:1009, 2000.

Appendix 5-1. Handout for Parents

To the parents of our patients:

Fever is a symptom that worries many parents, and it is a topic about which you will get a great deal of conflicting advice. Why? Because many years ago it was observed that a very few children with very high fevers appeared to suffer brain damage. These observations led to a fear that all fevers could be harmful, with higher fevers being worse. More recent research indicates that a moderate (102°F) or even high (104°F) fever is harmless to the great majority of children. It may even be that fever is beneficial, helping the body's immune system to recover from illness faster—that is, fever may be worse for the germs than for the child! In any case, we now understand that the body has an "emergency thermostat" that acts to keep body temperature below 107°C, the level at which damage might theoretically occur.

So, instead of an enemy to be feared and battled, consider that in children older than about 3 months of age, a fever (i.e., the child feels warm or hot) gives you a "heads-up," an opportunity to observe the child more closely for other signs and symptoms of illness. Many years of seeing both well and sick children have convinced me that how the child acts and looks to his or her parents is much more important than the degree of the fever as measured by any thermometer.

Call your doctor if fever is accompanied by:

- Severe pain.
- Difficulty urinating, breathing, talking, or making eye contact.
- A purplish rash.

OR

- Your child is under 3 months of age.
- Your child acts very ill.
- The fever lasts more than 4 days.
- The fever is measured above 105°F.

For fever alone, without other signs or symptoms, a child over 3 months old can be safely watched at home. Most of these fevers mean that the child's immune system is working to overcome a viral infection, which takes a few days.

Since fever by itself is not harmful, it is not necessary to take extreme measures such as undressing the child or sponging him or her with water or alcohol. Since your child may be more comfortable if the fever is lowered somewhat, acteminophen or ibuprofen may be given according to the directions on the bottle or as directed by your doctor. Aspirin should never be used for fever reduction in children because of the risk of Reye's syndrome, a rare but dangerous liver condition.

In conclusion—your observations as a caring parent of your child's degree of illness are much more important than any information you can obtain using a thermometer. Trust yourself and your observations. When in doubt, call your doctor.

Richard H. Schwartz

Otitis Media and Sinusitis

Acute otitis media (AOM) is one of the top three outpatient diagnoses in children between 6 months and 36 months of age. By 3 years of age, 50 percent of children can be expected to have had two or more office or clinic visits for AOM and 25 percent will have six or more visits to a physician for AOM or secretory otitis media (otitis media with effusion, or OME). Some 20 percent of all pediatric antibiotic prescriptions involves treatment for middle ear disease.

Acute bacterial sinusitis is also a common reason to prescribe antibiotics. In the past 30 years, we have come a long way in establishing precise criteria for diagnosis of acute otitis media (and distinguishing it clinically from OME), and acute sinusitis. Still, these diagnoses should be based on the 1997 clinical practice guidelines of the Centers for Disease Control and Prevention/American Academy of Pediatrics/American Academy of Family Physicians (CDC/AAP/AAFP) in order to reduce unnecessary antibiotic consumption for an erroneous diagnosis (Table 6-1).

Advances in the diagnosis of AOM include widespread use of pneumatic otoscopy with halogen bulb illumination and rechargable batteries, the availability of acoustic impedance (tympanometry) and acoustic reflectometry, an understanding of the natural history of persistent secretory otitis media, and good clinical practice guidelines for timing of referral for tympanostomy tubes.

We know that decongestant-antihistamine combination drugs are ineffective adjuncts for AOM. We have also followed the rise and fall (because of bacterial resistance to one or both components) of the popularity of trimethoprim-sulfamethoxazole and erythromycin-sulfisoxazole (Pediazole) as first- or second-line treatment for AOM. Controversies for the new millennium include how to deal with bacterial resistance to first-line antibiotics and reevaluation of treatment choices, use of alternative and/or complementary medical management of AOM, selective withholding of antibiotics for children older than 2 years, management strategies for the "otitis prone" child, and consideration of the use of second-generation fluoroquinolones for difficult-to-treat cases of acute otitis media. *There is no controversy over the fact that secretory otitis media should not be treated with antibiotics.*

Table 6-1

Principles of Judicious Use of Antimicrobial Agents for Otitis Media

> Classify episodes of otitis media as AOM or OME
> Antimicrobials are indicated for treatment of AOM
> Antimicrobials are not usually indicated for OME
> Diagnosis of AOM requires documented middle-ear effusion and signs of acute local or systemic illness
> Antimicrobial prophylaxis should be reserved for those with documented recurrent AOM, defined by ≥ 3 episodes in 6 months or ≥ 4 episodes in 12 months

KEY: AOM, acute otitis media; OME, otitis media with effusion.
SOURCE: Centers for Disease Control and Prevention and the American Academy of Pediatrics, 1998.

Otitis Media

Diagnostic Criteria for Acute Otitis Media

Every clinician caring for children should become adept at skillful examination of the eardrums of infants and children, including those with Down syndrome, who are among the most difficult to examine. The requisite skill to perform pneumatic otoscopy can be attained best at the side of an expert mentor and fine-tuned after visualizing hundreds of eardrums. Prerequisites for accurate diagnosis include:

1. A well-maintained halogen light source. The halogen bulb should be changed every 3 to 5 months with normal use; a charged new battery should be inserted every 3 years.
2. Properly designed 3-, 4-, and 5-mm otoscopic specula that can be inserted 5 to 6 mm into the ear canal. Smaller disposable aural specula are often unsuitable for infants and young children because of serious design flaws.
3. Skilled use of stainless steel blunt aural curettes, disposable plastic curettes, or aural lavage to remove ear wax and skin.
4. Firm restraint of a struggling infant or young child's arms, head, and thighs either in mother's lap or supine on the examination table.
5. Application of alternate negative and positive pressure (biphasic pressures are necessary) with the pneumatic otoscope.

Failure to follow any one of the prerequisites reduces diagnostic precision. More errors probably occur because of failure to develop expert otoscopic skills and to use precise criteria for diagnosis of AOM than are caused by the choice of antibiotic or the duration of therapy.

Diagnostic criteria for AOM such as redness of the tympanic membrane(s), blurring or oblit-eration of the cone of light (light reflex), and even limitation of mobility of the tympanic membrane have been repeatedly shown to correlate poorly with recovery of bacterial pathogens after tympanocentesis. Criteria that correlate better with bacterial pathogens include the combination of symptoms, and signs listed below.

SYMPTOMS

Generalized symptoms include irritability or cranky behavior, whining, crying, or screaming, anorexia, and sleep disturbance. Complaints of pain may be absent, especially during infancy. Only one-third of older children with minor complaints of earache have true AOM. Only two-thirds of infants and young children have demonstrable symptoms of pain in the face of tympanocentesis-proven AOM. Fever is also not necessary for the diagnosis. Fever is present in about one-third of children, more so in infants. Because OME can cause tugging at the ears, fussiness, anorexia, and even low-grade fever from a concomitant upper respiratory infection (URI), it is good practice to insist on visualizing the bulging of an opacified, poorly mobile tympanic membrane, even if this requires time-consuming removal of ceramen.

Localized symptoms include rubbing or tugging at the auricle, digging an index finger into the auditory meatus, verbal complaints of earache, saying "hurt," and complaints of fullness of the middle ear with diminished hearing acuity. Complaints of pain or crying, *when protracted and severe*, correlate best with pneumatic otoscopic sings of AOM.

SIGNS

The principal pneumootoscopic signs of acute otitis media include fullness or bulging of the tympanic membrane, opacification of the tympanic membrane; and reduced or absent tympanic membrane (TM) mobility (absolute immobility is not necessary).(Table 6-2) The color of the TM is now recognized to be of minor importance. The color may be predominantly pink or red, dull yellow, dull gray, or off white. Diffusion or absence of the light reflex (cone of light) is no longer used as criteria of AOM. All too frequently, the clinician visualizes a dull, thickened tympanic membrane in neutral or retracted position, vague or absent light reflex, TM blush, and absent mobility to positive pressure. This is not acute otitis media.

Fullness or bulging of the TM is the most important diagnostic sign. It means that the liquid in the middle ear cleft is under positive pressure, probably secondary to an intense microbe-initiated inflammatory reaction. *Without distinct fullness or bulging of the TM, a diagnosis of AOM cannot be made with certainty.*

Another important sign, present in approximately 2 percent of children with AOM, is spontaneous acute otorrhea from a ruptured eardrum or through a tympanostomy tube.

Pathogenesis

RISK FACTORS

Important variables related to the frequency of AOM in all children include exposure to cigarette smoke, frequency of nasal colonization of respiratory viruses, face-to-face and hand-to-mouth contact with peers and adults (especially those who touch other young children and neglect to wash their hands); the length and

angulation of the eustachian tube, and possibly the presence of chronically infected lymphoid tissue in the nasopharynx. Allergies to food or inhalants also play a role. Some otolaryngologists strongly believe that spillover gastroesophageal reflux is important in the pathogenesis of otitis media.

Some children are more likely than others to become otitis-prone—that is, to have had more than two separate episodes of AOM in the preceding 6 months or more than 3 episodes in the preceding 12 months (antibiotic failures do not count, nor does secretory otitis media) (Table 6-3). Otitis-prone children include those in child-care settings, those who had a first episode of AOM before the fourth month of life, highly food-allergic children, infants not breast-fed for at least 3 months, children with a strong family history of middle ear disease, those with chronic mucopurulent rhinorrhea, those living with or cared for by tobacco smokers, and babies who usually drink milk in a prone position. Children with cleft palate and or other selected craniofacial anomalies such as Down syndrome may be particularly susceptible to chronic secretory otitis media which may be associated with gastroesophageal reflux disease (GERD).

INFECTIOUS PROCESS

The infectious process is fairly straightforward. Respiratory syncytial virus, parainfluenza virus, and influenza virus are the most important

Table 6-2

Acute Otitis Media: Definition

1. Bulging position of membrane
2. Opacified tympanic membrane
3. Impaired mobility
4. Possibly also color change: gray/white, yellow, or red

Table 6-3

Factors Predisposing to Treatment Failure/Recurrence

1. Child-care center attendance
2. Bilateral acute otitis media
3. Otitis-prone child
4. First episode at age below 6 months
5. First-line antibiotic within past 30 days
6. Age below 2 years

respiratory viruses in the pathogenesis of AOM. These viruses multiply, elicit inflammatory mediators, cause swelling of the eustachian tube orifices, impede the ventilation and drainage functions of the eustachian tube, and damage the ciliated modified respiratory epithelial mucosa lining the middle ear cleft and eustachian tube. This sets the stage for nasopharyngeal bacteria, which enter the middle ear via the eustachian tube, adhere to the damaged mucosa, occasionally breach cellular defenses, and infect the cells. Depending on the virulence of the bacteria, there may be a sudden increase of inflammation with chemotaxis of polymorphonuclear leukocytes, phagocytosis, release of bacterial exoenzymes, and an outpouring of purulent material that causes the tympanic membrane to distend and produce the pain associated with AOM.

MICROBIOLOGY

Contrary to traditional opinion, investigators from Israel and the United States have proven repeatedly that only 10 percent, not the oft-repeated 30 percent, of middle ear cultures obtained by tympanocentesis are "sterile" when the diagnosis includes all necessary criteria for AOM. The five most important middle ear pathogens are *Streptococcus pneumoniae*, which causes approximately 40 percent of cases of acute otitis media; *Haemophilus influenzae* (20 to 30 percent); *Moraxella catarrhalis* (10 to 20 percent); *Streptococcus pyogenes* (2 to 5 percent, depending on age); and *Staphylococcus aureus* (1 to 4 percent). In many areas of the United States, resistance to amoxicillin because of production of beta-lactamase enzyme occurs in 30 to 60 percent of *H. influenzae* and 90 to 100 percent of *M. catarrhalis*. High penicillin-resistance (MIC > 2.0 μg/mL) occurs in from 8 to 10 percent of *S. pneumoniae* infections. The most important pathogens are the two streptococcal species, which can rapidly destroy the contents of the middle ear and enter the mastoid cavity. *H. influenzae* and *M. catarrhalis* rarely

spread beyond the confines of the middle ear. *Mycoplasma pneumoniae*, *Chlamydia*, and anaerobic bacteria are infrequent causes of AOM. Bullous AOM is caused not by *Mycoplasma* organisms but by highly virulent streptococcal bacteria that elicit a toxic reaction on the outer layer of the tympanic membrane.

Although there is usually concordance between results of cultures of the nasopharynx and simultaneous middle ear cultures, there are too many incongruous results to allow the results of nasopharyngeal culture alone to dictate antibiotic therapy. Concurrent purulent discharge from the conjunctivae in addition to AOM (conjunctivitis-otitis syndrome) is usually caused by nontypeable, *H. influenzae*. In the neonatal period, gram-negative enteric bacteria and group B streptococcus are important middle ear pathogens.

Otoscopic Examination of Neonates and Very Young Infants

Otoscopic examination of very young infants and young children with Down syndrome requires that a 3-mm aural speculum or occasionally a 2-mm speculum, inserted 3 to 5 mm past the auditory meatus, be used. Disposable plastic specula, as presently designed, do not meet this criterion. Moreover, these poorly designed specula often leak air during pneumatic otoscopy, impeding accurate assessment of mobility of the TM.

Acoustic Impedance and Acoustic Reflectometry

When the diagnosis of AOM is in doubt, use of an impedance instrument (tympanometry) or acoustic reflectometer with or without spectral gradient analysis can aid in the verification of the presence of middle ear effusion. These instruments, however, cannot differentiate between AOM and OME, also known as secretory otitis media. The acoustic reflectometer analyzes the frequency spectra of the reflected sound generated from the instrument and prints out a hard copy with a parallel port printer. This instrument, costing the physician from $40 (without spectral analysis or printed) to $300, has been shown to be about as sensitive as impedance testing. However, it is much less expensive, more portable, and easier to use. Wax impactions and the narrow ear canals of young infants reduce reliability; the instrument should always be used in concert with pneumatic otoscopy.

A modification of the acoustic reflectometer called EarCheck (MDI Instruments, Inc., Woburn, MA) is available for parents to use to detect acute or chronic middle ear effusion. These instruments furnish objective proof of otoscopic diagnoses in selected cases, as when the parent's diagnosis of AOM—based on symptoms of otalgia—and the clinician's diagnosis are discordant, or at the time of referral to an otolaryngologist for chronic secretory otitis media. Both instruments are invaluable for teaching purposes.

Treatment of Acute Otitis Media

As a general rule, the greater the virulence of the bacteria and the greater the pain and fever, the greater the importance of prescribing analgesics/antipyretics and antibiotics. There are more than twenty antibiotics that may be used for treating acute otitis media. Individual physician or parent preferences, previous experience, cost, taste, and ease and frequency of administration may influence one's choice of antibiotic (Table 6-4). Although amoxicillin remains the drug of choice for the treatment of AOM in most regions of the United States, there is a need for alternative antibiotic choices. In areas of the country where penicillin-resistant pneumococci are common, treatment can begin with amoxicillin 40 to 50 mg/kg/day up to 90 mg/kg/day in

Table 6-4

Suggested Therapy for Acute Otitis Media

Initial
    Amoxicillin 60–90 mg/kg/day (2 or 3 doses)
Failure of initial therapy
    Amoxicillin/clavulanate (7:1) 45 mg/kg/day
      (2 doses)
    Amoxicillin/clavulanate (14:1) 90 mg/kg/day
      (2 doses)
    Cefuroxime 30 mg/kg/day (2 doses)
    Ceftriaxone 50 mg/kg/day (2 doses IM)

two or three divided doses. Some physicians are now routinely giving 75 mg/kg/day. There have been no clinical studies comparing 40 mg/kg/day with 90 mg/kg/day. Several experts have recently recommended a truncated 5-day course of amoxicillin for non–otitis prone children who are above 3 or 4 years of age—a reasonable recommendation.

Amoxicillin is not a good choice if the child is allergic to antibiotics in the penicillin class, had taken it or another beta-lactam antibiotic in the past 30 days, or is very prone to develop acute otitis media. For penicillin-allergic children, an expanded-spectrum macrolide antibiotic such as azithromycin (10 mg/kg/day as a single dose on day one followed by 5 mg/kg/day on days 2 to 5) is a reasonable alternative to amoxicillin. It should be underscored however, that from 25 to 50 percent of penicillin-resistant *S. pneumoniae* infections are also resistant to macrolides and azolides, including azithromycin. A greater percent of penicillin-resistant pneumococci are co-resistant to trimethoprim-sulfamethoxazole. In addition, trimethoprim-sulfamethoxazole has lost some of its effectiveness against *H. influenzae*, and I have greatly reduced my use of this antimicrobial combination.

At present, from 20 to 40 percent of *Strep. pneumoniae* clinical isolates are drug-resistant strains. The most appropriate alternative antibiotics for the treatment of probable drug-resistant *S. pneumoniae* are amoxicillin/clavulanate suspension, 50 to 75 mg/kg/day in two divided doses of the 200 or 400 mg/5 mL; cefuroxime axetil suspension, dosed at 30 mg/kg/day in two divided doses, cefpodoxine proxetil suspension, cefdenir suspension; or ceftriaxone injection 50 mg/kg/day with a maximum volume per site of 1 mL. If the middle ear organism is thought to be *S. pneumoniae*, clindamycin, 20 mg/kg/day in two or three divided doses, is an excellent alternative choice. Cefuroxime axetil and cefpodoxime proxetil suspensions have a bitter taste. Mixing the suspension with an equivalent volume of chocolate or strawberry syrup improves compliance.

Results from several recent studies from Israel show excessive numbers of early recurrences of AOM after treatment with a single injection of ceftriaxone. For this reason, ceftriaxone should be injected for 2 or 3 days for a total dose of 100 to 150 mg/kg. This greatly increases both financial cost and the pain inflicted on the child, and it may be difficult to obtain reimbursement for the second day of treatment.

Investigational antibiotics with potential future usefulness in the treatment of AOM include those in the fluoroquindone, oxazolidinone, streptogramin, and ketolide class of investigational drugs. Trials with pediatric patients can be expected in the year 2000. Trials of an oral fluoroquindone suspension are already underway.

MANIPULATION OF RISK FACTORS

Risk factors that may be manipulated include removal from child care; elimination of tobacco smoking at home, at child care, and in the family car; continuation of breast-feeding for at least 3 months; a diet eliminating milk and soy as a trial; and avoidance of bottle feeding in the prone position. Suggested management strategies for the otitis-prone child, which I have not yet used, include conjugate pneumococcal polysaccharide vaccine, annual influenza immuniza-

tions for children older than 1 year, and a therapeutic trial of antireflux medications.

Antibiotic Prophylaxis for the Otitis-Prone Child

Although the current wisdom is to reduce the number of children who receive antibiotic prophylaxis for prevention of recurrent acute otitis media, there are some children who can truly benefit from a daily dose of antibiotic during the otitis season. Candidates for prophylaxis include children who have had at least three episodes of acute otitis media in the preceding 3 months and present for a fourth episode and children scheduled for tympanostomy tubes in the next month or two who cannot remain infection-free for that amount of time. Traditionally, prophylaxis meant sulfasoxazole, 30 mg/kg administered at bedtime, or amoxicillin, 13 mg/kg/dose to 30 mg/kg/dose. There are no recent studies of the efficacy of these antibiotics in prophylaxis in the era of high antibiotic resistance, so it's not clear if they are still as effective.

Management of the Acutely Draining Ear

Acute otorrhea indicates either a perforated tympanic membrane or sometimes simply liquefaction of cerumen associated with intensely inflammatory AOM. Otorrhea from a perforated drum may be spontaneous or flow out of a tympanostomy tube. The bacterial pathogens associated with acute otorrhea respond well to the usual oral antibiotics. When acute otorrhea is associated with patent tympanostomy tubes, several recent studies show good results following instillation of fluoroquinolone otic drops without coadministration of oral antibiotics.

Pain Management

When children with AOM whimper, cry, or scream because of pain and when pain interferes with sleeping, an analgesic should be ordered. Analgesics include acetaminophen syrup given at a dose of 15 mg/kg q4h; ibuprofen suspension, 10mg/kg q6–8h; acetaminophen with codeine syrup 1.0 mg/kg/dose of the codeine component; or paregoric syrup (one drop per pound of body weight) for young infants. Pain can also be reduced by physical means, as by applying a heating pad to cover the auditory meatus or warmed vegetable oil dropped into the affected ear canal(s). Topical anesthetic drops containing benzocaine in glycerin (Auralgan) can reduce the pain if the eardrum is intact, particularly if the bottle is warmed up under hot water prior to instillation of the drops. These commercially available eardrops can cause painful contact dermatitis on occasion and are contraindicated for acutely draining ears. If a clinician is experienced in performing a myringotomy or tympanocentesis, severe intractable pain can be immediately reduced following either procedure.

Tympanocentesis

The increasing frequency of drug resistant *S. pneumoniae* (DRSP) has caused a resurgence of interest in myringotomy and tympanocentesis, sadly underused and undermastered procedures. Following tandem failures of antibiotics such as amoxicillin followed by amoxicillin/ clavulanate or cefuroxime, or after failure of several doses of intramuscular ceftriaxone, tympanocentesis should be seriously considered. Tympanocentesis takes less skill than radial artery puncture or lumbar puncture. It is best performed after administration of an analgesic/ sedative or use of a topical anesthetic. Pain and memory of the event can be blunted by a mixture of acetaminophen and codeine syrup in a 4-oz bottle to which 2.5 mg/5 mL of diazepam is added by the pharmacist. The dose of codeine is 1 to 1.2 mg/kg body weight, given PO 20 min prior to the procedure. Midazolam, 0.1 mg/kg given by mouth, by rectum, or intranasally, is also employed. If midazolam is used, proper procedures for monitoring of vital signs and pulse oximetry should be followed (see Chap. 11 for more details on sedation and analgesia).

The target area for the tympanocentesis procedure is anywhere except the posterosuperior quadrant, preferably in the anteroinferior quadrant. Although most textbooks recommend the posteroinferior quadrant, it is theoretically possible to injure the round window in that location. The needle must be inserted with some force in order to enter the middle ear cleft through a thickened TM. A few drops of middle ear exudate should be obtained for culture and Gram stain.

Common mistakes include not performing the procedure when indicated, piercing the distal ear canal wall instead of the eardrum, and using a needle shaft that is too short or a bevel that is too long. I prefer a 17-gauge short-bevel needle with a sharpened cannula (obtainable from Bausch and Lomb, St. Louis, MO). Proper halogen illumination, meticulous cleaning of any wax or canal skin obstructing a clear view of the eardrum, and firm restraint are essential.

Reevaluation

After 48 to 72 h of receiving an appropriate antibiotic, the child should exhibit a decrease in otalgia or fussiness and a significant reduction in fever. Should the child continue to experience real pain (not just mild discomfort) and persistent fever, appear more ill, or display signs of acute mastoiditis, a prompt reevaluation visit is obligatory. The clinician should perform a careful examination with attention to signs of overwhelming sepsis, meningitis, mastoiditis, or unimproved acute otitis media. By the third day, the tympanic membrane usually returns to a more neutral position and appears less inflamed. If the child is still quite symptomatic and the tympanic membrane continues to bulge, a change of antibiotic as well as consideration of tympanocentesis is advisable.

If the clinical condition is improving, routine reevaluation is not needed for children older than 2 or 3 years of age and those with unilateral AOM and asymptomatic infants who are scheduled to return for routine health care within the next 3 months. In the clinically improving child with a past history of OME or in a young child with bilateral AOM, routine follow-up can usually be safely scheduled at 2 or 3 months.

Otitis Media with Effusion

EPIDEMIOLOGY

After a course of antibiotic therapy for AOM, approximately 50 to 70 percent of middle ears of young children will have OME. The mean duration of OME is 12 weeks; 90 percent will resolve by 90 days. Risk factors for protracted effusions are the same as those for otitis-prone children, most commonly attendance at child care centers and family propensity for OME. Children with Down syndrome, cleft palate, velocardiofacial syndrome, and fetal alcohol syndrome are particularly prone to chronic OME. Those with chronic nasal allergy, chronic adenoiditis, chronic sinusitis, cystic fibrosis, and dyskinetic cilia syndrome are also prone to middle ear effusion. The peak incidence of OME is seasonal, peaking in December through May in the mid-Atlantic states.

SYMPTOMS

OME may cause discomfort in the middle ear. Additional symptoms include inattention in school and a reduction in auditory acuity. Although the associated conductive hearing loss is usually mild or low-moderate, some children have significant conductive hearing loss, which may, if it is bilateral and lasts 4 months or more, interfere with communication and learning.

DIAGNOSIS OF OME

The tympanic membrane may be opacified and thickened and pink, gray, or white. Pneu-

matic otoscopy will reveal limited biphasic movement, and tympanometry or acoustic impedance will verify its presence. Impedance testing is complementary to pneumatic otoscopy, increasing both sensitivity and especially specificity when there is concordance between the two methods.

MICROBIOLOGY

Twenty percent of these effusions contain viable bacterial pathogens. However, the organisms tend to be low in numbers, and noninvasive *H. influenzae* or *M. catarrhalis* rather than *S. pneumoniae*. Moreover, antibiotic treatment has only a very modest efficacy in enhancement of draining the effusion.

HEARING LOSS

The conductive loss for children with effusions is in the shape of a bell curve. A few children with OME hear well at 20 dB while most have problems hearing pure tones or speech at the 30-dB level. The natural history of middle ear effusions has been well described. After an additional 30-day period, 50 percent of the effusions will resolve spontaneously; after 60 days, another 50 percent will resolve; and by 90 days, the cutoff point for the definition of chronic OME, all but 10 percent will resolve. Tympanometry or acoustic reflectometry are valuable adjuncts to aid in the diagnosis of OME.

MANAGEMENT

Children with OME should be followed over time; there is usually no need for antibiotic, decongestant, or antihistamine medications. Should the effusion(s) persist for 60 days or more, it may be worthwhile to suggest dairy-free and soy-free diets, proper bottle or breast position (no supine feeding), and elimination of irritants such as tobacco or wood smoke. Children with underlying problems—such as Down syndrome, cleft palate, velocardiofacial syndrome, fetal alcohol syndrome—and those with preexisting sensorineural hearing loss should be referred to an otolaryngologist at about the 60-day limit.

Otherwise normal children should be followed for another 30 to 60 days before otolaryngologist referral for a total of *120 days for minimally symptomatic bilateral effusions and at least 180 days for minimally symptomatic unilateral middle ear effusions.* Those who have very bothersome symptoms interfering with sleep, balance, hearing, and well-being should be referred earlier. Ask the parents of such children about behaviors such as inattention to language spoken from a distance or a need to increase the volume of the television sound, both of which may indicate significant conductive hearing loss.

An audiogram or otoacoustic emittance test should be obtained at or after the 60th day to quantify hearing acuity, sooner if there appears to be considerable hearing impairment. Should the threshold level for pure tones exceed 35 dB or should the child between the ages of 18 to 36 months have delay in language milestones, indistinct articulation of many words, or maladaptive behaviors attributed to chronic OME, a referral for tympanostomy tubes, laser-assisted myringotomy, *or* a therapeutic trial of a 7- to 10-day course of corticosteroids may be considered.

STEROIDS

The Agency for Health Care Policy and Research (AHPCR) guidelines for good clinical practice in the management of chronic OME do not support selective use of oral corticosteroids for chronic OME (metanalysis just missed clinical significance) (Table 6-1). Nonetheless, many physicians, including myself, claim success (defined as complete resolution of OME, restoration of hearing acuity, and no recurrence for at least 3 months) in about one-third of children so treated. The typical dose of prednisone, is 2 mg/kg body weight per day in three divided

doses for 3 days, followed by 1 mg/kg/day in two divided doses for 4 days. An alternative day schedule (days 9, 11, 13) can be used for the second week of therapy at 0.75 mg/kg/day to 1 mg/kg/day, morning dose only. If the 120-day cutoff falls in late April, May, or June, it would be advisable to wait a few more months, because summer may produce a spontaneous resolution of the effusion.

The role of immunotherapy (allergy shots) or alternative/complementary medicine in the management of chronic OME or recurrent AOM is uncertain.

SURGICAL MANAGEMENT

The standard initial surgical procedure for ventilation of the middle ear and/or reduction in frequency of episodes of AOM is insertion of tympanostomy tubes without adenoidectomy unless the adenoids are chronically infected, hypertrophic, and obstructing the eustachian tube orifice or the nasopharyngeal airway. Tympanostomy tubes usually function for 8 to 10 months, after which they become obstructed with debris or granulation tissue. Long-term tubes that have a toggle bolt design remain in place for several years; however, there is a higher incidence of permanent iatrogenic perforation of the tympanic membrane after this type of tube is surgically removed.

Adverse events associated with tympanostomy tubes include tympanosclerosis scarring of the TM (uncertain significance), persistent otorrhea, formation of granulation tissue at the orifices, and the rare iatrogenic implantation cholesteatoma. The risks of the untreated disease itself has similar consequences.

Complications of Acute Otitis Media

SUPPURATIVE COMPLICATIONS

Suppurative complications of AOM are uncommon. They include acute mastoiditis, Bell's palsy, thrombosis of the dural venous sinus or jugular vein, labyrinthitis, and intracranial extension of the infection. In the past 2 or 3 years there has been a resurgence of acute mastoiditis in some areas of the country for unknown reasons. The primary causative organisms are *S. pneumoniae* and *Streptococcus pyogenes*. *H. influenzae* and *M. catarrhalis* are rare causative agents. When the disease has progressed to subperiosteal abscess and coalescent mastoiditis, mastoidectomy is usually indicated.

Complications of Chronic Otitis Media with Effusion

Neglected or long-standing otitis media with effusion can cause problems in hearing, communication, and language acquisition in young children. When the tympanic membrane is chronically retracted, it may form a retraction pocket. If located in the posterosuperior quadrant, fibrous adhesions can, over time, wrap around the ossicular chain, causing ischemic erosion. Or a cholesteatoma may develop and slowly enlarge, damaging ossicles and middle ear function. The cholesteatoma may also cause a persistent perforation of the tympanic membrane and chronic foul-smelling otorrhea. Chronic otorrhea unresponsive to topical and systemic antibiotics should be evaluated for cholesteatoma.

Acute Sinusitis

Diagnosis

The paranasal sinuses are paired, air-filled cavities lined with modified respiratory epithelium that communicate with the ipsilateral nasal passage. Tiny ethmoid and maxillary sinuses are present at birth and grow proportionally with the size of the face.

The three key physiologic elements of the maxillary and ethmoid sinuses are (1) the patency of the respective ostia in the sinus cavity and in the ostiomeatal complex in the middle meatus of the nose; (2) the quantity and quality of the sinonasal secretions or exudate; and (3) the ability of the cilia to remove secretions from the sinus cavities and the nasal drainage pathways.

Acute ethmoid or maxillary sinusitis has two common presentations: severe and indolent. The former usually presents with high fever, stuffy nose, purulent nasal discharge as either anterior rhinorrhea or postnasal drainage, facial or eyelid swelling, headache or retroorbital pain, signs of toxicity, and an elevated polymorphonuclear leukocyte count. Acute bacterial ethmoid or maxillary sinusitis is usually caused by *S. pneumoniae* or *S. pyogenes*.

The indolent form of acute sinusitis is much more common and is estimated to occur after 6 to 7 percent of common colds (Table 6-5). It is characterized by thick, opacified nasal discharge that persists for 10 to 30 days after onset of common cold symptoms and does not improve after initiation of symptomatic measures. *The 10-day mark separates viral rhinosinusitis from acute bacterial sinusitis, and the 30-day mark separates acute sinusitis from subacute sinusitis.*

Acute bacterial frontal sinusitis is a special case. Because the frontal sinus develops in late childhood, this condition infrequently occurs before adolescence. It is most often caused by *S. aureus* and is sometimes not diagnosed until suppuration has spread to the frontal bone or brain. *Intense, well-localized frontal headaches*

Table 6-5

Criteria for the Diagnosis of Sinusitis

1. Nasal drainage for 10 or more days
2. Frequent daytime cough without wheezing
3. Nasal obstruction causing malaise

are the hallmark of frontal sinusitis. Nasal stuffiness may not be present.

Although acute bacterial sinusitis can occur in the first 6 months of life, it is infrequent and very difficult to diagnose clinically. Sinusitis often involves both maxillary sinuses and both ethmoid sinuses when computed tomography (CT) imaging is used. However, even short-duration purulent rhinorrhea is associated with positive CT scans in young children.

Pathogenesis of Acute Sinusitis

The pathogenesis of typical acute maxillary or ethmoid sinusitis is in many respects similar to that of AOM, but it is much more difficult to diagnose. Nasal allergies are the second most common predisposing condition following viral URIs. Barotrauma or disease of the teeth are less common antecedents of acute sinusitis in children.

While rhinovirus or coronavirus rhinitis invade only a small area of the nose and usually remains where it lands, other viral pathogens, particularly respiratory syncytial virus (RSV) sometimes extend to the maxillary and ethmoid sinuses. Common colds (rhinosinusitis) typically peak at 2 to 4 days and last from 5 to 7 days, while most cases of acute bacterial sinusitis begin after 7 to 10 days of viral URI symptoms. RSV, parainfluenza viruses, and influenza viruses are the most common primary viral causes of rhinosinusitis.

The natural history of rhinosinusitis (common cold) is well known. Secretions are typically serous for the first few days. They then may thicken, opacify, turn light green or yellow for a few days and finally become off white or watery. Following virus-mediated cellular damage, bacteria from the nasopharynx occasionally gain access to the sinuses. These bacteria adhere to the virus-damaged mucosal cells, invade them, incite an intense inflammatory process, and produce a purulent exudate. Secretions from true bacterial sinusitis usually remain thick and discolored for many days and do not

resume a watery appearance. Nasopharyngeal cultures do not help to predict the sinus pathogen.

The five major bacterial pathogens causing acute sinusitis are identical to those of AOM: *S. pneumoniae, H. influenzae, M. catarrhalis, S. pyogenes,* and *S. aureus.* Anaerobic bacteria, *Staphylococcus epidermidis,* and alpha-streptococcus species usually are considered as nonpathogens, although some authorities include them.

Ostiomeatal Complex

The sinus ostia, the openings into the nasopharynx, are the key to paranasal sinus infections. Because there is marked swelling surrounding these openings, the sinus exudate—which contains multiplying pathogenic bacteria, leukocytes, and cytokines—is unable to drain out of the sinus. This often causes a sensation of pressure and facial pain. Occasionally, it produces swelling of the eyelid, the malar area of the face and the ethmoid area adjacent to the nasal bridge.

An important warning sign is discoloration and true swelling of one or both eyelids because of obstruction to lymphatic and venous drainage of the eyelid area (inflammatory edema). Five major causes of edema in the nose and sinuses include (1) URIs; (2) allergies; (3) environmental irritants; (4) anatomic abnormalities, including adenoids, septal deviation, and a cystic distention of the middle turbinate bone (concha bullosa); and (5) GERD with spillover reflux.

Anatomic and Immunologic Causes of Acute Sinusitis

Less common underlying problems associated with acute sinusitis include those that cause mucosal swelling and those that cause anatomic obstruction. Causes of mucosal swelling include barotrauma, which may occur following an airplane flight or scuba diving; blunt facial trauma;

immune deficiency syndromes (particularly IgA deficiency); cystic fibrosis, ciliary dyskinesia, and certain dental procedures. Causes of anatomic obstruction include hypertrophic adenoids, deviated nasal septum, nasal bone spurs, nasal polyps (or, in rare cases, tumors), and retained intranasal foreign bodies.

Clinical Diagnosis

SYMPTOMS

The clinical diagnosis of acute bacterial sinusitis requires the following: (1) unremitting or worsening mucopurulent or mucus (less frequently serous) anterior or posterior nasal drainage for 10 or more days; (2) frequent *daytime* cough, usually without wheezing; (3) nasal obstruction causing malaise; and occasionally (4) fever (Table 6-5). These criteria are highly correlated with opacification or air/fluid levels seen on x-ray views of the ethmoid and maxillary sinuses and, most important, with recovery of bacterial pathogens after needle aspiration of the maxillary sinus. Sinus paracentesis will recover pathogens in the majority of such cases.

Additional symptoms of acute bacterial sinusitis in older children and adolescents include thick nasal crusts that block the sinus ostia and are finger-swept out of the nose in the early morning, frequent and quite annoying (to parents and classmates) backward snorting of mucopus from the nasopharynx into the oropharynx, and continual swallowing of thick, distasteful nasal secretions. The senses of taste and smell are blunted. Pain over the maxillary sinuses may be present during viral rhinosinusitis as well as bacterial sinusitis. Classic *symptoms* of acute sinusitis—such as headache, bad breath, and molar tooth pain—are insensitive and nonspecific and are usually absent or difficult to elicit in infants and young children.

SIGNS

Signs of acute sinusitis are often nonspecific and include anterior rhinoscopic visualization of a rivulet of mucopurulent material draining down the inferior meatus of the nasal passages. Actually the drainage originates in the middle meatus and spills over and is caught by the inferior meatus. Use of a topical vasoconstrictor nose spray prior to anterior rhinoscopy may permit visualization of the middle meatus, into which the frontal, anterior ethmoid, and maxillary sinuses drain. A rivulet of mucopurulent material draining from the nasopharynx down the posterior pharyngeal wall may also be noted on intraoral examination, especially if the child is gagged.

Transillumination of the frontal and maxillary sinuses is of no use in children younger than 8 years of age and, because of low sensitivity and specificity, is of questionable value even in older children. More sinister signs of acute sinusitis include eyelid swelling, and warmth and significant tenderness to slight pressure over the sinuses. These signs, which may present at any time after the onset of a simple upper respiratory infection, indicate the possibility of a serious sinus infection and should be evaluated promptly and treated with an appropriate antibiotic agent.

DIAGNOSTIC IMAGING

Radiography is not usually useful in milder forms of acute sinusitis but may be necessary in complicated or protracted cases. A well-taken history is usually adequate for diagnosis and sinus x-rays are often misleading. A sinus CT should be obtained when the patient is acutely ill or when surgery is under consideration. A single modified Waters view (occipitomental with open mouth) captures the maxillary and anterior ethmoid sinuses. In the most severe cases (for example, a patient in whom infection has spread to the orbit or an adolescent patient with severe frontal sinus symptoms or when central nervous system involvement is under consideration), it may be advisable to promptly obtain a CT study.

Positive findings on plain radiographic include: (1) complete or almost complete opacification; (2) presence of an air/fluid level in the maxillary sinuses; and (3) thickening of the mucosal lining more than 4 mm (Wald's criterion) or 6 mm (criterion for investigator trials of acute sinusitis). The latter is the least sensitive or specific of the three x-ray signs. Radiography or CT may also be useful when the diagnosis is really in doubt or when the patient has not responded well to several courses of antimicrobial agents.

Sinus Aspiration

Aspiration of the paranasal sinuses is rarely performed as an outpatient procedure in children. It is used for complicated sinusitis (i.e., an abscess that has spread to the eye, frontal bone, or brain). Aspiration may be required in an immunocompromised host, when fungal organisms are suspected, or when sinusitis has been particularly difficult to treat.

Management of Acute Sinusitis

Initial management of acute sinusitis in children includes use of measures to promote drainage and improve ciliary function; administration of a narrow-spectrum antibiotic; and adjunctive measures such as hypertonic saline nasal lavage; and use of antipyretic/analgesic drugs. First-line antibiotic choices for mild or moderate acute sinusitis include: amoxicillin (45 to 90 mg/kg/day in two or three divided doses), azithromycin (on day 1, a single dose of 10 mg/kg, followed, on days 2 to 5, by 5 mg/kg/day. Alternatively, clarithromycin (30 mg/kg/day in two divided doses for 10 days) or one of the broad spectrum oral cephalosporin drugs may be prescribed. I use cefuroxime axetil, amoxicillin-clavulanate, or ceftriaxone injections when a child with acute

sinusitis appears toxic (very ill), with hyperpyrexia, or when a beta-lactam antibiotic was taken within the previous 30 days.

Acutely ill children with severe frontal sinusitis should be comanaged with an otolaryngologist. In general, therapy should continue approximately 7 days beyond the point of substantial improvement or resolution of signs and symptoms. There is no evidence that longer treatment in otherwise uncomplicated cases is necessary or desirable.

When symptoms and signs of acute sinusitis continue unabated after 48 to 72 h of first-line antibiotics or when the child *worsens* after several doses of first-line antibiotic, the physician should first reevaluate the clinical situation. Alternative oral antibiotics that may be considered in selected cases of mild to moderate sinusitis include amoxicillin/clavulanate (45 to 80 mg/kg/day in two divided doses); cefuroxime axetil (30 mg/kg/day in two divided doses); cefpodoxime proxetil (10 mg/kg/day in two divided doses); or cefdinir (mg/kg/day).

For children with complicated acute sinusitis, including those with progressive inflammatory edema of the eyelids, high fever, or intense sinus pain, and for adolescents with severe acute frontal sinusitis, more intense, usually parenteral, antibiotic regimens are recommended. Subacute or chronic sinusitis may require amoxicillin/clavulanate, cefuroxime, and even ciprofloxacin in recalcitrant cases. Any worrisome CNS symptom such as unremitting severe headache should be evaluated with magnetic resonance imaging or contrast CT.

Topical Vasoconstrictors and Saline Nasal Lavage

Topical vasoconstrictor drugs include 0.05% oxymetazoline (one or two sprays or drops in each nostril for 3 days). Many otolaryngologists recommend nasal insufflation of normal saline or buffered hypertonic saline solution to wash out secretions and open the nasal passages. The nasal lavage is performed three or four times daily for the first 3 to 4 days of treatment. The utility of oral decongestants is open to question, but in the initial congestive stage of disease they may relieve symptoms. They have limited role, however, in subacute or chronic sinusitis.

Application of a warm cloth or a heating pad to the maxillary sinus areas may be of some benefit. Antihistamines and guaifenesin are of dubious value, though many clinicians prescribe them based on personal preference.

Subacute and Chronic Sinusitis

The diagnosis of subacute (longer than 30 days) or chronic sinusitis (i.e., symptoms lasting at least 12 weeks without improvement) is difficult. Otolaryngologists often think of the "big six" symptoms for chronic sinusitis. These are (1) persistent purulent nasal drainage either anteriorly or posteriorly—this often causes frequent loud snorting and swallowing the drainage; (2) a productive cough that occurs day and night; (3) nasal airway obstruction; (4) headache, facial pain, or toothache (in spite of a normal dental examination); (5) halitosis or a bad taste upon arising in the morning; and (6) behavior changes that includes general malaise.

Allergists, on the other hand, tend to think of sinusitis as a possible contributing cause for chronic cough and/or wheezing. In the evaluation of a wheezing child, many allergists order sinus radiograms or CT scans and prescribe prolonged courses of antibiotics for chronic sinusitis and gastroenterologists or pulmonologists consider and treat for gastroesophageal reflux disease.

The primary care clinician should consider treatment of subacute or chronic sinusitis with nasal steroids for 4 to 6 weeks. Many otolaryngologists use them successfully in conjunction with hypertonic nasal lavage. Evaluation for selected aeroallergens may be helpful in the evaluation of a child or adolescent with chronic sinusitis.

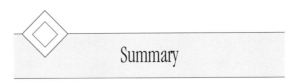

Summary

AOM and acute sinusitis are among the most common pediatric conditions for which antibiotics are prescribed. The diagnosis can be difficult and requires careful pneumatic otoscopy and/or anterior rhinoscopy, precise criteria for diagnosis, and moderate to high dosage of amoxicillin unless there are compelling reasons to chose an alternative antibiotic. Clinicians must be aware of the potential complications of these two conditions and possess a good knowledge of how to manage them.

References

1. Dagan R, Leibovitz E, Greenberg D, et al: Early eradication of pathogens from middle ear fluid during antibiotic treatment of acute otitis media is associated with improved clinical outcome. *Pediatr Infect Dis J* 17:776–782, 1998.
2. Berman S: Otitis media in children. *N Engl J Med* 332:1560–1565. 1995.
3. Block SL, Mandel E, McLinn S, et al: Spectral gradient acoustic reflectometry for the detection of middle ear effusion by pediatricians and parents. *Pediatr Infect Dis J* 17:560–564, 1998.
4. Bluestone CD, Klein JO: Clinical practice guideline on otitis media with effusion in young children: strengths and weaknesses. *Otolaryngol Head Neck Surg* 112:507–511, 1995.
5. Daly KA, Hunter LL, Giebink GS: Chronic otitis media with effusion. *Pediatr Rev* 20:85–93, 1999.
6. Pichichero ME: Changing the treatment paradigm for acute otitis media in children. *JAMA* 279: 1748–1750, 1998.
7. Block SL: Tympanocentesis: why, when, how. *Contemp Pediatr* 16:103–127, 1999.

8. Cracken GH: Treatment of acute otitis media in an era of increasing microbial resistance. *Pediatr Infect Dis J* 17:576, 1998.

9. Clement PA, Bluestone CD, Gordts F, et al:Management of rhinosinusitis in children. *Arch Otolaryngol Head Neck Surg* 124:314, 1998.

10. Wald ER: Sinusitis. *Pediatr Ann* 7:6811–6818, 1998.

11. O'Brian KL, Dowell SF, Schwartz B, et al: Acute sinusitis—principles of judicious use of antimicrobial agents. *Pediatrics* 101:174–177, 1998.

James A. Taylor

Urinary Tract Infections

There are few areas of clinical pediatrics that engender as much impassioned controversy as urinary tract infections (UTIs). There are significant disagreements regarding the diagnostic utility of urinalyses, proper technique of obtaining cultures, method of treatment for young children with UTI, role of circumcision, and necessity for radiologic evaluation of infected children. The crux of the controversy is this: UTIs, common infections in children, are easily diagnosed and usually resolve with a simple intervention. However, the potential consequences of an underdiagnosed or an undertreated UTI in a child, especially one with structural or functional abnormalities of the urinary tract, are devastating and may lead to renal scarring, hypertension, and/or chronic renal failure.

Although of similar pathophysiology, there are at least two distinct clinical presentations of UTIs. The classic child with UTI is the potty-trained girl with cystitis; on occasion there is clinical evidence of pyelonephritis in these children. However, with the increasing frequency of obtaining urine cultures in young children, it has become apparent that UTI is a common cause of fever among infants 0 to 23 months old. The management of these two groups of children is sufficiently different to be treated separately.

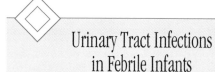

Urinary Tract Infections in Febrile Infants

Epidemiology

In the past, many UTIs in febrile children less than 2 years old were undiagnosed; undoubtedly these infections were frequently treated serendipitously with antibiotics prescribed for other reasons. However, when urine cultures were obtained on a representative sample of febrile infants less than 12 months old, the rate of UTI was 5.3 percent.[1] Previously, it had been thought that the incidence of UTI was higher in infant boys than girls; however, in this sample of 945 febrile children less than 1 year old only 2.5 percent of boys had positive cultures, versus 8.8 percent of girls. Beyond the difference in rates related to gender, there appear to be ethnic differences; 6.6 percent of Caucasian patients had UTI, as opposed to only 3.6 percent of African Americans. The highest-risk group comprises Caucasian females; in this study, the rate of UTI among Caucasian girls with a temperature above 39°C was 16.9 percent.[1] The rate of UTIs in febrile children 12 to 23 months of age declines, particularly among boys.[2]

Over 90 percent of UTIs in febrile infants are caused by *Escherichia coli*. Less common organisms include *Enterococcus*, *Pseudomonas*, *Staphylococcus aureus*, and *Enterobacter cloacae*. Approximately 3 to 5 percent of febrile infants below 12 months of age with UTIs will be bacteremic.

Most febrile infants with UTIs have pyelonephritis; ^{99m}Tc = dimercaptosuccinic acid (DMSA) scanning reveals evidence of renal parenchymal involvement in approximately 75 percent of patients less than 1 year old with positive urine cultures. Even with appropriate antibiotic treatment, 7 to 10 percent of these children will have some degree of renal scarring 6 months after the UTI. Renal scarring, particularly in children less than 3 years of age, is believed to be among the most common causes of hypertension and end-stage renal disease (ESRD) in children and adults. It is difficult to assess the risk of scarring causing hypertension or ESRD. However, in two critical reviews of the literature, estimates of the risk of developing hypertension or ESRD as a result of renal scarring were 10 to 20 percent and 5 percent, respectively.[3,4] The risk of renal scarring is thought to be doubled among children in whom there is a delay in diagnosis or treatment.

Between one-third and one-half of febrile infants with UTIs are found to have anatomic abnormalities of the urinary tract, such as vesicoureteral reflux (VUR), duplication, and obstruction. Untreated, these abnormalities result in a high rate of recurrent UTI and renal scarring. In particular, scarring with low-grade VUR occurs in approximately 13 percent of patients, while over one-half of patients with high-grade VUR develop scarring. This increased risk for scarring is thought to be caused by repeated UTIs; early recognition of VUR and the use of prophylactic antibiotics and/or surgical repair might prevent it. Thus, it is important to accurately diagnose and properly treat febrile infants with UTIs, not only to prevent renal scarring from the initial infection but also to identify those children with urinary tract abnormalities that might otherwise escape detection.

As with most discussions of circumcision, its role in preventing UTIs in boys is controversial. However, multiple studies, critical reviews, and metaanalyses have all reached the same conclusion: UTIs are more common in uncircumcised male infants. Combining evidence from multiple investigations, circumcision reduces the risk of UTI in boys less than 1 year of age by a factor of 4 to 10.[5] Despite this impressive relative risk, since UTIs are very uncommon in circumcised males (0.1 to 0.2 percent), it can be estimated that circumcision prevents 7 to 14 UTIs among the average group of 1000 male babies. To put these figures another way, it is necessary to circumcise 100 to 200 boys to prevent one UTI. Given the occasional complication from the procedure, the reduced risk of UTI is not a significant enough reason by itself to recommend circumcision.

Signs and Symptoms

Beyond the presence of a fever, there are few diagnostic clues that help identify which febrile infants might be at risk for UTIs. Symptoms such as vomiting, diarrhea, irritability, and poor feeding are common in young patients with UTIs; unfortunately, they occur with other infections and with similar frequency in children with negative cultures. A history of malodorous urine or abdominal tenderness on exam may be helpful diagnostic clues; however, these are both uncommon findings.

The height of the fever provides minimal information; infants with temperatures above 39.0°C are somewhat more likely to have UTIs than those with less fever. "Toxic appearing" patients are somewhat more likely to have a positive urine culture than those who are well-appearing despite their fever.

The febrile child less than 1 year old with another source for his or her fever is less likely to have a positive urine culture than a child with no identifiable cause for his or her elevated temperature. Thus, a careful history and physical examination can help to identify those febrile infants who are unlikely to have a UTI. Conversely, *for the child less than 2 years old with unexplained fever, culture of a urine specimen has a higher diagnostic yield than virtually any other laboratory test. This is particularly true for females, uncircumcised males, and those with temperatures above 39.0°C.*

Methods of Urine Collection

Suprapubic aspiration, transuretheral catheterization, and bagged specimens have all been recommended as the "best" way to collect urine in febrile infants being screened for UTI. Suprapubic aspiration can be technically difficult and painful; it also carries a small risk of complications. However, it may be less traumatic for male infants than collection by catheterization. Transuretheral catheterization is usually easily accomplished in young female children using a sterile 5 Fr feeding tube. In experienced hands, the procedure can be completed with only moderate discomfort to the baby. Catheterized collection also has the advantage that the urine can usually be collected in a timely manner.

Bagged urine specimens have typically been discouraged because of the possibility of contamination, leading to a falsely positive urine culture. This is a significant limitation, since infants with UTI are routinely subjected to expensive and uncomfortable radiologic procedures and are frequently admitted to the hospital for intravenous antibiotics. Cultures from bag urine specimens are 100 percent sensitive (meaning that all febrile infants with UTIs will have a positive culture) and have a specificity of approximately 70 percent. Thus, 30 percent of patients without an infection might be incorrectly diagnosed with UTI on the basis of a bag urine culture. Perhaps more importantly, given a 5 percent rate of UTIs among febrile infants, over 80 percent of positive cultures from bag urine specimens would be expected to be falsely positive. Thus, although the use of bag urine collection is a tempting option to parents and clinicians, especially when compared with the other techniques, this rate of false positives, potentially leading to other uncomfortable treatments and tests, is too high to recommend this procedure. Bag specimens that are discarded after a negative urinalysis and prior to culture may be an acceptable alternative in situations where UTI seems unlikely, such as in a circumcised boy. However, a small number of UTIs will be missed with this procedure. For the child whose bag urine specimen is found to have white blood cells and/or bacteria, another urine specimen, collected by transuretheral catherization, should be cultured. Finally, if a bag specimen is cultured and found to be positive, a second positive culture should be obtained prior to making a diagnosis of UTI.

Laboratory Tests

Quantitative bacterial culture is the definitive diagnostic test for UTI, with results from suprapubic aspiration considered the "gold standard." Any number of gram-negative bacilli cultured from a sample of urine collected by suprapubic aspiration is considered indicative of a true infection. Results from urine collected by transuretheral catherization are virtually as accurate as those collected via the suprapubic route. As compared with those from suprapubic aspiration, cultures from catheterized urines have a sensitivity of 95 percent and specificity of 99 percent.

Over 75 percent of febrile infants with UTIs have bacterial counts of greater than 10^5 colony-forming units (CFU) per milliliter of a single pathogen on urine collected by transuretheral catherization; over 90 percent have counts above 50,000 CFU/per milliliter. Thus, any febrile child whose urine specimen, collected by transuretheral catherization, grows more than 50,000 CFU per milliliter of a bacteria known to cause UTI should be treated as having an infection. Cultures with lower colony counts may be problematic. Colony counts of below 10,000 CFU per milliliter (obtained by transurethral catheterization) should be considered as contaminants unless the clinical picture is highly suggestive of a UTI (strongly positive leukocyte esterase or pyuria in a highly toxic child). Colony counts between 10,000 and 50,000 CFU per milliliter may be indicative of a true infection, particularly if the patient has pyuria. Conversely, DMSA scans on children with this degree of bacteriuria in the absence of pyuria are usually negative, suggesting that most of these patients do not have pyelonephritis and are, therefore, not at risk of renal scarring.[6]

The most time-honored method for evaluating urine for white cells and bacteria is through microscopy. The sensitivity of finding leukocytes on microscopy is 70 to 80 percent and has a specificity close to 80 percent. Quantifying the number of white cells per high-power field will alter the sensitivity and specificity of the test. Requiring a higher number of white cells per high-power field for the test to be considered "positive" decreases the number of false positives but increases the number of children with a "negative" urinalysis who actually have a UTI. Some have advocated quantifying the number of white cells per cubic millimeter; in research studies, this procedure has yielded sensitivities and specificities above 90 percent.[7] However, this test is not always available.

Indirect measurement of white cells is possible through the use of dipstick assessment of leukocyte esterase. Testing for white cells in this manner is virtually as accurate as microscopy, as well as having the advantage of being inexpensive and available at the bedside.

Microscopy can also be used to identify bacteria in the urine; finding bacteria has a sensitivity in the 80 to 90 percent range, with comparable specificity. However, experienced eyes are usually needed to differentiate bacteria from crystals and other debris. A more time-consuming but foolproof method is gram-staining a drop of unspun urine. The presence of bacteria in each high-power field indicates significant bacteriuria. As with leukocytes, dipsticks can provide an indirect measure of bacteriuria through the nitrite test. The nitrites present are produced by the reduction of dietary nitrates by gram-negative bacteria in the urine. Most gram-positive bacteria are not capable of reducing nitrates to nitrites. Nitrite is virtually always negative in patients without UTI; unfortunately, the sensitivity of this test is only about 50 percent.

Some experts advocate obtaining cultures only on urine with positive leukocytes and/or bacteria. If the decision to admit a febrile child to the hospital is based solely on the likelihood of UTI or if there is some other compelling reason to immediately make the diagnosis, formal urinalysis may be warranted. However, in the office setting, I find that the simplest strategy is to culture all urine obtained on febrile children via transuretheral catherization or suprapubic aspiration. For those children who have positive leukocyte esterase or nitrite tests, presumptive antibiotic treatment is initiated. For children with negative dipstick tests and in whom antimicrobial therapy is not otherwise indicated, the patient can be closely observed pending the results of the urine culture.

Treatment

Because of the potential of UTIs in febrile infants to lead to renal scarring, experts have recommended that these patients be aggressively treated with parenteral antibiotics. Clearly, there are circumstances when hospitalization and intravenous therapy are warranted. For example, inpatient treatment is definitely indicated when the patient is less than 3 months old, when there are signs or symptoms of urosepsis, when vomiting precludes oral antibiotics, or when noncompliance is likely.

Although there are theoretical advantages associated with parenteral therapy, a large clinical study has found that oral antibiotics may be equally effective.[8] In this multicenter trial, over 300 febrile infants with UTIs were randomized to receive either intravenous cefotaxime for 3 days followed by oral therapy for 11 days with cefixime, or oral cefixime alone for 14 days. There was no difference between groups in times to defervescence or initial clearing of the infection from the urine. Most importantly, DMSA scans 6 months after the episode found that the rate of scarring was similar in those receiving oral therapy alone and those who were initially treated with parenteral antibiotics. In the absence of other data, these results indicate that the majority of febrile infants over 3 months of age with UTI can be managed as outpatients and receive oral antibiotics.

If parenteral therapy is indicated, most children can be managed with a combination of ampicillin and gentamicin. Aminoglycosides should be used with caution in children who have decreased renal function. Data suggest that third-generation cephalosporins such as cefotaxime, ceftriaxone, or ceftazidime are acceptable alternatives to ampicillin and gentamicin. In the vast majority of patients, a response to therapy will be noted within 24 to 48 h. Once the patient has improved, he or she can be switched to an oral antibiotic based on the sensitivity pattern of the bacteria cultured from the urine.

Amoxicillin and trimethoprim-sulfamethoxazole have been the usual oral treatment for UTIs in children. Because of the growing resistance of many strains of *E. coli* to amoxicillin, trimethoprim-sulfamethoxazole would be the better choice in communities where this has been a problem. However, since cefixime alone has been shown to be as efficacious as the combination of parenteral and oral therapy, it should be considered as the initial drug of choice when a febrile infant with UTI is being managed with oral antibiotics. If a child with a UTI who is being treated with oral antibiotics does not become afebrile within 24 to 36 h, a second urine should be collected for testing and culture and the patient should be admitted to the hospital for intravenous therapy.

Regardless of the initial therapy, the choice of the definitive antibiotic should be based on the sensitivity pattern of the organism cultured from the urine. Combining results from several studies has shown that short-term therapy (1 to 3 days) is not as effective in young children as a longer duration of treatment (7 to 14 days).[4] For febrile infants with UTIs, the recommended total duration of treatment is 10 to 14 days.

A protocol for the diagnosis and initial management of the febrile infant with suspected UTI is presented graphically in Fig. 7-1.

Imaging Studies

Because of the frequency of abnormalities and consequences associated with these abnormalities, radiologic evaluation should be performed

Figure 7-1

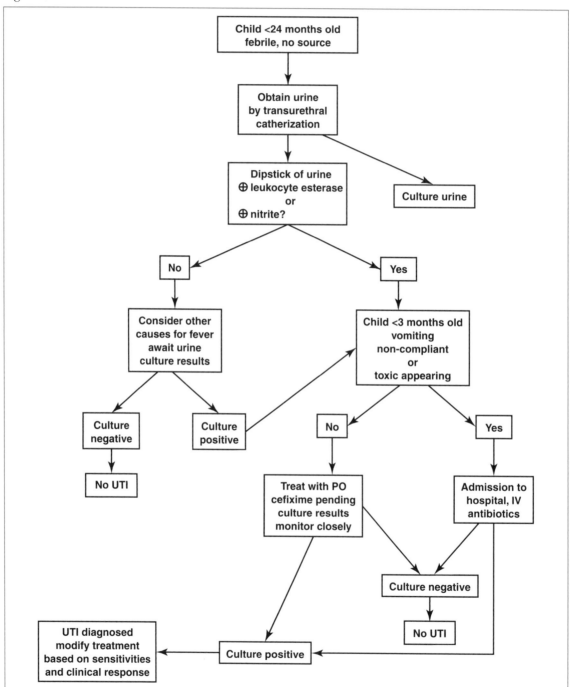

Suggested protocol for initial management of the febrile child below 24 months of age with suspected urinary tract infection.

on all febrile infants with UTIs. The two most commonly performed tests are renal ultrasound to identify children with obstructions and the voiding cystourethrogram (VCUG) to assess for vesicoureteral reflux (VUR). Radionuclide cystography can also be used to diagnose VUR. Although this technique has the advantage of less radiation than the traditional VCUG, less precise information is obtained. Thus although, radionuclide cystography can be used for following the course of VUR in a child, VCUG remains the preferred technique for the initial evaluation.

ULTRASOUND

Renal ultrasound has replaced intravenous pyelography (IVP) as the test of choice to detect obstructive lesions. Ultrasound has the advantages of being pain- and radiation-free. The test can be performed anytime after the diagnosis of UTI is made in a febrile infant. However, the yield is small; in one large study the results of ultrasound failed to alter the management of any of the children. Renal ultrasound is not a good method for determining VUR; less than 50 percent of cases of VUR are detected with this technique. With the advent of sophisticated prenatal ultrasound, it is likely that the vast majority of children with obstructive lesions will be identified in utero and the need for renal ultrasound obviated in many young infants.

VOIDING CYSTOURETHROGRAM

Conversely, despite the discomfort involved, the VCUG remains a powerful tool for identifying reflux in children with pyelonephritis. A VCUG should be obtained all febrile infants with UTI after the initial infection has been adequately treated. Because of the high prevalence of VUR in these patients, it is recommended that children receive prophylactic antibiotics while awaiting their VCUG.

The prevalence of VUR in children with UTI decreases with age; reflux is most common in infants less than 1 year of age. VUR also varies in severity and is graded on a I to V scale, with V being the most severe. Sometimes VUR is classified as low-grade (grade I or II, indicating no dilatation of the collecting system or ureter) or high-grade (grade III to grade V, indicating dilatation). This distinction has diagnostic implications; children with high-grade VUR are four to six times more likely to have renal scarring than those with low-grade VUR and 8 to 10 times more likely to have scarring than those with no VUR. The management of the child with VUR is discussed below.

Urinary Tract Infections in Older Children

The cumulative incidence of UTIs during childhood is approximately 3 to 8 percent in girls and 1 to 2 percent in boys. Almost two-thirds of UTIs among males occur in the first 1 to 2 years of life; conversely, only about 30 percent of infections in females occur during infancy. Thus, among older children, the vast majority of UTIs are in girls. In addition to the increasing predominance of females, the type of infection changes during later childhood. Unlike infants, who presumably usually develop pyelonephritis, cystitis predominates in older girls with UTIs.[9] Since cystitis rarely results in significant long-term morbidity and diagnosis in older children is easier, the management of UTIs in patients over the age of 2 years is usually much simpler than in infants.

Signs and Symptoms

Classically, clinical signs have been used to differentiate pyelonephritis from cystitis in older children with UTIs. The typical child with cystitis is a potty-trained girl who presents with dysuria, frequency, urgency and new-onset enuresis. These patients do not generally have systemic signs such as fever and do not have flank or back pain. Recurrences are common; approximately 30 percent of girls with one diagnosed UTI will have another symptomic infection. Fever and flank pain and/or abdominal tenderness in addition to dysuria and frequency are considered to be indicative of pyelonephritis. Children with pyelonephritis also frequently have leukocytosis and elevated erythrocyte sedimentation rates or C-reactive protein. Since pyelonephritis has been thought to be a more significant illness in terms of morbidity, many experts have stressed the importance of differentiating it from simple cystitis. Unfortunately, compared to the gold standard of DMSA scans, only about 50 percent of children with UTIs and systemic signs have evidence of involvement of the renal parenchyma.

Dysfunctional voiding—characterized by infrequent voiding, unihibited bladder contractions, bladder overdistention, and inadequate emptying of the bladder—is a significant risk factor for UTIs in potty-trained children. The majority of children with dysfunctional voiding are girls. In one series, 60 percent of children with the condition had at least one UTI, and VUR was present in 20 percent.[10] Chronic constipation with encopresis is also a risk factor for UTIs; up to one-third of girls with encopresis also have symptomatic infections.[11] There is no evidence that improper wiping techniques or bubble baths predispose a girl to UTIs.

Laboratory Tests

For potty-trained children, a clean-catch urine is usually sufficient for diagnosing UTIs; the minimal increase in precision of diagnosis associated with urine collected by transuretheral catherization does not justify the discomfort associated with the procedure in these patients. Because of the increased potential for contamination associated with clean-catch urines, colony counts above 50,000 to 100,000 CFU per milliliter are typically required to define a UTI. As with febrile infants, the vast majority of UTIs in older children are caused by *E. coli.*

The diagnostic utility of urine testing in potty-trained patients is similar to that among febrile infants. For the afebrile child with symptoms consistent with cystitis, dipstick evaluation for leukocyte esterase and nitrite is usually sufficient. The urine from patients with positive leukocyte esterase and/or nitrite should be cultured and the child started presumptively on antibiotics. For those older children with negative leukocyte esterase and nitrite on dipstick, the decision to culture the urine should be based on the rest of the clinical picture. For those with evidence of pyelonephritis, urine culture is indicated even if urine testing is negative because of the chance of a false-negative test.

Treatment

For uncomplicated cystitis sulfonamides, trimethoprim-sulfamethoxazole, nitrofurantoin, or cephalosporins are all reasonable first-line drugs. Because of increasingly resistant strains of *E. coli,* amoxicillin is less effective. The duration of treatment is controversial. Although several trials have shown short-course or single-dose therapy to be effective in adult women, analyses of data in children have suggested that lengths of treatment less than 3 days were not as effficacious as 7 to 10 days.[12] However, other investigators have reported that short (1- to 3-day) courses of trimethoprim-sulfamethoxazole result in cure rates of over 90 percent in children with cystitis.[13] On the basis of these data, "relatively" short, meaning 3- to 5-day, courses of treatment have been advocated. Regardless of the length of therapy, a follow-up culture is recommended after completion of the antibiotic course. Phenazopyridine (pyridium) may be helpful in alleviating the symptoms of bladder irritability. It should be given for no longer than 2 days at the dose of 4 mg/kg three times a day.

Older children with clinical evidence of pyelonephritis who are toxic-appearing or who have significant vomiting require hospitalization for intravenous antibiotics. Alternatively, in some children, it may be possible to avoid hospitalization through the use of long-acting third-generation cephalosporins, such as ceftriaxone. This medication can be administered intravenously or intramsucularly daily, pending a good clinical response and culture and sensitivity results. At this point, the child can be switched to an appropriate oral agent and complete a total of 10- to 14-day course of therapy. Many children with symptoms consistent with pyelonephritis may be managed entirely with oral antibiotics. Cephalosporins or trimethoprim-sulfamethoxazole are reasonable first-line therapies. Nitrofurantoin should not be used if pyelonephritis is suspected because high levels of the drug are not achieved in the renal parenchyma. Children being treated for pyelonephritis as outpatients should be followed closely; a follow-up urine culture 1 to 2 days after beginning therapy is useful in documenting an adequate response to treatment. Hospitalization is warranted for those patients in whom this repeat culture remains positive or when a rapid improvement in systemic symptoms is not noted.

Imaging Studies

It has been recommended by some that virtually all children with UTIs have a VCUG to detect VUR. The rationale for this recommendation is logical. VUR is common in children with UTIs but quite uncommon among those with no infections. VUR is particularly prevalent in the younger age group. In addition, there is some evidence, including animal data and longitudinal studies of selected patients, that VUR leads to recurrent infections. The corollary is also felt to be true: that in certain children cystitis can result in VUR. Recurrent UTIs in patients with VUR may be more likely to result in pyelonephritis and renal scarring than in those without VUR. There are data to suggest that antimicrobial prophylaxis in children with VUR may reduce infections and, theoretically at least, renal scarring. Thus, the aggressive approach of imaging all children with their first UTI to identify those with VUR who might benefit from early treatment may be warranted.

Unfortunately, the studies on which these recommendations are based have mixed results and methodologic flaws that limit their applicability. Two recent reviews have both concluded that current recommendations to identify and treat VUR in children with UTI to prevent renal scarring are based on inconclusive research.[14,15] Weaknesses in study design that were cited included small sample size, inclusion of specialized populations such as hospitalized patients or those referred for imaging, inclusion of children with more than one UTI, and inclusion of renal scarring that predated the index UTI.

Given the paucity of definitive data, it is difficult to make firm recommendations about which children with UTI should have a VCUG to detect VUR. The information presented here should be interpreted as broad guidelines based on the available evidence and pragmatic concerns. Ultimately, the decision on whether to obtain a VCUG is dependent on the parent's and clinician's aversion to risk versus their collective desire to avoid exposing the child to an uncomfortable and expensive radiologic procedure. My approach is outlined below.

For children less than 3 years old, I order a renal ultrasound and VCUG after their first documented UTI. These young patients have the highest probability of pyelonephritis, the highest rate of VUR, and most likely the highest rate of renal scarring associated with VUR. It is also difficult to follow these children clinically; obtaining urine cultures is problematic and differentiating UTIs from other illnesses in these patients can be quite hard. Imaging studies are also indicated in all males who have UTIs regardless of age.

As children grow older, the incidence of renal scarring as a result of UTIs probably declines. In one study, the rate of renal scarring after a UTI in patients who were 3 years old was 2.9 percent; for those who were 4 years old, no renal scars were noted during follow-up.[16] Given these data, the necessity of obtaining imaging studies in girls who are 3 to 5 years old at the time of their first UTI is debatable.

The prevalence of VUR drops precipitously in children over 5 years of age. Among asymptomatic children over 72 months old whose siblings have documented reflux, a group at high risk, the rate of VUR was 7 percent.[17] Thus, the risk of renal scarring in girls over 5 years old with their first UTI is minimal. Routine imaging is probably not necessary in such patients with uncomplicated cystitis. Most experts recommend VCUGs and renal imaging in older children with pyelonephritis, although there is little hard evidence on which to base this recommendation.

A few final caveats are needed. First, the designation of "first" UTI is somewhat misleading, since many infections in infants go undiagnosed. In assessing the risk of VUR and scarring in older children, a careful history may uncover the possibility of previous UTIs that were not detected. In such patients, a more aggressive approach to imaging is warranted. There is also anecdotal evidence suggesting that the rate of renal scarring is declining in children. This gratifying result may be due in part to early diagnosis and treatment of infections and VUR. Finally, it is likely that close clinical follow-up in children with UTIs is as important as the determination of VUR. The occurrence of new renal scars among children with VUR is frequently related to delayed diagnosis and treatment of new symptomatic infections. Conversely, prompt

recognition of a UTI may help minimize the risk of further damage to the kidneys.

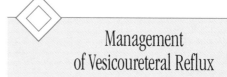

Management of Vesicoureteral Reflux

Although there continues to be controversy over its clinical significance, the goal of treatment of VUR, once identified, is more straightforward. The objective of therapy for VUR is to maintain a sterile urinary tract and, more specifically, avoid recurrent pyelonephritis where additional renal scarring is the most likely. Two modes of treatment are possible; antibiotic prophylaxis or surgical repair to prevent reflux.

Antibiotic prophylaxis has been shown to prevent recurrent UTIs in children with VUR. Nitrofurantoin or trimethoprim-sulfamethoxazole are appropriate agents to use for prophylaxis, and are administered on a once-a-day basis. Children on prophylactic antibiotics for VUR should have their urine frequently tested and cultured; symptomatic infections should be promptly treated. Breakthrough infections occur in approximately one-third of patients.

Surgical repair is effective in preventing VUR. Although the overall rate of UTIs is similar in medically and surgically treated children, there are some data to suggest that surgical repair reduces the incidence of pyelonephritis more effectively than antibiotic prophylaxis.[18] Surgical repair of VUR may be indicated in children above 6 years of age with bilateral grade IV reflux and those above 1 year of age with grade V reflux. For children with high-grade VUR who have repeated infections despite antibiotic prophylaxis or for those in whom grade III to IV reflux persists for several years, surgery is a reasonable alternative. Unfortunately, regardless of therapy, new renal scars occur in 15 to 35 percent of patients, with no difference in the efficacy of medical or surgical treatment.

The rate of resolution of VUR depends on the age of the child, severity of the reflux, and whether involvement is unilateral or bilateral. For children with grades I to II reflux, as many as 80 percent will have resolution within 5 years. Conversely, less than half of patients with unilateral grade IV reflux will resolve spontaneously. Those with bilateral grade IV reflux have an even lower rate of resolution. Similarly, older children with VUR are less likely to have resolution than those less than 5 years old. It is recommended that children with VUR have periodic imaging studies to ascertain if the reflux has resolved. Radionuclide cystography is usually adequate for follow-up studies.

References

1. Hoberman A, Chao H, Keller DM, et al: Prevalence of urinary tract infection in febrile infants. *J Pediatr* 123:17–23, 1993.
2. Shaw KN, Gorelick M, McGowan KL, et al: Prevalence of urinary tract infection in febrile young children in the emergency department. *Pediatrics* 102;e16, 1998.
3. Kramer MS, Tange SM, Drummond KN, Mills EL: Urine testing in young febrile children: a risk-benefit analysis. *J Pediatr* 125:6–13, 1994.
4. Downs SD: Technical report: urinary tract infections in febrile infants and young children. *Pediatrics* 103:e54, 1999.
5. American Academy of Pediatrics Task Force on Circumcision: Circumcision policy statement. *Pediatrics* 103:686–693, 1999.
6. Hoeberman A, Wald ER: Urinary tract infections in young febrile children. *Pediatr Infect Dis J* 16:11—17, 1997.
7. Hoberman A, Wald ER, Reynolds EA, et al: Pyuria and bacteriuria in urine specimens obtained by catheter from young children with fever. *J Pediatr* 124:513–519, 1994.
8. Hoborman A, Wald ER, Hickey RW, et al: Oral versus initial intravenous therapy for urinary tract infections in young febrile children. *Pediatrics* 104:79–86, 1999.
9. Rushton HG: Urinary tract infections in children: epidemiology, evaluation, and management. *Pediatr Clin North Am* 44:1133–1169, 1997.
10. Schulman SL, Quinn CK, Plachter N, Kodman-Jones C: Comprehensive management of dysfunctional voiding. *Pediatrics* 103:e31, 1999.
11. Loening-Baucke V: Urinary incontinence and urinary tract infection and their resolution with treatment of chronic constipation of childhood. *Pediatrics* 100:228–232, 1997.
12. Moffat M, Embree J, Grimm P, et al: Short-course antibiotic therapy for urinary tract infections in children. *Am J Dis Child* 142:57–61, 1988.
13. Petersen KE: Short-term treatment of acute urinary tract infections in girls. *Scand J Infect Dis* 23:213, 1991.
14. Garin EH, Campos A, Homsy Y: Primary vesicoureteral reflux: review of current concepts. *Pediatr Nephrol* 12:249–256, 1998.
15. Dick PT, Feldman W: Routine diagnostic imaging for childhood urinary tract infections: a systematic overview. *J Pediatr* 128:15–22, 1996.
16. Vernon SJ, Coulthard MG, Lambert HJ, et al: New renal scarring in children who at age 3 and 4 years had had normal scans with dimercaptosuccinic acid: follow-up study. *BMJ* 315:905–908, 1997.
17. Connolly LP, Treves ST, Connolly SA, et al: Vesicoureteral reflux in children: incidence and severity in siblings. *J Urol* 157:2287–2290, 1997.
18. Weiss R, Duckett J, Spitzer A: Results of a randomized clinical trial of medical versus surgical management of infants and children with grades III and IV primary vesicoureteral reflux (United States): the International Reflux Study in Children. *J Urol* 148:1667–1673, 1992.

Camille Haisley-Royster
Neil S. Prose

Skin Problems

Cutaneous diseases are commonly seen in primary care pediatrics, accounting for approximately 20 to 30 percent of pediatric visits to primary care physicians.[1] This chapter provides a practical approach to some of the most common pediatric skin problems.

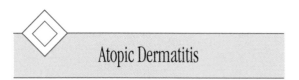

Atopic Dermatitis

Atopic dermatitis, or eczema, is the most common eczematous skin condition of childhood, with a prevalence of 10 to 15 percent. It is a chronic, fluctuating skin disease that is most common in infants and children and tends to improve with age.

Pathogenesis

The atopic phenotype is produced by the effect of environmental factors on a genetically susceptible individual. These children may have hay fever or asthma and often have a family history of these conditions. A number of environmental factors have also been implicated in the development of atopic dermatitis. These include house dust mites, dietary exposures, stress, and bacterial colonization.[2]

Clinical Description

The primary symptom of atopic dermatitis is intense pruritus. The rash is composed of scaling, crusted, erythematous patches and plaques affecting the face, neck and trunk. In infants, the lesions often present on the face. The elbows, knees and trunk are often involved, but sparing of the diaper area is characteristic and helps to distinguish this entity from psoriasis and seborrheic dermatitis. In childhood, the rash is frequently localized to the antecubital and popliteal fossae, neck, wrists and ankles. With chronicity, skin lesions may evolve into lichenified plaques characterized by thickening of the skin with increased skin markings and hyperpigmentation. African-American children may present with tiny follicle-based papules (Fig. 8-1, see Color Plate 9).

Associated clinical findings that are consistent with a diagnosis of atopic dermatitis include hyperlinear palms, periorificial pallor, xerosis/icthyosis, and keratosis pilaris.

Treatment

Treatment of atopic dermatitis consists of a regimen for dry skin care and the use of topical steroids and antihistamines (Table 8-1). Bath frequency is a controversial subject, but we usually recommend that patients bathe once daily with a mild soap.

EMOLLIENTS

An emollient should be applied after all baths and frequently throughout the day to avoid drying of the skin. Effective moisturizers include petrolatum, Aquaphor ointment, Eucerin cream and Theraplex emollient. Ointment formulations provide more moisture but are less esthetically pleasing than lotions or creams.

TOPICAL STEROIDS

In infants, mild topical corticosteroids such as hydrocortisone 1 or 2.5 percent ointment should be applied twice daily. As the condition improves, the use of the topical steroid may be reduced.

In older children, hydrocortisone ointment or another mild topical corticosteroid may be used, especially on the face. Patients with more severe disease may require short courses of a more potent agent, such as mometasone fuoroate (Elocon). However, these more potent formulations should not be used on the face. As the dermatitis improves, application of the topical

Table 8-1

Patient Information Sheet—Atopic Dermatitis

What is atopic dermatitis?
Atopic dermatitis or eczema is a common skin condition affecting primarily infants and children. It is manifest by an itchy skin rash that most frequently affects the face, neck, elbows, and behind the knees. However, it may also affect other areas of the skin.

What causes eczema?
Most affected children have a family history of eczema, hay fever, or asthma. Some environmental exposures, including dust mites and certain foods, may also contribute to the development of eczema.

How should I care for my skin while being treated for eczema?
• Baths should be taken once daily in lukewarm water with a mild soap (Unscented Dove, Tone, Basis).
• Baths should be followed by the immediate application of a moisturizer (Vaseline Petroleum Jelly, Eucerin, Aquaphor) to the skin. Moisturizer may be applied several times per day.
• Use prescription topical and oral medications as directed by your physician.

Will I always have eczema?
Eczema is a chronic skin care condition that can be controlled with a good skin care regimen and topical/oral prescription medications. Eczema improves with age and resolves entirely in the majority of patients.

steroid should be decreased and the use of an emollient continued. Topical corticosteroid side effects are rare, but patients should be monitored for development of striae, telangiectasias, or hypopigmentation of the skin.

ANTIHISTAMINES

Sedative antihistamines are particularly effective at suppressing the pruritus associated with atopic dermatitis. Because of the associated sedation, they should preferentially be given at bedtime. Choices include diphenhydramine, hydroxyzine, and cyproheptadine. Nonsedating antihistamines are not helpful in the control of pruritus in atopic dermatitis.

ANTIBIOTICS

Up to 90 percent of children with atopic dermatitis are colonized with *Staphylococcus*

aureus.[3] Exacerbations of atopic dermatitis, even with no signs of active infection, will often improve if the patient is treated with an antistaphylococcal agent, such as amoxicillin/clavulanate (Augmentin) or a first-generation cephalosporin. Superinfection of atopic dermatitis with methicillin-resistant *S. aureus* (MRSA) is an emerging problem.

Diaper Dermatitis

Diaper dermatitis denotes an erythematous, scaly eruption in the diaper area that may be due to several different etiologies.[4] The most common cause is an irritant contact dermatitis. Other causes include seborrheic dermatitis, cutaneous candidiasis, and psoriasis.

Pathogenesis

Irritant contact dermatitis results from the excessive heat and moisture in the diaper area combined with the effect of fecal and urinary enzymes on the skin. In this environment, the skin is often secondarily infected by *Candida albicans*.

Clinical Description

Irritant contact dermatitis usually affects the convex surfaces of the buttocks, lower abdomen, and upper thighs, sparing the creases. It is characterized by erythematous, mildly scaly, shiny patches.

Candidiasis is manifest by beefy red papules and plaques with satellite papules and pustules. Seborrheic dermatitis is characterized by well-circumscribed salmon-colored plaques with yellowish scale. In addition, involvement of the scalp, face, and flexural areas is often present. Psoriasis presents with well-defined scaly plaques that may involve the folds and is often resistant to treatment.

Patients with systemic signs such as failure to thrive, fevers, or lymphadenopathy should be evaluated for more serious conditions, such as immunodeficiency, histiocytosis X, or acrodermatitis enteropathica.

Treatment

Treatment of irritant contact dermatitis is aimed at decreasing the occlusion and moisture in the diaper area. This requires regular washing with a mild soap and water and frequent diaper changes. Mild topical steroids such as hydrocortisone 1% will decrease inflammation and aid in healing. Barrier ointments containing zinc oxide may also be helpful. In addition to the steroid cream, patients with a long-standing rash or with signs of candidal infection should be treated with a topical antifungal agent such as clotrimazole or spectazole.

Seborrheic Dermatitis

Seborrheic dermatitis is a common scaling dermatosis of infancy; it appears most frequently between the second and eighth week of life.[5] The etiology of this disorder is unclear but is thought to be multifactorial. The yeast *Pityrosporum ovale* may play a causative role.

Clinical Description

The eruption commonly begins on the scalp with thick yellow plaques with underlying erythema ("cradle cap"). The lesions may extend onto the centrofacial skin, neck, and behind the ears. The diaper area and flexures of the extremities are also often affected. Unlike atopic dermatitis, the lesions are usually not pruritic.

Psoriasis is less common in infants but may have similar presentation. As in diaper dermatitis, the presence of failure to thrive or lymphadenopathy may indicate underlying immunodeficiency, histiocytosis X, or acrodermatitis enteropathica.

Treatment

The treatment of seborrheic dermatitis should be based on the severity and extent of the eruption. Mild cases of cradle cap may be treated with frequent washing with a mild baby shampoo. More severe involvement may require antiseborrheic shampoos containing selenium sulfide or tar. A mild topical steroid such as hydrocortisone 1% may be applied sparingly to the scalp and skin as needed.

Hemangiomas

Hemangiomas are benign proliferative tumors of the endothelium that usually present within the first 4 weeks of life. Indications of the impending lesion such as macular erythema or telangiectasia may be present at birth.

Clinical Description

Hemangiomas may be superficial, deep, or mixed tumors. The superficial lesions are characteristically red, raised, well-demarcated papules or plaques (Fig. 8-2, see Color Plate 10). They are usually compressible and may partially blanch with pressure. The lesions are most often solitary and frequently present on the head and neck. Deep hemangiomas are soft, bluish nodules with overlying normal skin. Mixed hemangiomas present with both a superficial and deep component.

The lesion usually develops in the first month of life and undergoes a period of growth for the first 6 to 8 months. Thereafter, an interval of stability in size develops, which lasts from 6 months to 1 year. Subsequently, the hemangioma enters a period of involution. In 50 percent of cases, the hemangioma resolves by age 5, and 90 percent resolve by age 9. Most lesions resolve completely with minimal sequelae.

Treatment

The vast majority of hemangiomas resolve spontaneously without any complications and require no treatment. These patients may be followed using serial photographs to document resolution of the hemangioma.

Hemangiomas that may deserve further evaluation include periorbital lesions, lesions overlying the lumbosacral spine, large cervicofacial hemangiomas, multiple hemangiomas, and ulcerated hemangiomas.[6]

Periorbital lesions require referral to an ophthalmologist and close follow-up to assure that the lesion is not affecting vision. Such patients may require treatment with systemic corticosteroids or interferon-alpha to preserve vision. Radiologic evaluation with magnetic resonance imaging (MRI) or computed tomography (CT) may also be necessary to evaluate for orbital extension.

Hemangiomas overlying the lumbosacral spine may be associated with the tethered cord syndrome or other manifestations of spinal dysraphism. Tethered cord syndrome is initially asymptomatic. However, once symptoms develop, they are often irreversible. Evaluation of the lumbosacral spine by MRI is recommended.

Large cervicofacial hemangiomas may also be associated with underlying abnormalities, including subglottic hemangiomas and posterior fossa malformations. Subglottic hemangiomas often present with inspiratory stridor. These patients may require tracheostomy and treatment with corticosteroids. In addition, any large, rapidly growing hemangioma may be associated with high-output heart failure.[7]

Children who present with multiple small, monomorphous, cutaneous hemangiomas are at risk for visceral hemangiomas. The most frequently affected organs are the liver, larynx and gastrointestinal (GI) tract. Patients may develop GI bleeding, respiratory distress, enlargement of the liver, or cardiac failure. Radiologic evaluation with ultrasound or CT may be necessary, as well as treatment with corticosteroids or interferon-alpha.

Ulcerated hemangiomas most often occur in the diaper area and are painful. Patients with ulcerated lesions should be referred for treatment with the flash-lamp pulse-dye laser, as this results in improved healing.

After resolution, patients may have some remaining skin changes, including atrophy and excess sagging skin. This may be improved by plastic surgery. Hemangiomas on the lips and nose, in particular, may not resolve completely and may require further treatment to improve appearance.

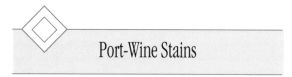

Port-Wine Stains

A port-wine stain is a congenital vascular malformation that is usually present at birth. Unlike hemangiomas, these lesions are usually persistent and grow in proportion with the child. The incidence of port-wine stains is approximately 0.5 percent of newborns.

Clinical Description

Port-wine stains are present at birth or develop soon thereafter. As the name suggests, the color is typically reddish purple and the lesion is macular (Fig. 8-3, see Color Plate 11). As the child ages, the surface may become more nodular and the color may deepen to a purplish hue. The most common location is on the face, but the stains may occur in other sites. Lesions in the V_1 distribution of the facial nerve may be associated with intracranial vascular malformations (Sturge-Weber syndrome). These patients often present with seizures during the first year of life and should be evaluated with MRI or CT to detect the characteristic "railroad track" calcifications that develop within the intracranial lesions. The calcifications often appear after the first year of life. Patients with facial port-wine stains in the V_2 distribution of the facial nerve are at risk of developing glaucoma and should have regular ophthalmologic evaluation. In addition, port-wine stains on the limbs may be associated with hypertrophy of the affected limb (Klippel-Trenaunay syndrome). Cobb syndrome

is a rare association of a lumbosacral port-wine stain with an underlying angioma of the spinal cord.

Treatment

Port-wine stains are usually persistent. Patients may be treated with the 585-nm pulsed tunable dye laser, which has a low risk of scarring.[8] Patients may also use makeup foundations such as Covermark or Dermablend to camouflage the lesion.

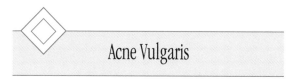

Acne Vulgaris

Acne vulgaris is one of the most prevalent skin conditions affecting children. It is most common during adolescence and is estimated to affect between 75 and 85 percent of teenagers, being slightly more prevalent in boys. Acne has a tendency to decrease in severity with age. However, many people continue to have problems with acne into adulthood.

Pathogenesis

Several factors are important in the development of acne. These include increased sebum production, abnormal keratinization of the pilosebaceous duct, and colonization of the skin by *Propionibacterium acnes.*[9] Sebum production increases during puberty because of the maturation of the sebaceous gland under the influence of androgenic hormones. Abnormal keratinization of the ductal epithelium results in obstruction of the canal with retention of sebum and proliferation of *P. acnes.* This bacteria are chemotactic for inflammatory cells and also lyse sebum to produce proinflammatory free fatty acids. The different treatments for acne are directed at correcting these pathogenic factors.

Clinical Description

Acne typically affects the face, back and chest, the areas of the skin with the highest concentration of sebaceous glands. Lesions may consist of open comedones (whiteheads), closed comedones (blackheads), pustules, and nodules (Fig. 8-4, see Color Plate 12). Postinflammatory erythema or hypo/hyperpigmentation usually resolves over several months. However, areas of depression in the skin ("ice-pick" scarring) may be permanent.

Treatment

The choice of treatment depends on the severity of the lesions. Topical therapy alone can be used in patients with mild to moderate acne. The choice of topical medication depends partly on the predominant acne lesion present. Topical medications should be applied to the lesions and the surrounding normal skin (Table 8-2).

TOPICAL RETINOIDS

The retinoid tretinoin and adapalene exert a comedolytic effect on the pilosebaceous unit, resulting in decreased formation of comedones. These agents may be used alone in patients with mild acne characterized by multiple open comedones. They may also be used in combination with topical or oral antibiotics in patients with inflammatory papules and pustules. Tretinoin is available as an 0.025, 0.05, and 0.1% agent in either a cream, gel, or microsphere (Retin-A micro) formulation. Adapalene is available as a water-based gel in a 0.1% concentration.

The primary side effect of these medications is the production of mild erythema and scaling

Table 8-2

Patient Information Sheet—Acne Vulgaris

What is acne?
Acne is a common skin condition affecting most teenagers. Patients typically develop "blackheads," pustules (pimples), and cysts on the face, chest, and back.

What causes acne?
Acne is caused by the effect of normal hormones, present at the time of puberty, on the oil glands in the skin. There is no good evidence that it is caused by any particular foods. However, it is important to eat a well-balanced diet. It is not caused by dirt on the skin.

How should you care for your skin while being treated for acne?
- Wash your skin gently with a mild, nonirritating soap (Dove, Purpose) once or twice daily.
- Use the prescription topical and oral medications as directed by your physician.
- Some acne medications increase your skin's sensitivity to the sun. Therefore, it is important to avoid excessive sun exposure and to use a sunscreen with a sum protection factor (SPF) of 15.
- Most medications take from 6 to 8 weeks to produce a positive effect. Some medications may also initially worsen your acne. Therefore continue to use the medications and do not become discouraged.

Will I always have acne?
In the majority of patients, acne tends to improve with age and frequently resolves after a few years. However, some patients may continue to have problems into adulthood and may require ongoing treatment.

of the skin. This may be minimized by starting with the lowest concentration of tretinoin (0.025%) and, initially, having the patient apply the medication every other day. The cream formulation is also less irritating than the gel. Adapalene has been found to pose a lower risk of irritation than tretinoin and is as effective as the 0.05% concentration of tretinoin.[10] These topical preparations may result in increased photosensitivity and patients should be advised to use sunscreens and avoid excessive sun exposure. To help decrease the risk of irritation, patients should wait at least 30 min after washing before applying the agent, preferably at bedtime.

AZALEIC ACID

Azaleic acid is a dicarboxylic acid produced by the yeast *P. ovale*. It has a comedolytic effect, similar in efficacy to that provided by the topical retinoids. In addition, it has been found to exert potent antimicrobial activity against *P. acnes* comparable to the effect of benzoyl peroxide.[11] It may be used alone in patients with mild acne with primarily open comedones or in combination with oral or topical antibiotics in patients with inflammatory papules or pustules.

Azaleic acid is formulated as a 20% cream and is applied twice daily if tolerated. The primary side effects are mild erythema and tingling after application. There is no increased photosensitivity.

BENZOYL PEROXIDE

Benzoyl peroxide and the other topical antibiotics are indicated for use in patients with inflammatory acne that includes closed comedones, pustules, and nodules. This medication is most often used in combination with a comedolytic such as a topical retinoid or azaleic acid.

Benzoyl peroxide is a highly effective antimicrobial agent producing a marked reduction in the colonization of the skin by *P. acnes*. It has

been found, in a number of clinical studies, to be as effective as topical erythromycin and clindamycin.[12] Benzoyl peroxide also exerts a mild comedolytic effect.

Benzoyl peroxide is available in several concentrations ranging from 2.5 to 10% and in a number of formulations including solutions, creams, and gels. It is potentially irritating and may produce erythema and scaling. Patients should be started at lower concentrations and the frequency of application and concentration increased as tolerated. If benzoyl peroxide comes in contact with clothing, it may produce permanent bleaching.

TOPICAL ANTIBIOTICS

The most commonly used topical antibiotics are erythromycin and clindamycin. A combination of benzoyl peroxide and erythromycin (Benzamycin) is also highly effective. These medications decrease surface colonization with *P. acnes*, decrease neutrophil chemotaxis, inhibit lipase activity of *P. acnes*, and are useful in inflammatory acne.

Topical antibiotics are available in a number of formulations including solutions, lotions, gels, and creams. Side effects are usually limited to irritation characterized by dryness, scaling, or erythema. Very rarely, topical clindamycin has been reported to cause pseudomembranous colitis.[13]

ORAL ANTIBIOTICS

Oral antibiotics are commonly used for patients who do not respond to topical medications or who have moderate to severe inflammatory acne. Oral antibiotics decrease *P. acnes*, reduce neutrophil chemotaxis and inhibit bacterial lipase. The most frequently used medications are erythromycin and the tetracyclines. Clindamycin and sulfamethoxazole-trimethoprim are used less frequently because of the increased risk of serious side effects.

The tetracyclines include tetracycline, doxycycline, and minocycline. Tetracycline is prescribed at a dose between 250 and 1000 mg/day; however, it should not be used in children less than 9 years of age because it may permanently stain developing teeth. The most common side effects are nausea, vomiting, and diarrhea. Doxycycline and minocycline are used at doses of 50 to 100 mg/day. Minocycline may result in vertigo and may cause bluish-gray hyperpigmentation at sites of prior inflammation or discoloration of the permanent teeth. It is also rarely associated with severe hepatitis and arthritis. All of the tetracyclines may cause increased photosensitivity, but this side effect is most significant with doxycyline.

Erythromycin is prescribed at a dose of 250 to 1000 mg/day. The primary side effects include nausea, vomiting, abdominal pain, and diarrhea.

Isotretinoin (Accutane)

Isotretinoin is a systemic retinoid that is very effective in the treatment of severe nodulocystic acne. It is used in patients with acne resistant to other modes of treatment and in patients who are at significant risk of scarring. Isotretinoin exerts its primary effect on the sebaceous gland by decreasing sebum production.[14] The recommended dosage range is 0.5 to 1 mg/kg/day for 4 to 5 months. The more common side effects are cheilitis, dry skin, conjunctivitis, epistaxis, and arthralgias/myalgias. More serious side effects include hypertriglyceridemia, depression, and increased liver enzymes. This medication is contraindicated in pregnancy because of its teratogenicity. All female patients of childbearing age are required to use reliable contraception from 1 month before initiating the medication to 1 month after completing isotretinoin. Liver enzymes, lipid levels and β-HCG should be monitored regularly during treatment.

Surgery

Permanent scarring may remain after treatment of acne. Laser resurfacing or dermabrasion may be useful in decreasing the scarring.

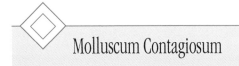

Molluscum Contagiosum

Molluscum contagiosum is a viral infection of the epidermis that occurs most commonly in children and adolescents. The etiologic agent is a DNA virus of the Poxviridae family, the molluscum contagiosum virus.

Clinical Description

Molluscum contagiosum is characterized by the development of erythematous, pearly, umbilicated papules on the face, trunk, or extremities (Fig. 8-5, see Color Plate 13). Ten percent of patients may have an associated patchy dermatitis affecting the surrounding skin. Infection occurs by contact with an affected person and transmission has been reported during contact sports, such as wrestling. Diagnosis is usually based on the characteristic clinical appearance. However, atypical presentations may require biopsy, which demonstrates the characteristic intracytoplasmic inclusion bodies.

Treatment

Molluscum contagiosum often resolves without treatment; the duration of the lesions varies from 2 to 18 months.[15] If treatment is desired, options include gentle curettage, brief application of liquid nitrogen, or application of topical cantharidin. The topical anesthetic lidocaine (EMLA) may be applied under occlusion 1 to

2 h prior to treatment to decrease the discomfort that may be associated with curettage or liquid nitrogen application.[16]

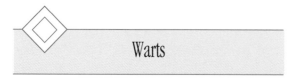

Warts

Verrucae are caused by infection of the skin with the human papillomavirus (HPV). They may be inoculated by trauma and may be transferred from one skin site to another.

Clinical Description

Various subtypes of human papillomavirus cause different clinical types of verrucae.[17] The common wart (verruca vulgaris), which occurs most frequently on the hands, is typically a rough, hyperkeratotic, yellowish to brownish papule (Fig. 8-6, see Color Plate 14).

Verruca plana are usually small, flat topped, flesh-colored, slightly hyperkeratotic papules that occur on the arms, legs, and face and may present a linear distribution.

Plantar warts often occur on pressure points on the foot and may be painful. These lesions are hyperkeratotic and, on paring, often reveal small black dots representing thrombosed capillaries.

Treatment

The majority of warts in children will regress spontaneously within 2 years. Therefore, if it is decided to treat the warts, therapy should be chosen to minimize pain and scarring.

TOPICAL MEDICATIONS

Salicylic acid is a keratolytic agent that is typically used to treat plantar warts and common

warts on the hands. It is available in concentrations ranging from 10 to 50% and in a number of different formulations including solution, plaster, and gel. The medication is applied to the wart daily with attention to avoiding normal skin, where it may cause irritation.

Tretinoin cream (Retin-A, Avita) may be used to treat verruca plana.[18] It is thought to produce an irritant effect, resulting in the immune system's recognition of the wart and its subsequent regression.

CRYOTHERAPY

Cryotherapy may be used as a first-line treatment or, if topical medications fail, to result in resolution of the wart. The most frequently used agent is liquid nitrogen ($-196°C$). This method of treatment may produce pain and there may be secondary swelling, erythema, or blistering. Periungual warts should be treated with caution to avoid damage to the nail matrix, with resultant nail deformity. Liquid nitrogen may be applied with a cotton applicator, which is less threatening to children than a metal cryosurgery container. It should be applied for 5 to 10 s to produce a ring of frosting of 1 to 2 mm around the wart. Liquid nitrogen is more effective if the application is repeated, allowing for two freeze-thaw cycles. Application may be repeated at 3- to 4-week intervals until the wart resolves.

ALTERNATIVE TREATMENTS

If the warts do not regress with the treatments discussed above, consideration may be given to treatment with the pulse-dye laser. Although initial case series had suggested that cimetidine might be effective in prompting regression of warts, recent clinical trials have found cimetidine to be no more effective than placebo.[19]

Tinea Capitis

Tinea capitis is a fungal infection of the scalp caused by dermatophytes of the genera *Microsporum* and *Trichophyton*. It primarily affects school-aged children. In the past, most cases of tinea capitis in the United States were caused by the fluorescent dermatophyte, *Microsporum canis*. However, currently the most common cause of tinea capitis in the United States is *Trichophyton tonsurans*, which is not fluorescent under the Woods lamp.[20] This disorder occurs most commonly in African-American children.

Clinical Description

Tinea capitis commonly presents as scaly, round, or irregular patches of broken hairs on the scalp. *Black-dot tinea capitis* refers to patches of alopecia studded with black dots representing broken hairs and is primarily caused by *T. tonsurans* (Fig. 8-7, see Color Plate 15). The lesions may be solitary but are often multifocal. Tinea capitis may also present as an inflammatory, isolated, boggy plaque called a kerion. In children, with appropriate treatment, the kerion usually heals without producing permanent alopecia. Tinea capitis is often associated with prominent occipital and cervical lymphadenopathy. Patients may also develop annular scaly patches of tinea corporis on the face and trunk due to shedding of fungal elements from the scalp.

Diagnosis

Definitive diagnosis may be obtained by culturing scale or hair from the infected areas. Hyphae and spores may also be detected on examination of a potassium hydroxide preparation from an area of scaling.

Treatment

Tinea capitis requires treatment with a systemic agent. The most frequently prescribed medication is griseofulvin. The initial dose is 15 to 20 mg/kg/day of the microsized griseofulvin suspension for 6 weeks, which should be taken with a fatty meal to enhance absorption. In healthy children, when the medication will only be administered for 1 to 2 months, we do not routinely obtain complete blood counts.

In children with kerion, a brief course of prednisone (dose of 1 mg/kg to a maximum of 40 mg) may decrease the inflammatory response and reduce the risk of scarring. The addition of a 2.5% selenium sulfide shampoo twice weekly helps to decrease shedding of spores. Because of the high asymptomatic carrier rate for dermatophytes, we recommend that children return to school on commencing treatment.

Terbinafine, a new allylamine antifungal, has been found in clinical trials to be as effective as griseofulvin with shorter treatment duration.[21] However, this medication is not yet available as a suspension and has not yet been approved for use in children.

Tinea Corporis

Tinea corporis is an infection of glabrous (non-hairy) skin due to invasion of the stratum corneum by dermatophytes. It most commonly occurs on the face (tinea facei) but may also occur on the trunk and extremities.

Pathogenesis

Fungi of the genera *Trichophyton*, *Microsporum*, and *Epidermophyton* may all cause tinea corporis. The infecting organism is most often *Trichophyton rubrum*; however in infants, *T. tonsurans* is also frequently encountered.[22] Risk factors for infection include exposure to an infected animal, exposure to a family member with tinea capitis, and immunodeficiency.

Clinical Description

The appearance of lesions in children is similar to the presentation in adults. The lesions are classically scaly, erythematous patches with raised annular, advancing, borders (Fig. 8-8, see Color Plate 16). Lesions may be solitary or multiple. Infection with a zoophilic organism such as *Microsporum canis* often results in inflammatory lesions with follicle-based pustules. Lesions that have been previously treated with corticosteroids may have an atypical appearance, with less scale and erythema (tinea incognito).

Diagnosis

Tinea corporis may be diagnosed by examination of scale from a lesion with potassium hydroxide under a microscope. Pustular lesions may be unroofed and the contents examined with potassium hydroxide to demonstrate hyphae. Scale from the lesion may also be cultured.

Treatment

If tinea corporis is suspected or diagnosed, the scalp should be examined for evidence of tinea capitis. If tinea capitis is diagnosed, treatment with systemic antifungals is required. If lesions are limited to the skin, treatment with topical antifungals is usually successful. The most frequently used medications are the azoles and include clotrimazole, miconazole, econazole, or oxiconazole. These agents are applied once to twice daily for 2 to 4 weeks until lesions are

clear. The new allylamine antifungal terbinafine, applied twice daily, is also effective.

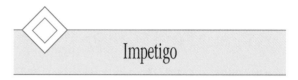

Impetigo

Impetigo is the most common bacterial skin infection in children. It occurs in two forms: (1) nonbullous impetigo caused by *Staphylococcus aureus* or group A β-hemolytic streptococcus (GABHS, or *Streptococcus pyogenes*) and (2) bullous impetigo caused by *Staphylococcus aureus*.

Pathogenesis

Nonbullous impetigo occurs after inoculation of the pathogenic bacteria into traumatized skin. Bullous impetigo is primarily due to *Staph. aureus*, phage group II, which produces a toxin, exfoliatin, that causes intraepidermal cleavage and bullae formation. Impetigo is more common with increased humidity, increased temperature, and poor hygiene. It is also more common in chronic skin conditions like atopic dermatitis.

Clinical Description

Impetigo occurs most frequently on the face and extremities. Facial lesions are often periorificial. Nonbullous impetigo presents as small vesiculopustules that rupture to form erythematous plaques with a characteristic honey-colored crust. Bullous impetigo presents with flaccid bullae that easily rupture to form shiny, circular, erythematous macules with a rim of scale. Regional adenopathy and leukocytosis may accompany skin lesions; however, systemic symptoms are rare.[23]

Complications of impetigo include acute poststreptococcal glomerulonephritis (APSGN). This is caused by nephritogenic strains of group

A β-hemolytic streptococcus. It occurs most frequently in children ages 3 to 7 years and an average of 18 to 21 days after the episode of impetigo. Rheumatic fever has not been reported to occur after impetigo.

Treatment

The options for treatment include topical and oral antibiotics. Mupirocin is a by-product of fermentation of *Pseudomonas fluorescens*. It exerts a bactericidal effect by inhibiting bacterial protein synthesis via inactivation of isoleucyl-tRNA synthetase. Several studies suggest it is as effective as erythromycin with fewer side effects.[24] Mupirocin is applied three times daily for 7 to 10 days. It is effective against *Strep. pyogenes* and *Staph. aureus*, including multiply resistant strains.

Twenty years ago, most cases of nonbullous impetigo were due to GABHS and were treatable with penicillin. However, over the past two decades, studies have shown that the vast majority of cases are now due to *Staph. aureus* that is frequently resistant to penicillin.[25] Appropriate treatment options include erythromycin and first-generation cephalosporins such as cephalexin.

Patients with recurrent impetigo may have colonization of the nares by *Staph. aureus*. Treatment with mupirocin intranasally four times a day may eliminate colonization.

Pityriasis Rosea

Pityriasis rosea is a common, scaly, self-limited dermatosis primarily affecting young adults and children. It affects males and females equally and most commonly occurs in the fall and spring.

Pathogenesis

The etiologic agent of pityriasis rosea has long been suspected to be viral. This was based on the associated clinical features as well as prior identification of virus-like particles in cells from skin lesions. Most recently, studies have identified human herpesvirus 7 DNA in the skin of patients with pityriasis rosea.[26]

Clinical Description

Pityriasis rosea may begin with the appearance of a pink macule or papule that subsequently enlarges to a 2- to 10-cm oval patch (Fig. 8-9, see Color Plate 17). This lesion, the herald patch, is usually solitary and may not be noticed by the patient. It occurs primarily on the neck or trunk. The herald patch is a sharply defined, oval plaque with an elevated border and fine white scale. Some 5 to 14 days later, the patient develops a secondary widespread, bilateral, symmetrical eruption of 0.5- to 1.5-cm pink, oval patches with a "collarette" of fine white scale. The long axis of these lesions is distributed along the skin cleavage lines on the trunk, producing the characteristic "Christmas tree" pattern. Lesions usually present on the trunk and proximal extremities with sparing of the face and distal extremities. However, the eruption may present in an "inverse" pattern affecting the face and distal extremities. This presentation occurs more frequently in African-American children. Rarely, patients may have oral involvement, with erythematous macules, vesicles, or ulcer-ations.[27]

In 5 percent of patients, preceding myalgias, arthralgias, headache and fever, or upper respiratory infection may be noted. The eruption may be pruritic but is often asymptomatic. Patients may continue to develop crops of new lesions for 2 to 3 weeks, which then heal and resolve over 2 to 3 months, often with postinflammatory hypo- or hyperpigmentation.

Differential Diagnosis

The herald patch may initially be diagnosed as tinea corporis. However, the diagnosis becomes clear with the appearance of the secondary eruption. The generalized eruption of pityriasis rosea resembles secondary syphilis. However, syphilis often involves the palms and soles, and a history of preceding chancre is often present. In nummular eczema, the individual lesions are more often round and lack the characteristic "Christmas tree" distribution. Guttate psoriasis is characterized by multiple oval pink papules with silvery white adherent scale.

Diagnosis

The clinical appearance and progression of the eruption suggests the diagnosis. In patients with atypical presentations, a skin biopsy may be helpful. The presence of a superficial perivascular infiltrate, focal spongiosis, and mounds of parakeratosis are consistent with pityriasis rosea.

Treatment

Treatment of this eruption is aimed at controlling pruritus. Topical antipruritics, such as Sarna lotion or Aveeno baths, are effective. Mild topical corticosteroids and oral antihistamines may also provide some relief but will not hasten resolution of the lesions.

Contact Dermatitis

Contact dermatitis is an eczematous eruption of the skin due to exposure to an exogenous material. It is classified into irritant (more common) and allergic contact dermatitis. The incidence of allergic contact dermatitis is lower in children than in adults.

Pathogenesis

Irritant contact dermatitis is a nonimmunologic reaction due to exposure of the skin to an inherently irritating substance. Acute irritant contact dermatitis is caused by contact with a potent substance such as an acid. The subacute and chronic forms are caused by repeated exposure to less potent irritants such as saliva, urine, or detergents.

Allergic contact dermatitis is a type IV delayed immunologic reaction due to contact with an allergen. The first step in development of this reaction is sensitization. After exposure, the allergen is presented by the Langerhans cells in the epidermis to T lymphocytes. This results in proliferation of T lymphocytes that are programmed to respond to the allergen. Subsequent reexposure to the allergen results in activation of the T lymphocytes (the elicitation phase) with release of inflammatory mediators.

Clinical Description

Acute irritant contact dermatitis due to contact with a potent chemical produces rapid onset of well-defined erythema, edema, vesiculation, and possibly ulceration at the site of contact. Subacute or chronic irritant dermatitis presents as patches of erythema, crusting, and scaling that may be associated with pruritus or a burning sensation. In children, this may occur around the mouth with the use of a pacifier, where the occlusion, moisture, and chronic contact with saliva produce the irritation. Irritant contact diaper dermatitis occurs because of repeated exposure to irritants in feces and urine in the context of the increased moisture and occlusion in this location. Irritant diaper dermatitis presents as erythematous patches and papules with sparing of the inguinal skin folds in the diaper area.

Allergic contact dermatitis occurs 8 to 24 h after exposure to the allergen. In the United States, the most common causes are poison ivy and poison oak. The allergen is found in the oleoresin of the plant and is composed of pentadecylcatechols and heptadecylcatechols. Other trees in this family that may produce the same reaction include poison sumac, cashew, and mango. Distinct linear lesions with erythema, edema, vesiculation, and pruritus are characteristic of reactions to plants and are produced by the leaves brushing against the skin.

Other common causes of allergic contact dermatitis include nickel, which often is due to exposure to jewelry or metal fasteners on clothing (Fig. 8-10, see Color Plate 18). Erythematous, scaly, pruritic patches on the ears, neck, or lower abdomen are characteristic. With chronic rubbing of the lesions, the skin may become thickened, with increased skin markings producing lichenification.

Ingredients in topical medications, including neomycin in topical antibiotics and benzocaine in topical anesthetic products, may also produce sensitization.

Diagnosis

Diagnosis is based on the clinical history and presentation. The distribution of lesions may be a helpful clue in determining the sensitizing allergen. Patch testing may also be a useful aid in diagnosis and treatment of suspected cases of allergic contact dermatitis. Patch tests are applied to normal skin and read 48 h later. Tests must be interpreted carefully to determine the clinical relevance of any positive reactions.

Treatment

In irritant contact dermatitis, further contact with the eliciting substance should be avoided. In subacute and chronic forms, a mild topical corticosteroid may be helpful. Attempts should be made to decrease contact with excessive saliva. Diaper dermatitis may be improved by keeping the area clean and dry by cleansing with a mild soap and increasing the frequency of diaper

changes. In cases with secondary candidal infection, a topical antifungal medication should be applied.

Allergic contact dermatitis also requires avoidance of the offending allergen. Children should be taught to recognize poison ivy, poison oak, and poison sumac. In addition to avoidance, allergic contact dermatitis is treated with topical corticosteroids. The potency of the corticosteroid employed depends on the severity of the inflammatory reaction and the anatomic location of the lesions. *Rhus* dermatitis frequently requires treatment with potent topical steroids such as fluocinonide. Severe cases may require a brief taper of systemic corticosteroids.

References

1. Tunnessen WW Jr: A survey of skin disorders seen in pediatric general and dermatology clinics. *Pediatr Dermatol* 1:219–222, 1984.
2. Rothe MJ, Grant-Kels JM: Atopic dermatitis: an update. *J Am Acad Dermatol* 35:1–11, 1996.
3. Abeck D, Mempel M: Staphylococcal aureus colonization in atopic dermatitis and its therapeutic implications. *Br J Dermatol* 139:13–16, 1998.
4. Singalavanija S, Frieden IJ: Diaper dermatitis. *Pediatrics* 16:142–147, 1995.
5. Janniger CK: Infantile seborrheic dermatitis: an approach to cradle cap. *Cutis* 51:233–235, 1993.
6. Esterly N: Hemangiomas in infants and children: clinical observations. *Pediatr Dermatol* 9:353–355, 1992.
7. Enjolras O, Gelbert F: Superficial hemangiomas: associations and management. *Pediat Dermatol* 14:173–179, 1997.
8. Ashinoff R, Geronemus RG: Flashlamp-pumped pulsed dye laser for port-wine stains in infancy: earlier versus later treatment. *J Am Acad Dermatol* 24:467–472, 1991.
9. Cunliffe WJ: The sebaceous gland and acne— 40 years on. *Dermatology* 196:9–15, 1998.
10. Cunliffe WJ, Caputo R. Dreno B, et al: Clinical efficacy and safety comparison of adapalene gel and tretinoin gel in the treatment of acne vulgaris. *J Am Acad Dermatol* 36:126–134, 1992.

11. Gollnick H, Graupe K: Azaleic acid for the treatment of acne: comparative trials. *J Dermatol* 1: 27–39, 1989.

12. Burke B, Eady EA, Cunliffe WJ: Benzoyl peroxide versus topical erythromycin in the treatment of acne vulgaris. *Br J Dermatol* 108(2):199–204, 1983.

13. Parry MF, Rha CK: Pseudomembranous colitis caused by topical clindamycin phosphate. *Arch Dermatol* 122:583–584, 1986.

14. Orfanos CE, Zoubolis ChC: Oral retinoids and the treatment of seborrhea and acne. *Dermatology* 196:140–147, 1998.

15. Overfield TM, Brody JA: An epidemiologic study of molluscum contagiosum in Anchorage, Alaska. *J Pediatr* 69:640–642, 1966.

16. Ronnerfalt L, Fransson J, Wahlgren CF: EMLA cream provides rapid pain relief for the currettage of molluscum contagiosum in children with atopic dermatitis without causing serious application site reactions. *Pediatr Dermatol* 15:309–312, 1998.

17. Jablonska S, Majewski S, Obalek S, et al: Cutaneous warts. *Clin Dermatol* 15:309–319, 1997.

18. Janniger CK: Childhood warts. *Pediatr Dermatol* 50:15–16, 1992.

19. Yilmaz E, Alpsoy E, Basaran E: Cimetidine therapy for warts: a placebo-controlled, double blind study. *J Am Acad Dermatol* 34(6):1005–1007, 1996.

20. Frieden I and Howard R: Tinea capitis: epidemiology, diagnosis, treatment and control. *J Am Acad Dermatol* 31:S42–S46, 1994.

21. Haroon TS, Hussain I, Aman S, et al: A randomized double blind comparative study of terbinafine for 1, 2 and 4 weeks in tinea capitis. *Br J Dermatol* 135(1):86–88, 1996.

22. Silverman RA: Pediatric mycoses, in Elewiski BE (ed): *Cutaneous Fungal Infections*, 2nd ed. United Kingdom, Blackwell Science, 1998, pp 261–271.

23. Darnstadt GL, Lane AL: Impetigo: an overview. *Pediatr Dermatol* 11:293–303, 1994.

24. Barton L. Friedman AD, Sharkey AM, et al: Impetigo contagiosa: III. Comparative efficacy of oral erythromycin and topical mupirocin. *Pediatr Dermatol* 6:134–138, 1989.

25. Coskey RJ, Coskey LA: Diagnosis and treatment of impetigo. *J Am Acad Dermatol* 17:62–63, 1987.

26. Drago F, Ranieri F, Malaguti F, et al: Human herpesvirus 7 in patients with pityriasis rosea: electron microscopy investigations and polymerase chain reaction in mononuclear cells, plasma and skin. *Dermatology* 195:374–378, 1997.

27. Allen RA, Janniger CK, Schwartz RA: Pityriasis rosea. *Cutis* 56:198–202, 1995.

Monica S. Vavilala
Frederick P. Rivara

Chapter

9

Trauma

Injuries are the most frequent cause of pediatric death and acquired disability. The commoness of the problem and the potential for adverse outcome makes injury an important issue that pediatricians and other child health providers deal with on a daily basis. The purpose of this chapter is to give the practicing clinician a framework in which to consider and understand the management of pediatric trauma as well as to discuss some aspects of trauma prevention. It is not meant to serve as a primary reference for the definitive treatment of pediatric trauma.

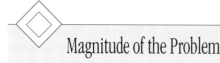

Magnitude of the Problem

Approximately 20,000 children and adolescents die from injuries each year in the United States, as shown in Table 9-1. Motor vehicle injuries account for almost one-half of these pediatric trauma deaths. However, motor vehicle injuries do not represent a homogeneous problem but are made up of a number of different subgroups.

MOTOR VEHICLE INJURIES

Motor vehicle occupant injuries account for nearly 5000 deaths each year. The risk of occupant death is greatest for teens, in whom the risk of death per mile driven is higher than for any other age group. This is due to a combination of risk-taking behavior and inexperience; alcohol use in this age group actually accounts for a much smaller portion of motor vehicle fatalities than for young and middle-aged adults.

PEDESTRIAN INJURIES

Pedestrian injuries are another important cause of fatal injury in the pediatric age group. Among very young children, these usually represent tragic back-over injuries in the driveway, usually inflicted by a family member. Among school-aged children 5 to 9 years old, pedestrian injuries are among of the most common causes of death and serious head injury for most locales. These injuries represent a mismatch between the skills of the child to cross the street and expectations by society and parents on tasks at this age. The evidence clearly indicates that children at this age do not have the skills to cross the street reliably every time.

BICYCLE INJURIES

Bicycle injuries can occur with traffic and without, although most of the serious and fatal injuries result from being struck by a car. One-third of emergency department visits, two-thirds of hospitalizations, and three-fourths of deaths related to bicycling are from brain injury.

Table 9-1

Injury Deaths in the United States, 1996

MECHANISM	AGE IN YEARS			
	0–4	5–9	10–14	15–19
All injuries	3,759	1,770	2,482	11,642
Motor vehicle occupant	514	359	531	3,566
Pedestrian, traffic-related	225	264	234	279
Bicycle, traffic-related	4	81	112	65
Drowning	533	223	225	388
Suffocation	532	57	77	67
Fire and flames	515	223	111	109
Falls	55	30	21	94
Poisonings	57	18	34	190
Unintentional gunshot	17	27	94	238
Homicide	752	179	335	2924
Suicide	0	4	298	1817

SOURCE: National Center for Injury Prevention and Control. (www.cdc.gov/ncipc)

FALLS

Falls in children are a common occurrence but a relatively uncommon cause of death. Most studies indicate that serious injury is unlikely in falls of less than 10 ft, with the exception of falls by children under 1 year of age which can result in serious injuries even from short distances. Barlow, in a study of falls from heights in New York City, found that the LD_{50} was approximately five stories.[1]

FIRES AND BURNS

Fires and burns continue to pose a terrible problem in the United States, although the death rates have decreased substantially in recent years. Most deaths related to fire are due to smoke inhalation, not incineration in the fire. Burn mortality is related to age, with children under age 1 having a substantially higher mortality than older children, adolescents, and adults. Mortality is also related to the presence of smoke inhalation and, of course, percent of the total body surface area involved with full-thickness burns.

FIREARMS

Gunshot wounds affect children in many ways, both as victims and as survivors of other family members who are shot. Young children and school-aged boys are primarily killed by accidental gunshot wounds. Suicide among teens primarily involves guns. Finally, among young minority males, homicide involving guns represents a major if not the most common cause of death.

DROWNING AND POISONING

Drowning and poisoning are mentioned here because they are often included in discussions of pediatric trauma, although they are not discussed in this chapter. Poisonings represent a success story in pediatrics in that the rate of unintentional poisoning deaths to children under age 6 have plummeted in this country. Drowning continues to be a major problem, especially for young children and teens.

NONFATAL INJURIES

Mortality rates are only the tip of the proverbial iceberg in relation to pediatric trauma. Less than 10 percent of hospitalized pediatric trauma patients die. In turn, an even smaller portion of those with medically treated injuries are hospitalized. Studies indicate that as many as 25 percent of children receive medical care for injuries each year in the United States. The causes of these injuries are quite different from those resulting in death or even hospitalization. The most common are injuries due to falls or those due to sports and recreational activities. Burns and motor vehicle–related injuries are much less common.

Emergency Department Evaluation

It is essential that child health care providers be familiar with the issues surrounding the medical evaluation and treatment of the acutely injured child. This is because children have anatomic and physiologic characteristics that differ from those of adults. It is, therefore, vital that practitioners recognize what is normal and what is not for a given age. The differences in parameters of cardiac and respiratory function are described in Table 9-2. The unique anatomic and physiologic features also makes taking care of pediatric trauma patients challenging.

The concept of having a designated "pediatric trauma team" comprising an anesthesiologist, surgeon, neurosurgeon, and nurse responding to critically ill children in the emergency department has been proposed in an attempt to

Table 9-2

Pediatric Vital Signs Appropriate for Age

	PULSE RATE (BEATS PER MINUTE)	BLOOD PRESSURE (MMHG)	RESPIRATORY RATE (BREATHS/MIN)
Infant	100–160	70–90	30–40
Child	80–100	80–100	20–30
Adolescent	60–90	100–120	12–20

improve patient outcomes. Most recently, although Vernon et al. have documented shorter times for patient evaluation, they were unable to show improved survival with the institution of such a team at a pediatric level one trauma hospital.[2] Although there has also been discussion centered around whether "regionalization" of care to pediatric trauma hospitals versus adult trauma hospitals improves outcome, improvements in pediatric trauma care will probably come from improving the various aspects of the critical care of children rather than developing regional trauma centers specifically for children.[3]

Whether in a tertiary care center or a small community hospital, there is no substitute for preparation of both personnel and equipment when the arrival of an injured child is anticipated. This includes designation of duties based on clinical experience and familiarity with pediatric resuscitation equipment. The color-coded Broselow tape, bags, and carts contain treatment guidelines based on estimated patient size and are currently used in many centers and are extremely helpful to both nurses and physicians. The Broselow tape can be used upon arrival of the child to estimate weight, medication doses, and equipment appropriate for age. It is very user-friendly. We have recently purchased the tape, cart, and bags and have found them to improve our ability to efficiently procure equipment during resuscitation. [The Broselow tape, bags, and cart can be obtained from Armstrong Medical Company (Lincolnshire, Illinois)].

The general approach to pediatric trauma follows that of the adult. In order of priority, it includes the primary survey, secondary survey, and finally definitive care of all injuries.[4] The primary survey detects and simultaneously treats life-threatening injuries. Only then is a secondary survey performed: a thorough head-to-toe physical examination to address other injuries in need of treatment. During the definitive phase of therapy, injuries are managed by the appropriate or nonoperative treatment modality and a disposition is made. To avoid confusion and conflicting decision making, it is vital that one person be in charge and direct the care of the injured child.

Primary Survey and Resuscitation

The primary survey consists of managing the patient's ABCDEs (Table 9-3). It is key to remember that the primary survey and resuscitation are performed simultaneously. Although the principles outlined below apply to all injured children, it is critical to understand and follow the steps described by the pneumonic ABCDE in assessing and managing the child with major trauma. *Errors in management usually occur because the ABCDE's are not followed appropriately.*

Table 9-3

Primary Survey

A	Airway with cervical spine
B	Breathing
C	Circulation
D	Disability (neurologic status)
	Level of consciousness
	A = alert
	V = responds to verbal stimuli
	P = responds to painful stimuli
	U = unresponsive
E	Exposure (undress, check temperature, prevent heat loss)

Source: Adapted from Committee on Trauma, American College of Surgeons: *Advanced Trauma Life Support Course*, Chicago, ACS, 1998.

Airway Maintenance and Cervical Spine Immobilization

The first priority and most important maneuver to master in treating the injured child is to maintain the airway. However, spinal injury must be assumed at this stage and the child's cervical spine must be immobilized as the airway is evaluated. If the child has upper airway obstruction, the airway must be opened, with the head and neck placed in neutral position. Although there are three ways to open the airway, only the chin-lift or jaw-thrust techniques are acceptable in the setting of trauma. Performing a head tilt will extend the spine and may worsen both airway obstruction and injured spine. A correctly sized oropharyngeal airway should be used when airway obstruction is not relieved by the above-mentioned maneuvers. Oropharyngeal airways are available in infant, small, medium, and large sizes. The use of nasal airways is discouraged because of their potential for tissue disruption, bleeding, and facial trauma.

VENTILATION

Upper airway obstruction that is not relieved by the steps outlined above requires the use of positive-pressure ventilation, which should be applied using the appropriately sized face mask. The head and neck must be in neutral position. Because all trauma victims are considered to have a "full stomach" and hence to be at risk aspiration of gastric contents, cricoid pressure must be applied gently during intubation or mask ventilation. *Although it is not necessary for clinicians to know how to intubate patients, it is critical for them to be facile in the use of mask ventilation.*

Bag-mask ventilation may be performed using either the one-handed or two-handed technique. With the former, one hand is used to hold the face mask and the other to inflate the bag attached to the circuit and face mask. With the head in neutral position, oxygen is delivered to the patient using positive pressure. Pressure gauges or rise of chest wall with positive pressure can estimate adequacy of oxygen delivery. *Often, inability to move air forward is due to a lack of appropriate fit of mask over the face and inadequate jaw thrust.*

Pulse oximetry should be used to assess oxygenation. Some facilities are equipped with capnographs that measure end-tidal CO_2. These devices can be used to estimate adequacy of ventilation. If the end-tidal CO_2 is 35 mmHg, then the arterial Pa_{CO_2} will usually be 5 mmHg greater, or 40 mmHg.

TRACHEAL INTUBATION

Indications for tracheal intubation include an inability to maintain an airway, hypoxia or hypercarbia refractory to treatment with passive supplemental oxygen, hemodynamic instability (including cardiorespiratory failure), and inability to protect the airway because of decreased mental status.[5] Mechanism of injury and prehospital course are also important qualifiers to the overall assessment of probability and extent of injury and need for tracheal intubation.

There are a number of ways to calculate tracheal tube size. Commonly, when the age of the child is unknown, the child's fifth distal phalanx can be used to approximate the internal diameter of the tracheal tube. Alternatively, the general formula for children older than 2 years of age can be used:

$$\text{Tracheal tube internal diameter in millimeters} = \frac{[16 + \text{age (years)}]}{4}$$

Children might require a tube size 0.5 mm smaller or larger than calculated. Tracheal tube placement should always be confirmed by chest auscultation. The presence of CO_2 on an indicator does not guarantee proper placement, because small amounts of air in the stomach after positive-pressure ventilation may falsely indicate tracheal placement. Conversely, absence of CO_2 does not exclude proper placement, because the presence of CO_2 requires an intact cardiorespiratory function. Chest auscultation is also necessary to assess depth of tracheal tube placement. A useful formula to approximate tracheal depth is:

$$\text{Depth of tracheal tube at patient's gum line in millimeters} = 3 \text{ times tracheal tube size in millimeters}$$

ALTERNATE METHODS OF VENTILATION

Patients with structural facial abnormalities or syndromes are prone to have difficulty with mask ventilation and intubation. If a difficult airway is suspected or anticipated, it is imperative to obtain consultation from the anesthesiologist and/or otolaryngologist. Although there is ample experience and a wide literature regarding the use of various alternative strategies to maintain the airway in the adult, this is lacking in children. Needle cricothyrotomy kits are available from various commercial vendors and can be used. Alternatively, needle cricothyrotomy can be performed using a large-bore cannula into

the trachea below the obstruction and connecting this to oxygen at 15 L/min via a Y connector. One can ventilate the lung by alternately occluding the open end of the Y connector for 1 s of inspiration and leaving it open for 3 s of expiration. Hypercarbia, hypoxia, and subcutaneous emphysema are potential complications. Surgical cricothyrotomy is difficult to perform for children in an emergency setting; the risk of complications is high.

Breathing

By observation and auscultation, one can answer the question "Is the child breathing?" Determine respiratory effort and work of breathing by assessing the child's color and respiratory rate. If the child is breathing adequately, deliver supplemental oxygen via a face mask and monitor the patient using pulse oximetry in an extremity. It may be necessary to warm the extremity or search for more than one site to obtain consistent saturation readings if the child's extremities are vasoconstricted because of shock. Symmetrical chest expansion, absence of tracheal deviation and bony crepitus, and good aeration decrease the likelihood of hemopneumothoraces. The presence of fractured ribs on chest radiograph increases the likelihood of underlying pulmonary injury.

Even though chest radiographs are helpful to confirm tracheal tube placement and to diagnose pulmonary injury, interventions that are lifesaving should be based on clinical evaluation and index of suspicion and not be delayed for confirmation by radiographs. These conditions include tension pneumothorax, hemothorax, sucking chest wounds, flail segment, and pericardial tamponade.

Circulation

In this segment we focus on assessing the cardiac output and perfusion of the injured child.

Signs of hypovolemic shock include cool extremities, pallor, sweating, capillary refill longer than 2 s, and tachycardia. Children with significant blood loss can compensate for that loss for a long period of time. *Tachycardia might be the only clinical finding until the circulating blood volume decreases by 25 percent. Only in advanced stages do blood pressure and urine output decrease. Therefore any child presenting with persistent tachycardia and normal blood pressure should be suspected of having hypovolemia and/or ongoing blood loss.*

VASCULAR ACCESS

Vascular access poses the biggest challenge in dealing with shock in children. Two reasonable and expeditious attempts at large-bore peripheral vascular access should be made by experienced personnel. Should attempts at intravenous access fail, as they often do because of peripheral vasoconstriction, an interosseous needle (13 or 18 gauge) should be inserted approximately one fingerbreath below the tibial tuberosity after sterile prep and used until definitive vascular access is available. This should be done within 5 min of arrival in the emergency department if peripheral venous access is unsuccessful. Interosseous access is contraindicated in children over 6 years of age because of the thickness of the cortex and in the presence of ipsilateral proximal extremity fracture. The proximal tibia and distal femur are preferred sites. Central venous access should be attempted only by experienced personnel. Should attempts at percutaneous vascular access and interosseous needle placement fail, a venous cut-down should be attempted.

FLUID ADMINISTRATION

Fluid and or blood may be necessary in boluses of 20 mL/kg to improve perfusion, decrease heart rate, and increase blood pres-sure. Fluid therapy is guided by repeated assessment of hemodynamics and circulatory status. *The most common mistake made by physicians in the emergency department is to giving too little fluid rather than too much.* A type and cross-match and laboratory evaluation assessing electrolytes and coagulation must be immediately sent. If typed and cross-matched blood is unavailable, type O blood that is not cross-matched may be given. At our institution, 16 units of type O blood (8 units of O-negative and 8 units of O-positive) are available for such situations. If there is a choice, females should be given O-negative blood.

There is generally no role for vasopressor therapy in the emergency department setting. Because hypovolemia is usually the cause of hypotension, the emphasis should be on restoring intravascular volume with crystalloids or colloids rather than with vasopressors.

Disability

This refers to a rapid neurologic assessment and has two components: "AVPU" and pupillary exam. The clinician is asked to decide whether the patient is alert, responsive to voice, responsive to pain, or unresponsive (AVPU). The pupillary exam tests for reactivity and symmetry. Unlike the AVPU scale, which is used in the primary survey, the Glasgow Coma Scale (GCS) is used in the secondary survey. The adult GCS scoring system is modified for the preverbal child (Table 9-4).

Exposure

Exposure is important to allow a thorough examination. However, the injured child is susceptible to hypothermia and clinicians must remember to take the temperature and try to keep the child warm. Furthermore, once the ABCs are secured and stabilized, the child

Table 9-4

Glasgow Coma Scale and Modification for Young Children

GLASGOW COMA SCALE		CHILDREN'S COMA SCALE	
RESPONSE	**SCORE**	**RESPONSE**	**SCORE**
Eyes		Eyes	
Open spontaneously	4	Open spontaneously	4
Verbal command	3	React to speech	3
Pain	2	React to pain	2
No response	1	No response	1
Best motor response		Best motor response	
Obeys verbal command	6	Spontaneous or obeys verbal command	6
Localizes pain	5	Localizes pain	5
Withdraws in response to pain	4	Withdraws in response to pain	4
Abnormal flexion	3	Abnormal flexion	3
Extension posturing	2	Extension posturing	2
No response	1	No response	1
Best verbal response		Best verbal response	
Oriented and converses	5	Smiles, oriented, interacts	5
Disoriented and converses	4	Interacts inappropriately	4
Inappropriate words	3	Moaning	3
Incomprehensible sounds	2	Irritable, inconsolable	2
No response	1	No response	1

should be turned to examine the back for evidence of injuries. Unless the cervical and thoracic spines are radiographically and clinically cleared of fractures, the child must be "log rolled." Similarly, the child must be moved with the use of a long log roller.

LABORATORY STUDIES

Once the resuscitation phase is completed, a series of laboratory tests and radiographs may be obtained. The need for these tests will depend on the mechanism of injury and the findings on the primary survey. Some of the specifics of what test to order is institution-dependent.

SECONDARY SURVEY

A thorough head-to-toe examination follows the primary survey to identify the injuries necessitating definitive treatment. This should be done only after the initial resuscitation has been completed and initial diagnostic studies obtained.

DEFINITIVE CARE

In the definitive care phase of treatment, all injuries are managed by the appropriate operative or nonoperative strategies. Select patients might be candidates for transfer to specialty facilities.

Traumatic Brain Injury

Brain injury is important for a variety of reasons. It is far and away the most common cause of death from pediatric trauma. In most centers, it accounts for 85 percent or more of the deaths among children who are brought to emergency departments with trauma. It is also the most important cause of long-term disability from injury.

Initial stabilization of the trauma patient was discussed above. One critical issue in the care of children with brain injury is the preservation of cerebral perfusion pressure. Experimental and clinical data indicate that hypoxia and hypotension adversely affect neurologic outcome in brain-injured patients. Unfortunately, most of these data come from studies of adults. In one study of children with severe head injury, patients who had decreased oxygen delivery from hypotension had a three- to fourfold increased risk of death compared to those without hypotension.[6]

In the past, one of the common medical responses to patients with severe brain injury was intubation and hyperventilation. However, there is increasing evidence that hyperventilation not only does not improve the outcome after closed head injury but may actually lead to poorer survival and higher risk of neurologic sequelae. In a randomized controlled trial of hyperventilation in patients with severe head injury, 18 percent of hyperventilated patients with initial motor Glasgow Coma Scale scores of 4 to 5 had good recovery or moderate disability compared to 48 percent of the control group that was not hypoventilated.[7] Hyperventilation decreases intracranial pressure by decreasing cerebral blood flow; in areas of injured brain, this decrease in blood flow may be deleterious.[8,9]

IMAGING

One major area of concern is whether or not to obtain a computed tomography (CT) scan on a child with brain injury. All would agree that a child in coma or with focal neurologic signs should be assessed with CT as soon as possible, since the possibility of a focal lesion is significantly increased in that group. But what about a child with a mild head injury or the child with a history of loss of consciousness who now is seemingly well? Should such a child have a cranial CT scan? Although the experts vary in their recommendations, the literature is actually fairly consistent.

Table 9-5 summarizes the studies that have examined the prevalence of positive CT scans in

Table 9-5

Prevalence of Positive Findings on Computed Tomography among Children with Closed Head Injury

Author (Year)	GCS Score 15 (N)	% ICH	Required Hematoma Evacuation	GCS Score 13–15 (N)	% ICH	Required Hematoma Evacuation
Rivara, 1987	NA	NA	NA	51	15.7%	0
Quayle et al., 1997	266	6%	1 of 16	NA	NA	NA
Dietrich et al., 1991	195	5.6%	NA	233	8.2%	NA
Hahn and McAllen	739	NA	5.8%	791	NA	5.4%
Davis, et al., 1994	168	7%	0	NA	NA	NA
Nay, et al., 1999	1,170	1.5%	2	NA	NA	NA

KEY: GCS, Glasgow Coma Scale; ICH, intracranial hemorrhage; NA, not available.

those examined after mild head injury, including isolated loss of consciousness. A number of conclusions can be drawn from these studies. First, the risk of intracranial hemorrhage (ICH) in such children is *not* zero; the studies consistently find a rate of ICH of approximately 5 percent. Second, some of these children do require intervention such as craniotomy to treat the intracranial hemorrhage. Third, clinical predictors of which children will have positive CT scans have relatively low sensitivity and specificity.[10] Vomiting as a sign has very limited usefulness in all studies. Most studies find that most other clinical signs are little better.[11,12]

The studies also appear to be in agreement that children with head injury and a negative CT scan can be discharged home from the emergency department if there are not other injuries that require inpatient care. The risk of new hemorrhages or subsequent problems is very low in these children. Davis and colleagues found only one new bleed in 400 children with mild head injury and negative initial CT scans.[13]

A number of questions remain unanswered. Perhaps the most important is the significance of a small cerebral contusion or extraaxial hemorrhage in an asymptomatic child with a prior loss of consciousness. Many physicians do not examine children with CT scans after a mild head injury because most (although not all) of those with positive CT scans will not require operative intervention. Is it thus unnecessary to know about these lesions, either for issues related to immediate care or for long-term consequences? The answers to these questions are for the most part unknown, creating a dilemma for the clinician. Carefully done prospective cohort studies do reveal that children with mild head injury have few long-term sequelae, although the number of children with mild injury and abnormal head CT scans in this study was small.[14]

So what should a physician do when confronted with a child with a loss of consciousness after a head injury? Almost all would agree that if the neurologic exam is abnormal (including increased sleepiness and decreased coherence),

a CT scan is appropriate. At our institution and similar institutions where CT scans are readily available around the clock, all such children are assessed with CT.

We recommend obtaining a CT scan and arranging for neurosurgical evaluation in all such patients. If there is a history of loss of consciousness but the neurologic exam is normal, there are two options: CT or admission to hospital. In the absence of readily available CT, we recommend admission to the hospital for observation. If a CT is performed, it is normal, and there is no other reason for hospitalization, the child can be discharged home. But because patients with large scalp lacerations and/or skull fractures or who are less than 3 months of age are at higher risk of having an intracranial injury, they should be imaged. As a general rule, when CT is indicated and readily available, it is preferable, in terms of resource consumption, to obtain the CT rather than admit the child to the hospital for observation.

A note of caution about discharge instructions to parents: Many physicians issue warnings about signs of impending trouble from a brain injury, asking parents to return to the emergency department if these signs or symptoms appear. This practice is not supported by any data. The ability of parents to accurately monitor children at home for signs of trouble is unknown and should never be used in lieu of further diagnostic assessment in the emergency department prior to discharge.

SEIZURES

Overall, about 2 to 5 percent of patients will have a seizure after head trauma. This is related to the severity of the head injury. As many as 35 percent of patients with initial GCS scores less than 8 experience seizures. The vast majority of these occur within the first week after injury. There is evidence that treatment with phenytoin in the first week decreases the risk of these early seizures but has no effect on the risk of seizures beyond the first week.[15] Thus, for inpatients with coma and with intracranial pathology, we load with phenytoin in the emergency department (20 mg/kg) and place these children on maintenance does of phenytoin of 6 to 8 mg/kg for the first week following injury and then discontinue the medication.

Cervical Spine

Among the most important injuries to diagnose in any trauma patient are neck injuries. Most patients with significant trauma will arrive in the emergency department on a backboard with a cervical collar in place. What should the physician do to rule out a fracture of the cervical spine?

Spine injuries are relatively infrequent in children. The exact incidence is not known but is probably around 1 percent of all children admitted to the hospital for care of an injury. One estimate places the incidence at 21.2 per million population per year in children and adolescents under the age of 19. Half of all children with spinal cord injuries die at the scene of the injury. Approximately one-half of patients with cervical spine injury have concomitant head injury, and the presence of head injury substantially increases the risk of spine injury. Among children with cervical spine injury, about 10 to 15 percent occur to those under age 8, one-quarter to those aged 8 to 12, and 60 to 70 percent to those over 12.

Younger patients have injuries predominantly to the upper cervical spine, while older children have a more adult pattern with injuries to the lower cervical spine. This is related to the fulcrum of cervical motion. In young children, the cervical spine has maximal movement at C1 to C3. Past age 12, this moves down to the area of C5 to C6, resulting in injury to the lower part of the spine.

Cervical spine fractures can occur without neurologic deficit, and neurologic deficit can occur without fracture. Neurologic deficit without fracture has been termed *SCIWORA* (spinal cord injury without radiologic abnormalities).

SCIWORA was a diagnosis made in the era before magnetic resonance imaging (MRI). Most of these children will have radiographic abnormalities on MRI. SCIWORA can occur in the cervical or thoracic spine. The onset of neurologic deficit is delayed in about one-quarter of children with SCIWORA. These children often have brief sensory of motor deficits initially, with later onset of more severe signs. The majority of SCIWORA injuries appear to be due to flexion or hyperextension and to ligamentous stretching or disruption without bony injury. Nevertheless, children with these spinal cord injuries need to be treated with spine immobilization because injury can occur.

IMAGING

The largest question for the physician caring for the child is deciding which children require radiographs of the cervical spine. Complete plain radiographic assessment of the cervical spine includes anteroposterior and lateral views down to the cervicothoracic junction and views of the odontoid. Much has been written about the need (or lack of need) to obtain cervical spine x-rays, but few studies have actually been conducted to provide useful data.

Rachesky et al. reviewed the 7-year experience at two hospitals in Tucson. Cervical spine radiographs were obtained on 2133 children, of whom 25 (1.2 percent) had evidence of a cervical spine injury on x-ray. No single clinical predictor alone had a sensitivity of 100 percent in predicting positive x-rays. However, all children who had cervical spine injury had either neck pain or were in a motor vehicle crash and had head trauma.[16]

Dietrich reviewed 50 children admitted to the hospital with cervical spine fractures; 30 of 31 (97 percent) children who were alert complained of neck tenderness.[17] Jaffe studied children seen in the emergency department for assessment of spine injury as well as children referred for care of cervical spine injury. In this highly selected series, 59 of 206 children had cervical spine injuries. A clinical algorithm was developed that included eight variables: neck pain; neck tenderness; limitation of neck mobility; history of trauma to the neck; and abnormalities of reflexes, strength, sensation, or mental status. Positive findings in any one of these eight variables correctly identified 58 of 59 children with cervical spine injury, yielding a sensitivity of 98 percent and specificity of 54 percent.[18] These data must be interpreted with caution. The number of studies is obviously limited and the number of cervical spine injuries actually studied is small. None of the studies would eliminate more than one-third of radiographs if the protocol were followed; treating physicians must ask themselves whether this cost savings is worth the risk.

In some children, especially small children, radiographic examination of the spine can be difficult with plain films. CT has been used to facilitate examination; more recently some institutions have used spiral CT, which has the advantage over plain films of speed and accuracy. In children who are receiving a CT for evaluation of head trauma, it makes sense to keep the child on the table for a few minutes longer and obtain a CT of the cervical spine as well.

The spine cannot be "cleared" by radiographic examination alone. This requires physical examination in an awake child in whom the presence of pain and tenderness can be assessed. If the child is not awake, continued use of a cervical collar may be indicated.

Spinal Shock

Understanding the physiology and recognizing the presentation of spinal shock will help the practitioner differentiate it from the more commonly seen septic shock. Spinal shock results when the spinal cord is injured, resulting in loss of sympathetic innervation to the heart and loss of vasomotor tone. This means that, instead of the usual hypotension and tachycardia seen with hypovolemic and septic shock, hypotension presents with bradycardia. To treat this condition, fluid therapy alone is not sufficient. This is one of the few instances in which vasopressors are used for treatment of the trauma victim.

Spinal shock refers to the condition after spinal cord injury. Muscle flaccidity and loss of reflexes are present initially. Apparent absence of any spinal cord function may be only temporary and, weeks to days later, spasticity may supersede flaccidity in areas where spinal cord function does not return. We treat patients with suspected spinal cord injury with methylprednisolone for at least 24 h.

Abdominal Trauma

The majority of abdominal injuries are blunt injuries and occur as a result of motor vehicle accidents. Trauma to the liver and spleen accounts for 30 to 50 percent of injuries, while injuries to the kidneys, pancreas, and hollow viscera are seen in less than 10 percent of cases. Lumbar flexion-distraction injuries and compression fractures are also reported to occur with blunt abdominal trauma. Children restrained by lap belts who present with abdominal or flank ecchymosis are at high risk of pancreatic and other intraabdominal injuries. Additionally, children with lap-belt ecchymosis account for a very high proportion of hollow viscus and lumbar spinal injuries (Chance fracture).[19,20] Penetrating abdominal trauma, seen in older children and adolescents, usually results from stab wounds or gunshot wounds. In these cases, gastrointestinal injury is the rule and solid-organ injury is the exception, occurring in approximately 10 percent of cases.

Victims of blunt abdominal trauma who are unstable are taken to the operating room for exploratory laparotomy. Because of advances in imaging technology, hemodynamically stable patients are frequently observed in an intensive care unit setting after evaluation with computed tomography (CT) or, less frequently, transabdominal ultrasound (US). The use of diagnostic peritoneal lavage in this setting has been replaced by less invasive and more sensitive techniques (CT and US). Akgur et al. compared the sensitivity and specificity of utilizing US versus diagnostic peritoneal lavage and found greater accuracy in detecting free intraperitoneal fluid by comparison with CT.[21] In cases of penetrating abdominal trauma, exploratory laparotomy is the rule. These children may or may not undergo diagnostic peritoneal lavage. All in all, there is no consensus as to how these children should be managed, and individual centers have differing protocols.

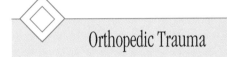

Orthopedic Trauma

Extremity injuries are common in children and growth plate injuries are more common in children than in adults. The Salter-Harris classification describes various fractures through the growth plate. Care of the injured extremity first involves control of actively bleeding sites, followed by palpation of pulses and a neurologic examination. Underlying vascular injuries must be ruled out; children may need arteriography to delineate the extent of vascular injury.

Orthopedic consultation should be obtained for all displaced fractures or when there is any question of neurovascular integrity. Imaging the extremity and sometimes the contralateral extremity for comparison is the rule. Pelvic fractures may be splinted and the patient immobilized for comfort prior to orthopedic consultation. Inferior vena cava and ureteric

injuries must be ruled out when pelvic fractures are present.

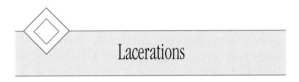

Lacerations

Lacerations are commonly seen in pediatric practice. They may be simple or complex and may or may not require referral to a specialist. All lacerations should be thoroughly inspected after irrigation with saline for extent, depth, and underlying fractures, and a history of immunizations should be taken. Lacerations that are greater than 6 h old are best left open unless they are large or when the risk of hemorrhage outweighs the risk of infection.

In general, antibiotics are not indicated unless there is concern for wounds that might extend to joints, synovial sheaths, or other important structures, requiring surgical exploration. Therefore, for lacerations of the volar aspect of the hand and fingers, or soles of feet, and for immunocompromised patients and those contaminated wounds or wounds more than 6 h old, antibiotics should be prescribed.

Skin closure may be achieved by using adhesive strips, glue, and/or sutures. Suturing remains the most common treatment modality. A relatively new product is 2-octyl cyanoacrylate (Dermabond topical skin adhesive; Ethicon, Inc.), recently approved for use in children who have simple lacerations not under tension; it is gaining in popularity. Advantages include decreased emergency department time and resource utilization and no need for sedation and monitoring after the procedure. Adhesive strips can be used for abrasions or minor lacerations. Many children will require sedation for laceration repair (see Chap. 11 "Sedation and Pain Control") in addition to topical anesthesia with TAC (tetracaine-adrenaline-cocaine) or LET (lidocaine-epinephrine-tetracaine). The timing of suture removal depends on the wound site. In general, face and scalp lacerations should be removed after 5 to 7 days and extremity sutures should be removed after 10 to 14 days.

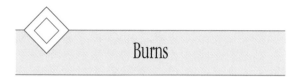

Burns

Burns are an important pediatric trauma problem because of their frequency, the morbidity associated with their care, and the high likelihood of scarring and impairment.

The type of burn incurred is generally dependent on the child's developmental status. Thus, nonmobile infants are scalded when hot liquid are spilled on them or when they are placed in contact with hot surfaces. Curious toddlers pull on cords, pots, and cups or step on hot coals. Mischievous school-aged children experiment with gasoline, and teenagers play with fireworks. Here we address issues related to the initial care of the burned child and to wound management.

RESUSCITATION

As discussed earlier, the first priority is given to the ABCs. The presence of soot in the mouth; singed nasal hairs, eyebrows, or face; neck burns; and hoarseness or stridor increase the chance that significant airway burns have occurred. When inhalational injuries and carbon monoxide poisoning have occurred, prophylactic tracheal intubation must be strongly considered. It is important to remember that variations in presentation, management, and complications occur depending on whether the burn is chemical or electrical and whether or not inhalational injury occurred.

Most clinicians are familiar with estimating the percentage of body burned (total body surface area, or TBSA) and the "rule of nines" and with estimating depth of burn injury. It is impor-

tant to remember, however, that burn depth can be estimated only grossly in the emergency department setting. As a rule, children who sustain a 10 percent or greater body burn and those with second-degree or greater burns should be referred to a burn center. Children who sustain circumferential burns or burns involving the face, hands, soles of feet, or perineum should also be referred to a burn center.

Intravenous fluids are usually initiated in patients who have greater than a 10 percent burn. Several formulas have been proposed to estimate fluid requirement in children. What is most important, here is to realize that the fluid requirement is greatest during the first 24 to 48 h and that these formulas serve only as guidelines to managing intake and output. Each patient is unique, and adequacy of resuscitation should be assessed by looking at hemodynamics, including urine output. At our institution, we use the Parkland formula for the first 24 h: 4 mL/kg per 100 mL TBSA. Isotonic crystalloid (normal saline, lactated Ringers), one-half over the first 8 h; one-quarter over the next 8 h. Maintain urine output between 0.5 and 1.0 mL/kg/h.

WOUND CARE

For patients presenting to the emergency department with minor burn wounds, the mainstay of treatment is to provide wound dressing and analgesia. There is, however, controversy regarding whether to leave blisters intact or to debride them. Although there are no data addressing this issue, proponents who leave blisters intact cite pain as the main problem with debridement, and those who support blister debridement cite risk of infection as the reason to intervene. Therefore, the final decision to debride or not is variable and should be made in consultation with a burn specialist. One strategy is to debride blisters larger than 2 cm when first seen and to debride smaller blisters after the first 48 h after healing has begun.

Burn wounds should be carefully inspected for extent of injury and infection. They should be cleaned and dressed. Silver sulfadiazene is the most widely used topical treatment of burn wounds.

PAIN CONTROL

Pain control is a major issue in burn care and many treatment modalities have been used to alleviate pain in children, including guided imagery, hypnotherapy, relaxation, and pharmacology. Of these, the mainstay of treatment is the use of opioids. Unfortunately, the amount of pain that children experience is all too often underestimated, especially during dressing changes. Individualized pain medication needs should be anticipated and given before the procedure starts. Tolerance develops in those patients receiving opioids over a period of time, and the need for large doses of opioids should not lead to a fear of dependence and to under-dosing. It is important to remember that burned patients will need background, breakthrough, and incident pain control (Table 9-6).

It is frequently difficult to separate anxiety from pain in young children. Tachycardia and hypertension occur under both conditions. Pre-verbal children are the most challenging sub-population of patients. Intubated children are also challenging because they are often para-lyzed; this does not mean that they are sedated. Both recall and the "awake but paralyzed state" are conditions we must avoid by adequately providing sedation and/or analgesia. The doses of drugs commonly used for sedation are provided in Table 9-7. A more extensive discussion of pain control and sedation is provided in Chap. 11.

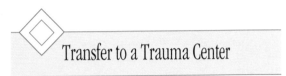

Transfer to a Trauma Center

The first tenet in practicing medicine is *primum no nocere* or "first do no harm." It is therefore important to be familiar with the ability of one's medical facility to deal with pediatric trauma. The availability of consultants with appropriate levels of expertise in taking care of children, functioning equipment, and trauma designation dictate whether or not these patients are best served at the facility. Should you decide to transfer a patient to a trauma center, initial stabilization of the patient should occur as described above. The transferring physician should speak to the accepting physician and both should decide on a mode of transfer: ground versus air; ALS (Advanced Life Support) versus BLS (Basic Life Support). Once the ABCs are secured, the patient is ready to be transported.

Table 9-6

Commonly Used Parenteral Opioid Equivalents

OPIOID	POTENCY	ROUTE	DOSE (MG/KG)
Meperidine	0.1	IM, IV	0.5–1.0
Morphine	1	IM, IV	0.05–0.1
Hydromorphone	5	IM, IV	0.01–0.02
Fentanyl	100	IV	0.001–0.002

Table 9-7

Doses of Drugs Commonly Used For Sedation

DRUG	ROUTE	DOSE (MG/KG)
Barbiturate		
Methohexital	Rectal	20–30
Benzodiazepines		
Diazepam	Oral	0.1–0.3
	Intravenous	0.1–0.3
	Rectal	0.2–0.3
Midazolam	Oral	0.5
	Intravenous	0.05–0.15
	Rectal	0.5
Ketamine	Oral	3–10
	Intravenous	1–3
	Intramuscular	2–10
Opioids		
Morphine	Intravenous	0.05–0.3
	Intramuscular	0.05–0.3
Meperidine	Intravenous	1–3
	Intramuscular	1–3
Fentanyl	Intravenous	0.001–0.005 (1–5 µg/kg)

Trauma Prevention

As physicians, our goals are to prevent morbidity and disability from pediatric trauma. With the most severe injuries, such as brain injuries and burns, these goals can be only partly realized. Prevention of the injuries from occurring must therefore receive our attention and energy.

Physicians can be involved in prevention at a number of different levels. Suggested educational interventions can be provided for families in the office, emergency department, and hospital setting. The physician can also be active in interventions in the community, joining others as members of a coalition to address a particular injury problem. Finally, the physician can become involved at a state or national level,

usually with legislative or regulatory interventions to prevent injuries.

In the office, injuries are best prevented by approaching them according to the developmental stage of the child and being specific with the advice given. Parents are much more likely to do something useful to decrease the risk of injury if told of one or two specific actions rather than being told to "childproof" the home. Table 9-8 illustrates the most common injuries occurring at different ages, along with the advice that should be provided for prevention.

For young infants, the most important measures are car-seat use, lowering the tap-water temperature, and installing smoke detectors. Young infants need to be in rear-facing car seats in the back seat of the car. Such children should *never* be placed in a front seat when there is an airbag. Lowering the tap-water temperature to 125°F or lower can prevent scald burns in these

Table 9-8

Developmental Approach to Injury Prevention:
A Guide to Office Counseling

Newborn to 1 year
  Car seats
  Tap-water temperature
  Smoke detectors in kitchen and bedrooms
1 to 4 years
  Bathtub safety: no unsupervised bathing
  Poison-control number on phone
  Toddler and booster-seat use
5 to 9 years
  Bicycle helmets
  Pedestrian safety
  Booster-seat and seat-belt use
10 to 14 years
  Seat belts
  Multipurpose sports helmets
  Safe storage of guns
15 to 19 years
  Seat-belt use
  Safe storage of guns
  Drinking and driving

children. Smoke detectors in the child's bedroom as well as outside the kitchen are an extremely cheap way to protect a family from fire death.

When children are a bit older, parents should be cautioned about the use of baby walkers. These can pose a serious risk of injury from falls down steps or burns when these infants roll around the kitchen. In addition, these devices have been found, if anything, to slow development; there is no evidence that they help the infant to walk earlier.

The toddler should graduate to a forward-facing car seat still secured in the *rear seat* of the car. Poisonings become a risk at this age and can be avoided by the use of childproof caps on all medications and removing access to household poisons. These children are at increased risk of drowning, especially from swimming pools. Any pool should be protected with a four-sided fence and participants in any boating activities should always wear life jackets.

The young school-aged child is at risk for pedestrian and bicycle injuries. Pedestrian injuries can be prevented by assuming that the child does not have the developmental skills to cross streets safely alone until about age 9 or 10. The most serious bicycle-related injuries are to the head; helmets decrease the risk of brain injury by 88 percent.

Older children and young teens continue to be at risk of motor vehicle injuries and should always be properly restrained with a lap-shoulder belt. They are at risk of bicycle related head injuries and of drowning, although usually in open bodies of water and not in pools. Males in particular are also at risk from play with guns, leading to unintentional shooting deaths. Home ownership of guns is a very sensitive issue for most families; however, many are receptive to the idea of safe storage of guns in a gun safe or lock box.

Teenagers are at greatest risk of motor vehicle–related injuries. Seat-belt use at this age is going to depend on building a habit of use earlier as well as continued modeling by parents and older siblings. Suicide and homicide occur all too commonly at this age. It is important to realize that most of these are committed with guns. Safe storage of guns has the potential to decrease access to guns among suicidal adolescents as well as prevent theft of guns in home burglaries.

Conclusions

Pediatric trauma is an important problem for the child health care provider because of its incidence and potential for death and long-term disability. Although definitive care of trauma will rest with the surgeon, understanding how to treat trauma as well as how to prevent it is a necessary skill in pediatric practice.

References

1. Barlow B, Miemirska M, Gandhi RP, Leblanc W: Ten years experience with falls from a height in children. *J Pediatr Surg* 18:509–511, 1983.

2. Vernon DD, Furnival RA, Hansen KW, et al: Effect of a pediatric trauma response team on emergency department treatment time and mortality of pediatric trauma victims. *Pediatrics* 103: 20–24, 1999.

3. Knudson MM, Shagoury C, Lewis FR: Can adult trauma surgeons care for injured children? *J Trauma* 32:729–737, 1992.

4. Committee on Trauma, American College of Surgeons: *Advanced Trauma Life Support Course.* Chicago, ACS, 1993, pp 261–281.

5. Jo Rice L, Britton JT: Airway management, in Eichelberger MR (ed): *Pediatric Trauma: Prevention, Acute Care and Rehabilitation.* St. Louis, Mosby–Year Book, 1993, pp 162–168.

6. Pigula FA, Wald SL, Shackford SR, Vane DW: The effect of hypotension and hypoxia on children with severe head injuries. *J Pediatr Surg* 28:310–314, 1993.

7. Muizelaar JP, Marmarou A, Ward JD, et al: Adverse effects of prolonged hyperventilation in patients with severe head injury: a randomized clinical trial. *J Neurosurg* 75:731–739, 1991.

8. Brain Trauma Foundation: Guidelines for the management of severe head injury. *J Neurotrauma* 13:639–734, 1996.

9. Lang EW, Chesnut RM: Intracranial pressure and cerebral perfusion pressure in severe head injury. *New Horiz* 3:400–409, 1995.

10. Rivara F, Tanaguchi D, Parish RA, et al: Poor prediction of positive computed tomographic scans by clinical criteria in symptomatic pediatric head trauma. *Pediatrics* 80:579–584, 1987.

11. Nagy KK, Joseph KT, Krosner SM, et al: The utility of head computed tomography after minimal head injury. *J Trauma* 46:268–270, 1999.

12. Quayle KS, Jaffe DM, Kuppermann N, et al: Diagnostic testing for acute head injury in children: when are head computed tomography and skull radiographs indicated? *Pediatrics* 99:E11, 1997.

13. Davis RL, Mullen N, Makela M, et al: Cranial computed tomography scans in children after minimal head injury with loss of consciousness. *Ann Emerg Med* 24:640–645, 1994.

14. Hahn YS, McLone DG: Risk factors in the outcome of children with minor head injury. *Pediatr Neurosurg* 19:135–142, 1993.

15. Hahn YS, McLone DG: Risk factors in the outcome of children with minor head injury. *Pediatr Neurosurg* 19:135–142, 1993.

16. Rachesky I, Boyce WT, Duncan B, et al: Clinical prediction of cervical spine injuries in children. Radiographic abnormalities. *Am J Dis Child* 141: 199–201, 1987.

17. Dietrich AM, Ginn-Pease ME, Bartkowski HM, King DR: Pediatric cervical spine fractures: predominantly subtle presentation. *J Pediatr Surg* 26:995–999, 1991.

18. Jaffe DM, Binns H, Radkowski MA, et al: Developing a clinical algorithm for early management of cervical spine injury in child trauma victims. *Ann Emerg Med* 16:270–276, 1987.

19. Anderson PA, Rivara FP, Maier RV, Drake C. The epidemiology of seatbelt-associated injuries. *J Trauma* 31:60–67, 1991.

20. Sturm PF, Glass RBJ, Sivit CJ, Eichelberger MR: Lumbar compression fractures secondary to lapbelt use in children. *J Pediatr Orthop* 15:521–523, 1995.

21. Akgur FM, Aktug T, Olguner M, et al: Prospective study investigating routine usage of ultrasonography as the initial diagnostic modality for the evaluation of children sustaining blunt abdominal trauma. *J Trauma* 42:626–628, 1997.

22. Andrews JS: Conscious sedation in the pediatric emergency department. *Curr Opin Pediatr* 7:309–313, 1995.

Abraham B. Bergman
Kenneth W. Feldman

Chapter

Child Abuse

One of the most difficult tasks in medicine is having to deal with children whose injuries have been inflicted by others. It is not that extensive knowledge or complex skills are required. Rather, the situation is challenging because the emotional stakes are high, considerable energy may be required to control the physician's own abhorrence of the abusive act and a feeling that no good may result from one's efforts. In this chapter we attempt to show that most primary care clinicians can capably deal with the vast majority of abused children and that this involvement need not entail extensive legal involvement. For this to happen, it is imperative that there be a clear understanding of what the clinician can contribute and, more importantly, what the clinician cannot contribute in cases of child abuse.

Child abuse can be broadly or narrowly defined. As used in this chapter, the term covers physical injury, sexual abuse, physical neglect, and emotional abuse. Though little is said here about emotional abuse, it assuredly produces infinitely more cumulative morbidity in children than does physical abuse. Besharov says that "emotional abuse is an assault on the child's psyche, just as physical abuse is an assault on the child's body."[1] Unless there is devastating brain injury, the injuries inflicted by physical abuse eventually heal. The act or acts of sexual abuse do not produce permanent physical injury. Rather, the damage to the child in such cases comes from having to grow up in an environment where basic trust and protection do not exist. We deal with physical abuse not because it is more important but because it is definable, and procedures exist for dealing with it. We observe abuse of the psyche in much the same way as physicians observed pneumococcal pneumonia in the era prior to antibiotics. One hopes that feasible approaches for dealing with emotional abuse will someday emerge. For now we deal with what we can.

Historical Perspective

Physical abuse was not "discovered" as a medical entity until 1946, when John Caffey, a pediatric radiologist, described a series of children with multiple fractures of the long bones along with chronic subdural hematomas.[2] The entity was not recognized by clinicians for another 20 years. A vivid recollection in the mind of one of us (ABB) is that of a case conference during internship in 1959 where a child with multiple fractures of different ages was discussed. The radiologist said, "trauma," but he was ignored. The discussion among the clinicians centered not on whether but which particular metabolic bone disease was affecting the child. In 1962 a group of clinicians in Denver led by Henry Kempe coined the term *battered child*[3] and instituted a successful campaign throughout the United States to mandate the reporting of child abuse and neglect.

It was not until the 1970s, however, when child protection teams became available in most medical centers, that most physicians began to recognize and report child abuse. At the same time sexual abuse began to be recognized; and in the 1980s partner abuse was "discovered" by physicians. All of these violent behaviors had, of course, existed all through history. They emerged into the open, however, only after societal values changed and the behaviors were deemed to be unacceptable.

The clinician's responsibility in abuse is limited and straightforward—to make the diagnosis, treat the child's injuries, and make a report to the proper authorities. Though more is said below, in most cases the diagnosis is not difficult. Not included in the clinician's job description is acting as a police officer (i.e., conducting an investigation of who inflicted the injuries) or social worker (i.e., deciding who should care for the child). Neither should the clinician rush to judgment and assume the role of avenging angel. Furthermore, just as important as diagnosing injuries is identifying those that are unintentional (accidental) and differentiating poor parental judgment from true neglect. For example, the lack of a functioning smoke alarm or not restraining a child properly in a car are both unwise, but such actions do not warrant intervention by state authorities. On the other hand, an infant who fails to gain weight from not receiving enough calories probably does require state protection.

Epidemiology

The true incidence of child abuse is difficult to ascertain. So much depends on the criteria used for diagnosis, the frequency with which the diagnosis is reported to authorities, the criteria used by investigative agencies to substantiate abuse, whether the reports are recorded in an accurate registry, and whether the registry is available to investigators. The importance of accuracy of a registry is exemplified by a retrospective study of infant deaths in North Carolina, a state with an excellent medical examiner system. It that study, 60 percent of the homicides determined to be due to abuse were not coded as such by the health department's vital records system.[4] In reality, child abuse is the main cause of death by trauma in infants under 12 months.

From the perspective of the practitioner, the incidence numbers mean little. What is important to know is that although cases of abuse do not arise every day, anyone practicing primary care is apt to see one or two children a year who are physically or sexually abused. Physicians who practice in emergency departments and among families living in poverty will see more such children.

Origins of Child Abuse

The likelihood of an individual child being abused is enhanced or diminished depending on the culture in which the child is raised, the characteristics and behaviors of the child itself, the social stresses on the family, and the background and personality of those who care for the child. Bittner and Newberger have formulated a model for understanding child abuse that takes these factors into account (Table 10-1).[5]

Sociocultural Factors

Children are safer in environments where they are valued, rather than being regarded more as property. This value transcends poverty. In some cultures there are individuals, usually middle-aged or older women, who are known to "look after" children in troubled living situations. We often see this in black and Hispanic communities. In contrast, children are more vulnerable where corporal punishment is rampant and where visitors to the home are discouraged. Thus children in poor white families living in isolation are at relatively high risk. Abuse is seen more frequently in military populations, where relatively young parents cope with the stresses of child rearing far away from family support systems.

Child Characteristics

Some children are more difficult to care for than others. Those born prematurely, who are handicapped, who are developmentally delayed, or who are hyperactive may often require more patience than a caretaker may possess. Children's temperaments, of course, vary, and temperament can also contribute to the risk of abuse. The combination of an exuberant, independent child and a controlling caretaker with little tolerance is risky. Most serious injuries occur in very young children. About two-thirds of reported cases of physical abuse involve children below age 5. Brain injuries and fractures are most common in infants; burns and abdominal injuries in toddlers.

Perpetrator Characteristics

The public perception of a "child abuser" is that of a fiend with fangs and a tail who preys upon children. Although there are instances of calculated cruelty, (e.g., multiple cigarette burns) they are fortunately rare. The majority of physical abuse is intended as discipline and occurs as a sudden, impulsive act of violence. The perpetrator "loses control" and lashes out. The seriousness of the injury depends on the degree of force used and the age of the child. If a caretaker is unemployed, feels worthless, and has grown up in a culture of violence, the setup for abuse is present. Alcohol is a great potentiator of violence. The most frequent triggering events are, in infants, crying that will not stop ("Damn it, shut up!"), or, in toddlers, toilet accidents ("I'll teach you to crap on the floor!") and refusal to eat ("You damn well are going to eat that food on your plate!") Older children are punished for a variety of real or perceived transgressions. The caretaker may attribute willfulness or malice to the child's actions and expect obedience that is

Table 10-1
Model for Understanding Child Abuse

Sociocultural Factors

Values and norms concerning violence and force; acceptability of corporal punishment
Inegalitarian, hierarchical social structure; imbalanced interpersonal relationships
Values concerning competition versus cooperation
Exploitative, alienating economic system; acceptance and encouragement of permanent poor class
Devaluation of children and other dependents
Institutional manifestations of the above factors in areas such as law, health care, education, welfare system, sports, and entertainment

Family Stresses

Parent-produced stresses
  Low self-esteem
  Abused as child
  Depression
  Substance abuse
  Character disorder
  Ignorance of child rearing
  Unrealistic expectations
Child-produced stresses
  Physical difference (e.g., handicapped)
  Mental difference (e.g., retarded)
  Temperamental difference (e.g., difficult)
  Behavioral difference (e.g., hyperactive)
  Foster child
Social-situational stresses
Structural factors
  Poverty
  Unemployment
  Mobility, isolation, poor housing
  Parental relationship patterns of discord and assault, domination/submission

Parent-child relationship
  Attachment problems
  Perinatal stress
  Punitive child-rearing style
  Scapegoating
  Role reversal
  Excess or unwanted children
  Triggering situation
  Discipline argument
  Family conflict
  Substance abuse
  Acute environmental problem
  Lack of money
  Maltreatment
  Injury
  Inability to provide care
  Poisoning
  Psychological problems

beyond the developmental capacity of an infant or child.

A change has taken place in over the past 30 years in the types of abuse that present to a clinician. The originally described "battered baby" was an undergrown infant with multiple fractures of different ages, sometimes with a subdural hematoma, the injuries having been inflicted by the infant's mother. Fortunately such victims of chronic abuse are now seen only rarely, a tribute to the increased diagnostic skills of physicians and the presence in all states of protective services. Now we are more likely to see acute injuries in previously healthy infants and children.

There has been no diminution in the incidence or severity of severe abuse, including homicide. Our community (Seattle) is probably typical. We have seen between four and eight child homicides a year for over 25 years.

There has also been a shift in the gender of perpetrators. Serious injuries are now more apt to be inflicted by men, especially those who are not the fathers of the children, the "baby-sitting boyfriends." The relatively few women who inflict serious injuries are apt to have obvious psychiatric impairments, either through illness and/or drugs and alcohol. Several related factors have contributed to this gender shift, such as more children in single-parent families, reduced economic status of single-parent families, lack of affordable child care, and reliance on inappropriate caretakers. Cohabiting males who are drafted into child care duties while the mother works is a "setup" for adversity. Questions about child care arrangements should be a part of health supervision visits.

The connection between physical abuse and domestic violence should be recognized. Questions about domestic violence should be a part of child abuse investigations and vice versa. Common features of the perpetrators include poor self-image, need to assert power, history of being abused as a child, poor impulse control, and problems with drugs and/or alcohol.

Diagnosis

The diagnosis of abuse in most cases is straightforward. The main obstacles to accurate diagnosis are reluctance on the part of the clinician to entertain the possibility of abuse and a focus on treatment of the injury without considering how it occurred. The reluctance to consider abuse occurs more often when the clinician and family know each other and the family is middle or upper class. Multidisciplinary protection teams exist in most pediatric medical centers. Referral to such centers is indicated when the diagnosis is in doubt and/or assistance with the psychosocial and legal aspects are needed.

The first words of the history provided by the parents or caretaker are important and should be recorded verbatim. If abuse is suspected, it is important not to challenge the history or point out inconsistencies if the story changes. Further verbal evidence should be documented; hearsay evidence may be admitted in court if properly elicited and preserved.[6] Visible injuries should be documented by photographs.[7] If a good camera is not available or if lighting is poor, a sketch may be more reliable than a photograph.

Table 10-2 lists circumstances in the history that strongly suggest abuse. *The most crucial*

Table 10-2

Caregiver Risk Factors Making Abuse More Likely

Explanation of injury is not plausible
Explanations are inconsistent or change
The seriousness of the child's condition
   is understated
There is delay in obtaining treatment
Caregiver cannot be located
Male caregiver is not the child's father
History of domestic violence
History of substance abuse

points are an explanation of the injury that is not plausible or explanations that change and are inconsistent. When there is uncertainty, the clinician should not feel obliged to come up with an immediate determination about the cause of the injuries as long as the injuries are treated and the safety of the child is assured. Consultation with other specialists—such as radiologists, ophthalmologists, orthopedic surgeons, neurosurgeons, and burn surgeons—is often helpful. It is just as important to designate an injury as accidental when this is the case, and thus clear caretakers of suspicion, as it is to identify an injury that is intentionally inflicted.

Sadly, it is now common for abuse to be alleged in bitter custody disputes. It is well to remember that clinicians do not serve as agents for protective services workers, lawyers, or police officers; we work on behalf of our patients.

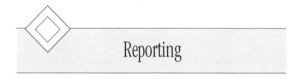

Reporting

When there is reason to believe that an injury may have been inflicted, laws in all states mandate a report to protective services or a law enforcement agency. The law does not require the diagnosis of abuse to be certain, just that there is reasonable cause to suspect abuse. Our practice is to report all serious injuries (i.e., when hospitalization occurs) to both the police and protective services. In cases of "poor parenting," where injuries have not been inflicted, we tend to refer to public health nurses. Nurses can make both physical and psychosocial assessments and are generally more readily welcomed into homes than protective services workers.

Families need to hear directly from physicians when the diagnosis of abuse is being considered and when a report to protective services is made. The "confrontation" is not as scary as it seems. More often than not the air is cleared

and the clinician can concentrate on treating the child. Words like these can be used:

> "I do not believe that these injuries occurred by a fall from the couch. *Someone* injured your child. I am required therefore, under the law, to make a report to the authorities, who will investigate further and try to sort matters out." The term *someone* is used advisedly. We can only say that the child's injuries were inflicted; not who inflicted them.

The natural expectation is that upon delivery of such news, the parents will rise up in wrath, but this rarely occurs. The more common reaction is sullen sadness. That is because often the person who inflicted the injuries is not present. But even when he or she is present, because the diagnosis is usually not a surprise, resignation is the most common response. What happens afterwards depends on what resources are available. Ideally, a team approach is best. The clinician makes the diagnosis and cares for the child's injuries. A social worker undertakes more extensive evaluation of the family, especially the care arrangements for the child, and serves as liaison with other agencies (police and protective services).

If a child is not judged to be in a safe setting and might be harmed, we delay informing the caretaker of a protective services report. In cases of sexual abuse also, for which the child's history is the most significant part of the evidence, authorities should interview the child before caretakers are informed.

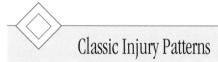

Classic Injury Patterns

Bruises

Bruises associated with excessive punishment are the most common manifestation of abuse. Accidental bruises are, of course, omnipresent in active toddlers. The difference between bruises of abuse and those that toddlers normally sustain lies in their location and the age of the child. Normal bruising appears in prominent surfaces over bones, such as forearms, elbows, hips, brows, and shins. Bruises on the buttocks, back, flank, genitalia, and the dorsal surfaces of the hands and feet are less likely to be accidental. Likewise, nonmobile infants rarely inflict bruises on themselves. In a study of 973 children under age 3 during well-child visits, our Seattle colleagues found that 21 percent had accidental bruises. However only 0.6 percent of infants younger than 6 months had bruises, compared with 19.3 percent of those aged 9 to 11 months and 49.4 percent of 18- to 23-month olds. Similarly, only 2.2 percent of children who were not walking had bruises, compared with 52 percent of those who walked. The authors concluded that abuse should be suspected if bruises are found on infants younger than 9 months who are not mobile and when they are seen in atypical areas such as the abdomen, hands, or buttocks of older children.[8]

Although the color of bruises evolves, the timing remains an inexact science. The only validated color dating is the absence of yellowing prior to 18 h after the onset of injury.[9] In addition to being struck, shaken, or thrown, injuries can be inflicted by objects such as belts, cigarettes, hangers, etc. The mark left on the skin may suggest that object used in the attack, such as a belt (Fig. 10-1, see Color Plate 19).

Skeletal Trauma

Most abusive fractures are caused by twisting or pulling an extremity, producing injury to the metaphysis, or by shaking a child so hard that the flailing limbs cause traction on the ends of the long bones (Fig. 10-2). In addition to metaphyseal fractures, skeletal injuries highly associated with abuse are fractures of the posterior ribs, scapula, spinous processes, and sternum. Spiral fractures of the femur and humerus before the age of walking also suggest abuse.

Figure 10-2

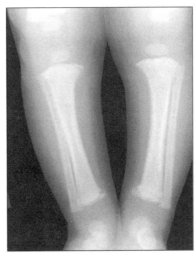

Metaphyseal fractures. This child somewhat over 2 months of age, also had facial bruising and an immersion burn of the buttocks as well as multiple fractures of the ribs and arms. Both tibial plateaus have metaphyseal chip fractures medially and bucket-handle fractures are present distally. Early periosteal new bone formation reflects initial healing of the fractures. This type of fracture results from traction on the metaphysis through the stronger joint ligaments and is virtually specific for inflicted injury.

Head Injuries

Most abuse deaths involve injuries to the brain. Debate continues as to whether these serious brain injuries occur as a result of being shaken or whether a hard impact is also necessary. It matters little; the forces required in either case are extreme. The results of head trauma include subdural and subarachnoid hemorrhage and primary brain injury, including diffuse axonal injury. Secondary effects of brain swelling and hypoxic/ischemic events can add to the injury, causing herniation, infarction, and brain death. These injuries are usually accompanied by retinal hemorrhages. (Fig. 10-3, see Color Plate 20). Uncomplicated skull fractures and epidural hemorrhages are usually *not* associated with abuse. Can a subdural hematoma or diffuse axonal damage be produced by a 2-ft fall off a couch or bed, a common story when such children are admitted to the hospital? Falls of less than 10 ft are unlikely to produce serious or life-threatening injuries in infants and children.[10] When confronted with such a story from parents or caretakers we say: "Anything is possible. The sun might also rise in the West, but it's highly unlikely. The type of injury your child sustained is similar to that seen in a high-speed motor vehicle crash or a 5-story fall onto cement."

Abdominal Injuries

Abdominal injuries are the second most common cause of child homicide, occurring as a result of a hard blow from a fist or a foot. Because the symptoms are nonspecific (vomiting, abdominal distention) and bruising is rarely present, the diagnosis is often delayed or missed. Injuries to the intestine, either rupture or hematoma, are more common than solid-organ trauma.

Burns

Tap-water scald burns constitute a significant proportion of serious abuse. They usually occur in the course of punishment for fecal soiling. The buttocks and legs are immersed in hot water while the caretaker holds firmly onto the trunk. A well-demarcated circumferential burn results. Depending on how the child is held, and how it reacts, the feet may be spared. Petechiae or finger marks on the trunk may occur where the child was restrained during immersion. Burns from contact with hot solids or smoldering objects such as cigarettes are more likely to have been inflicted if they are found on usually unexposed body parts.

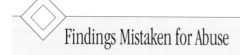

Findings Mistaken for Abuse

To the consternation of all concerned, a number of conditions are mistakenly suspected to be

abuse and reported to the authorities. To the uninitiated, Mongolian spots, the concentration of melanocytes over the sacrum and buttocks prevalent in dark-skinned children, are sometimes mistaken for bruising (Fig. 10-4, see Color Plate 21). Likewise, emergency medical and law enforcement personnel happening upon infants who have died misinterpret postmortem livedo, where blood settles to the dependent portions of the body at the time the heart stops beating and circulation ceases.

Folks remedies practiced mostly by recent immigrants are also mistaken for abuse. Among the most common are coining (*Cao Gio*) (Fig. 10-5, see Color Plate 22) and cupping (Fig. 10-6, see Color Plate 23).

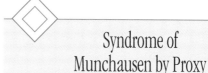

Syndrome of Munchausen by Proxy

Munchausen by proxy syndrome (MBPS), where a parent, usually the mother, systematically fabricates information about their child's health or intentionally makes the child ill, is an especially dangerous form of child abuse. If a child escapes death or serious injury, he or she is subjected is severe emotional trauma, the scars of which are difficult to erase. In July 1997, a moving article by Mary Bryk appeared in *Pediatrics* describing how her mother inflicted terrible injuries on her over an 8-year period. She said:

> My earliest memory of abuse is between the ages of 2 and 3. I was in the high chair with the tray pulled tightly to my chest. I could barely breathe, let alone move. My left leg was tied to the leg of the high chair with a dish towel. My hands were bound to prevent me from pulling at my mother's hair. She was very angry at me for fighting her. Her words were always the same and repeated frequently over the next several years: 'I'm doing this for your own good. The doctor wants me to do this treatment to make you better.' As the blows of the hammer were hitting my foot, all I

could understand was the pain. I came to believe it was my fault she was angry. I was not a good girl. I needed to try harder to please her so she would love me.11

Another chilling portrayal of MSBP has been provided by Southall and colleagues, who videotaped mothers attempting to smother infants brought to a hospital for evaluation of recurrent apnea.[12]

In addition to actively inflicting injuries or producing illnesses, MSBP presents in a wide variety of forms. Examples are fabricating the symptoms and signs of illness, doctor shopping, perceiving a well child to be ill, and enforcing invalidism on a child who is well, or has a minor illness. The victims are the quintessential "vulnerable children," where the parent has a deep-seated need for the child to be ill.

The American Professional Society on the Abuse of Children has recommended making separate diagnoses for a child who is the victim of illness falsification and for the motivation of a parent to falsify illness. The initial judgment about the child's need for protection should be based on the gravity of the child's injury or risk of injury, while the prognosis for remediation and treatment will depend on the caretaker's diagnosis.

MSBP frequently goes unrecognized; when it is found, intervention is difficult. Unlike the perpetrators of physical abuse, Munchausen parents may appear respectable and earnest to judges who have little knowledge of the entity. Fathers are typically passive and uninvolved, and mothers produce reams of documents to demonstrate how attentive they have been. Confrontation usually results in the child being taken to more gullible physicians. Counseling has little effect because of the lack of insight and deep-seated need for attention demonstrated by the mothers. *MSBP should be considered a medical emergency.* Even with all the attendant difficulties, victims of MSBP are at higher risk than victims of beatings or burnings; thus efforts at intervention should be made. Because of the complexity of the issues involved, consultation with a child

protection team should be strongly considered when the diagnosis of MSBP is considered.

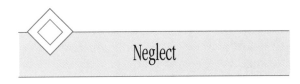

Neglect

Many more reports to protective services are made for neglect than for abuse. The criteria for reporting and for intervention, however, vary between individuals and from place to place. The distinction between "poor parenting" and true child neglect is not clear and begs the question as to when the power of the state (i.e., protective services intervention) should be invoked. The issue is especially sensitive in dealing with families of different cultures and social classes, where the norms of child care may differ. Another "gray zone" is medical neglect, where children do not receive the treatment prescribed by physicians.

As mentioned previously, when we have questions about child care, and there are not acute issues at hand, we tend to refer families to public health nurses for investigation. The most common reasons for neglect referrals are maternal substance abuse, especially in the neonatal period; acute mental illness; and failure of the infant to thrive. Children need to be fed, clothed, housed, protected from harm, and sent to school. When these responsibilities are not carried out, the state is obliged to ascertain the reasons and help provide remedies. The key is not so much concern about parental behavior but rather whether there are tangible signs that the child is adversely effected by the behavior.

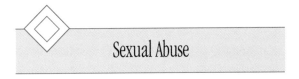

Sexual Abuse

Sexual abuse is defined as activity with a child under the age of consent that is carried out for the sexual gratification of an adult. The vast majority of instances occur with a family member or other person known to the child; stranger-offenders are rare. Accurate incidence data are virtually impossible to obtain; many cases are never reported, and as many as half the reports of sexual abuse to protective services are not verified. This is because (1) young children themselves cannot give a history, (2) confirmatory physical and/or laboratory findings are rare, and (3) caretakers are often oversensitive to nonspecific signs such as diaper rash, enuresis, and dysuria. Also, the allegation of sexual abuse has become all too common in child custody disputes. That there are many unsubstantiated cases, however, does not negate the fact that sexual abuse is not rare, and that several instances a year are apt to be seen in any primary care practice.

Initial Examination

Excellent guidelines for the evaluation of child sexual abuse have been developed by the American Academy of Pediatrics.[13] Needless to say, when a child with suspected sexual abuse is brought for evaluation, the emotional stakes are high. It is important for the clinician to display a calm, competent demeanor and attempt, insofar as possible, to put the child at ease. The clinician should not take orders from caretakers or law enforcement officials about the type of examination to carry out; the child's interests are paramount.

The purposes of the examination should be to identify and treat injuries or associated medical conditions and to evaluate and assist the patient and family in a time of emotional crisis. This includes assessing the safety of the child. As in physical abuse, initial statements are important. The history provided by the adult and especially a verbatim report from the child should be documented if possible. The medical findings should also be documented and forensic evidence collected.

The examination should be conducted with good light and magnification. An otoscope without a speculum will suffice for a screening examination. If abnormalities are suspected, the child should be referred for expert examination and photographic documentation. It should be remembered, however, that even in the face of penetrating genital trauma in girls, it is more common than not for the genital examination to be normal.[14]

A referral for medical care and counseling should be made, as well as a report to protective services. Terms like *history of sexual abuse*, or *concern of sexual abuse* should be used for the diagnosis. *Rape* is a legal term, not a medical diagnosis, and should not be used in the medical record.

Triage Decisions

If there is a *clear* report by a child or a witness that genital contact occurred within the prior 72 h, a medical/forensic examination as soon as possible is appropriate. The child should not bathe before the examination, and the clothing worn at the time of abuse should not be changed. If the clinician is unequipped to handle forensic samples and to maintain a chain of evidence, the child is best referred to a setting like an emergency department where these procedures are done. On the other hand, if there is a vague report or concern that abuse occurred within the prior 72 h, the decision for an emergency exam must be made on a case-by-case basis.

If there is a clear report that abuse occurred but that the last contact was more than 72 h prior and there are no physical signs or symptoms, a medical/forensic examination is not indicated on an emergency basis. The patient should be referred to a designated sexual assault center or counselor for crisis support, with the medical evaluation scheduled after counseling.

Dealing with the Legal System

Most physicians are understandably wary about dealing with the legal justice system. Reporting abuse to protective or police authorities may lead to a sizable investment of time and effort away from one's ordinary medical duties. However, some basic knowledge about how the legal system works may minimize the "hassle" and further the interests of our child-patients. Above all, it is important not to be intimidated and to appreciate the different perspectives of the legal and medical worlds. For beginners, it is prudent to accept the premise that a *legal proceeding is not a dispassionate search for the truth but rather an adversarial exercise.* Both sides try to bring out anything that helps their case and suppress anything that harms their case.

In child abuse, a clinician is most apt to be asked to give testimony in a criminal trial of the supposed perpetrator or to appear in a family court dealing with placement of a child. One may be asked to testify as a treating clinician, as an expert witness, or both. There is a difference. The physician who treated the patient is obliged to respond. More often than not, however, a written report or a copy of the hospital or office chart will suffice. There is rarely any dispute about the injuries incurred by the child, just about how they occurred. Insist that you will add nothing in oral testimony that is not already written in the chart. Such insistence my obviate a court appearance. If you do have to appear, most courts will try to accommodate a physician's schedule.

Expert Witness

If you are called as an expert witness, you "call the shots." That means you discuss beforehand what you might say, when you are available to appear, and your fee. When travel and waiting times are included, it is rare to be able to spend less than half a day in court testimony. Sometimes lawyers on both sides of the case say that they cannot talk to you beforehand because they are "too busy." That means they are not taking the interests of their clients seriously. We insist on speaking to them beforehand. Every lawyer wants to know what their witnesses plan to say and no one wants a hostile medical witness. Not surprisingly, the most experienced and prestigious attorneys tend to be the most solicitous of a physician's time. Less experienced attorneys may need education about the medical issues.

The term *expert* has different interpretations in the medical and legal worlds. To clinicians, the profile of an expert might be a medical school professor who has written 40 papers on some narrow subject. Most courts, on the other hand, will consider any physician who has read about, attended lectures on, and dealt with cases of child abuse during residency to be an expert. Generally, any pediatrician is considered to be an expert on children.

Subpoenas

Subpoenas sound imposing and with their arcane language are meant to be intimidating. Do not fall for this. Subpoenas are a way for lawyers to cover their backs by "documenting" that they have prepared their case. Above all, pay no attention to the dates and times for a court appearance listed on the subpoena. If you do, you will be sitting in an empty courtroom. Ignore attempts at intimidation. Once again, any lawyer who is serious about obtaining the testimony of a clinician will call to make arrangements beforehand, provide information about the inevitable court schedule changes, and fit the appearance into a mutually convenient time.

When testifying, stick to what you know, which is usually the medical diagnosis, and not who inflicted the injuries or where the child should be placed. Avoid sounding partisan: "Just the facts, doctor." Trials invariably take place many months or even years after the child has been seen in the hospital or office. Always have the hospital or office record in your hands and do not hesitate to refer to it. The quality of concurrent documentation is paramount. Attempting to recall details not recorded in the chart is risky.

The two most common questions asked of medical witnesses are: "What was the mechanism for producing the injury?" and "When did the injury occur?" Sometimes these questions can be answered easily—because of belt marks, a blow to the abdomen, blunt trauma to the head, bathtub immersion immediately prior to admission—but sometimes they are difficult. Invariably lawyers want more precision than physicians are able to provide. Again, do not be badgered. If you do not know, say so!

The timing of bruises and old fractures is notoriously imprecise; you must usually provide ranges rather than exact times. Consult a radiologist, pathologist, orthopedist, neurosurgeon, and/or ophthalmologist, but incorporate their views into your own. In other words, a primary care physician can interpret x-rays or retinal photographs to the jury.

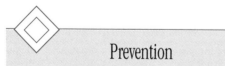

Prevention

Efforts to prevent child abuse are professed much and practiced little. The pathetic stories of battered babies punctuate newspaper and television news programs. Indignant "calls for action" by politicians and the appointment of blue-ribbon task forces are as ubiquitous as elevator background music, but little happens. The incidence of serious child abuse has not diminished. The tragedy is that even though we know

how to reduce the incidence of child abuse, that knowledge is not put to use. Following are some suggestions on prevention that can be employed at both the community and individuals levels.

Community Intervention

Henry Kempe and his Denver colleagues had three main objectives in the mid 1960s when they began to raise the consciousness of American physicians about child abuse. Two of their objectives were achieved: recognition of child abuse and establishment of protective services in all 50 states. Another objective was not achieved; deployment of "home visitors" to assist troubled families before abuse took place. Olds and colleagues convincingly demonstrated that regular home nursing visits to high-risk families reduce the incidence of abuse and other disorders of parenting.[15] Parenting education programs are helpful, but unfortunately they tend to attract "the converted." Community outreach to high-risk families who do not attend meetings or bring their children for health supervision visits are imperative. Crisis-care programs that provide immediate assistance to parents in times of crisis, and therapeutic preschools for children who have already been abused are other important components of community child abuse services.

Individual Intervention

There is much that can be done on an individual basis to identify infants at risk for abuse and to provide supportive services. The key is be sensitive to the clues and be willing to intervene. Table 10-3 is a high-risk checklist prepared describing behaviors that should "raise the red flag" in the prenatal period, delivery room, maternity ward, and physician's office. These behaviors are not specific for child abuse but are risk factors and warrant surveillance for disturbances of parenting. Once again, the best

Table 10-3

Child Abuse and Neglect—High-Risk Checklist for Infants

A. Prenatal observation and data
  1. —— The mother conceals the pregnancy (e.g., no prenatal care)
  2. —— Abortion is unsuccessfully sought or attempted.
  3. —— Relinquishment for adoption is sought, then reversed.
  4. —— No "nesting" behavior (e.g., preparation of layette).
  5. —— Unwed mother without emotional support.
  6. —— History of severe marital discord.
  7. —— History of serious mental illness, institutionalization, current depression, or repeated foster homes for either parent.
  8. —— History of drug addiction or alcoholism in either parent (very high risk if the mother is currently addicted)
  9. —— History of violent behavior or prison sentence in either parent.
  10. —— History of previous abuse or neglect of another child[a]
B. Delivery room observations
  1. —— Rejection of the baby (e.g., mother does not want to see him or touch it)[a]
  2. —— Premature baby.
  3. —— Infant born by cesarean section.
C. Maternity ward observations
  1. —— Lack of claiming behavior or maternal attachment by 48 h of age. (e.g., mother does not want to hold feed, or name her baby; no signs of cuddling, rocking, eye contact, or talking to the baby).[a]
  2. —— Disparaging remarks about the baby (e.g., that it is ugly, defective, a disappointment, mean, bad, etc.).[a]
  3. —— Repulsion at the baby's drooling, regurgitation, urine, stools, etc.
  4. —— The mother feeds her baby in a mechanical or other inappropriate way.
  5. —— A postpartum depression (this may mean the mother is overwhelmed).[a]
  6. —— Mother attempts to sign out of the hospital against medical advice.
  7. —— Prolonged separation of the baby from the mother due to neonatal complication or any severe illness requiring hospitalization in the first 6 months of life.
  8. —— Inadequate visiting patterns if the mother is discharged before the baby.[a]
  9. —— Reluctance to come in for the baby when discharge approved.[a]
  10. —— Spanking of the newborn baby or overt anger directed toward it (e.g., for crying or fussiness).[a] (Note: This behavior carries the gravest risk of any of the factors mentioned.)
D. Physician's office observations
  1. —— Lack of holding the baby.[a]
  2. —— Holding but no signs of attachment (e.g., no eye contact, talking, cuddling, etc.)[a]
  3. —— Rough handling.[a]
  4. —— Hygiene neglect.[a]
  5. —— Spanking of a young infant.[a]

[a]Most serious factors.
SOURCE: Modified by persmission from Schmitt BD: *New Child Protection Team Handbook*, 6th ed. New York, Garland, 1978.

initial intervention when risk factors are identified is involvement of a public health nurse. Until more than lip service is paid to prevention, child abuse will continue unabated.

References

1. Besharov D: *Recognizing Child Abuse: A Guide for the Concerned*. New York, Free Press, 1990, p 114.

2. Caffey J: Multiple fractures in the long bones of infants suffering from chronic subdural hematoma. *Am J Roentgenol* 56:163–173, 1946.

3. Kempe CH, Silverman FN, Steele BF, et al: The battered-child syndrome. *JAMA* 181:105–112, 1962.

4. Herman-Giddens, ME, Brown,G, Verviest, S, et al: Underascertainment of child abuse mortality in the United States. *JAMA* 282:463–467, 1999.

5. Bittner, S, Newberger EH: Pediatric understanding of child abuse and neglect, in Newberger, EH (ed): *Child Abuse*. Boston, Little Brown, 1982, pp 137–157.

6. Meyers JE: The role of the physician in preservation of verbal evidence of child abuse. *J Pediatr* 104:409–411, 1986.

7. Ricci LR: Photographing the physically abused child. *Am J Dis Child* 145:275–281, 1991.

8. Sugar NF, et al: Bruises in infants and toddlers: those who don't cruise rarely bruise. *Arch Pediatr Adolesc Med* 153: 399–403, 1999.

9. Schwartz AJ, Ricci LR: The aging of bruises: a review and study of color changes over time. *Pediatrics* 97:254–256, 1996.

10. Williams RA: Injuries in infants and small children resulting from witnessed and corroborated free falls. *J Trauma* 31:1350–1352, 1991.

11. Bryk M, Siegel PT: My mother caused my illness: the story of a survivor of Munchausen by proxy syndrome *Pediatrics* 100:1–7, 1997.

12. Southall DP, et al: Covert video recordings of life-threatening child abuse: lessons for child protection. *Pediatrics* 100:735–760, 1997.

13. American Academy of Pediatrics Committee on Child Abuse and Neglect: Guidelines for the evaluation of sexual abuse in children. *Pediatrics* 87: 254–260, 1991.

14. Adams JA, et al: Examination findings in legally confirmed child sexual abuse: it's normal to be normal. *Pediatrics* 94:310–317, 1994.

15. Olds DL, Eckenrode J, Henderson CR, et al: Long-term effects of home visitation on maternal life course and child abuse and neglect: 15 year follow-up of a randomized trial. *JAMA* 278:644–652, 1997.

Suggested Readings

Helfer ME, Kempe RS, Krugman RD (eds): *The Battered Child*. Chicago, University of Chicago Press, 1997.

Kleinman PK: *Diagnostic Imaging of Child Abuse*. Baltimore, Williams & Wilkins, 1987.

Reece RM (ed): Child Abuse: Medical Diagnosis and Management. Philadelphia, Lea and Febinger, 1994.

Plate 1
White Spots
and cavitation

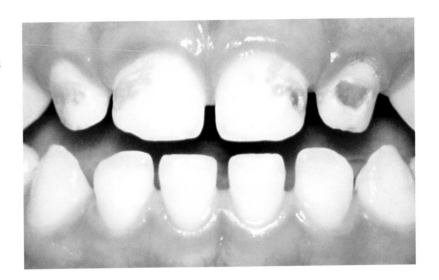

Plate 2
Cavitation

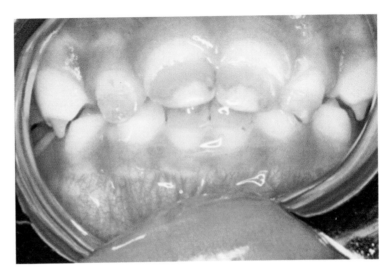

Plate 3
Enamel Hypoplasia

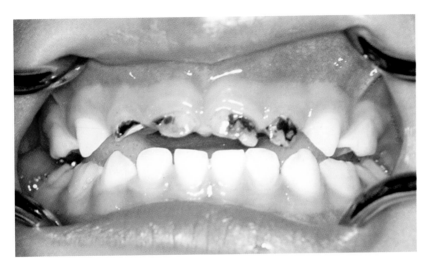

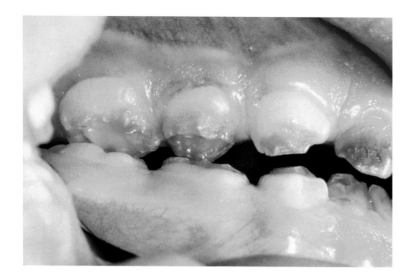

Plate 4
Enamel Hypoplasia

Plate 5
Mild flurosis

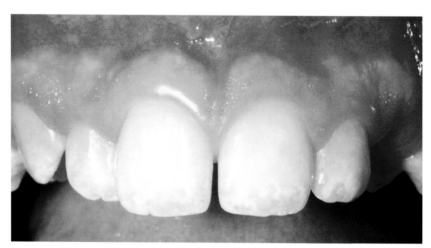

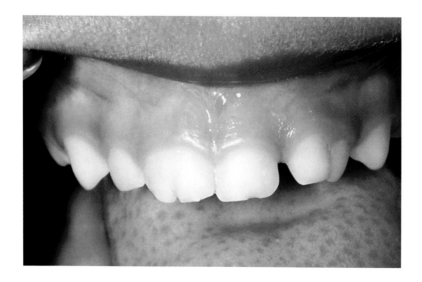

Plate 6
Fusion/Gemination

Plate 7
Bohn's Nodule

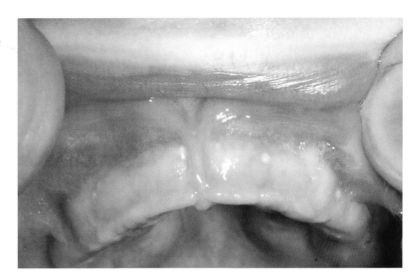

Plate 8
Dental lamina cyst

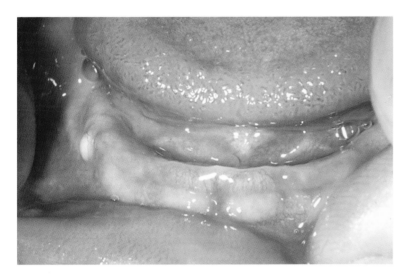

Plate 9
Atopic dermatitis. Multiple tiny follicular based papules in the antecubital fossa of an African-American child

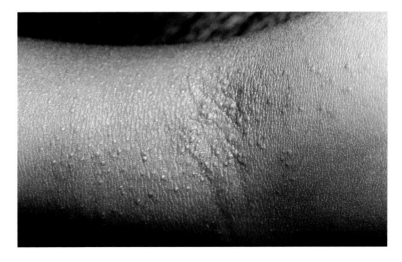

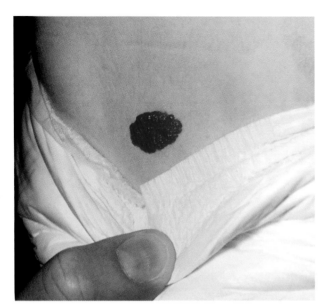

Plate 10
Superficial hemangioma. Well circumscribed, bright red plaque on lower back.

Plate 11
Port wine stain. Large irregular, purplish macule over sacrum. This lesion was associated with a tethered spinal cord.

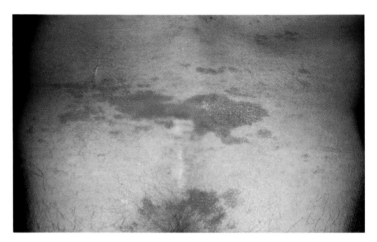

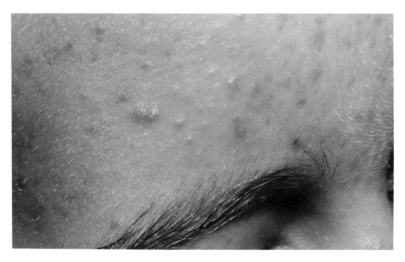

Plate 12
Acne vulgaris, moderately severe. Multiple erythematous papules and closed condones on the forehead.

Plate 13
Molluscum contagiosum. Multiple pearly, skin colored, umbilicated papules with a giant molluscum centrally.

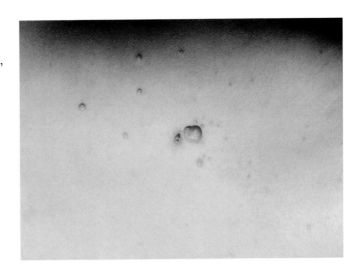

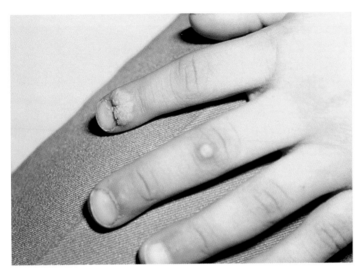

Plate 14
Verruca vulgaris. Large hyperkeratotic papule on the proximal nailfold.

Plate 15
"Black-dot" tinea capitis. Circular patch of alopecia with "black-dots" produced by broken hairs.

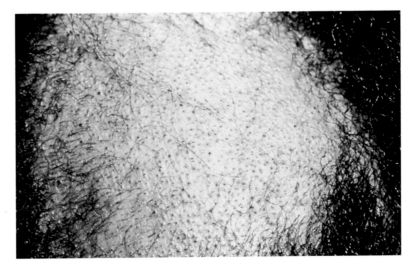

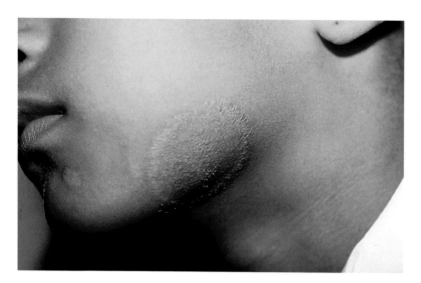

Plate 16
Tinea corporis. Large annular, erythematous, scaly plaque on jawline with smaller annular plaque on chin.

Plate 17
Pityriasis rosea. Herald patch on left shoulder surrounded by secondary eruption of smaller erythematous scaly patches.

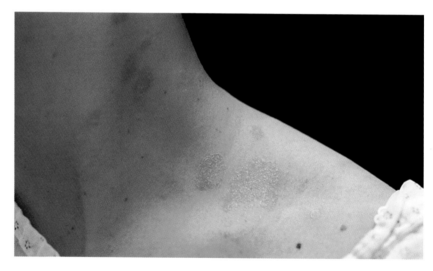

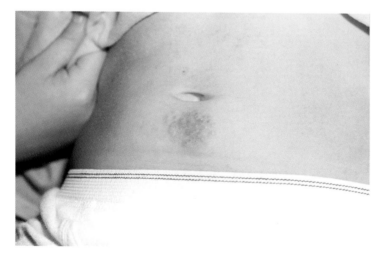

Plate 18
Contact allergic dermatitis due to nickel subacute. Multiple hyperpigmented papules localized to area of contact with metal snap on jeans.

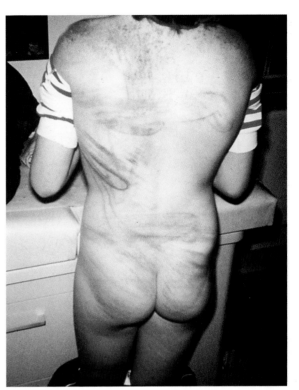

Plate 19
Belt marks. A seven year old child was whipped with a belt.

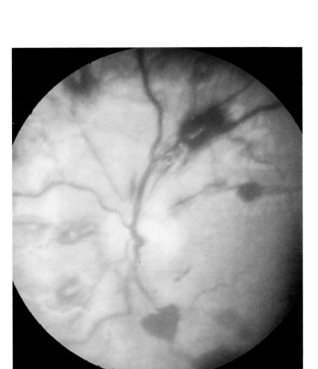

Plate 20
Retinal hemorrhages in an abused six month old infant.

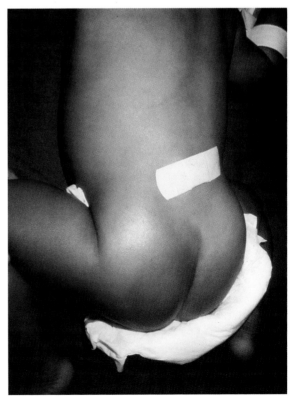

Plate 21
Mongolian spot: Typical steely blue/black pigmentation is seen over the buttocks and in patchy areas of the back of a black child. Mongolian spots are present in over 2/3 of Asian, Hispanic, Native American, and black infants.

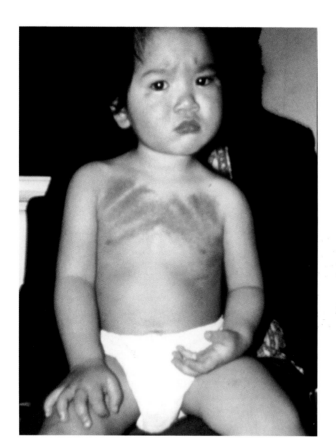

Plate 22

Cao Gaio (coin rubbing). Used to treat congestion. The lesions are produced by rubbing a warm oil onto the skin and firmly abraiding the skin with a coin.

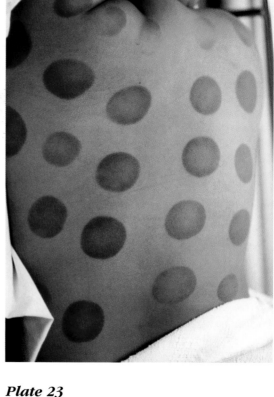

Plate 23

Cupping: An 11 year old Cambodian child with cough fever chest film had been treated by cupping. Alcohol is set on fire in a glass. When the fire goes out the glass is inverted onto the skin. The vacuum created is intended to draw out the chest congestion.

Plate 24

An 8-year-old girl with classic allergic shiners or dark circles beneath the eyes.

Sam R. Sharar

Chapter

11

Sedation and Pain Control

The clinical scenarios that require prompt and effective sedation and pain relief in children are easy to imagine—and often difficult to forget—for two reasons. First, these scenarios occur frequently and in multiple clinical practice settings, including acute traumatic injury (e.g., suturing of a facial laceration in a toddler, computed tomography (CT) of a school-aged child with recent closed head trauma), inpatient care (e.g., intravenous catheter insertion, bone marrow aspiration), and the outpatient setting (e.g., wound care procedures in the clinic, home analgesia for cutaneous burn pain or oncologic pain). These scenarios are further complicated by the fact that they commonly occur in adult-oriented institutions, where the infrequent experience and unfamiliarity with pediatric sedation and analgesia breeds a "discomfort level" about sedating children. Second, focused didactic teaching about sedation and pain management

in children is notoriously absent in many family medicine and pediatrics training programs. This deficiency is often exacerbated by the frustrating search to find published management "protocols" for pediatric sedation and analgesia, particularly when the need for them arises urgently.

These two shortcomings often result in situations where expectations thrust upon the primary clinician by nursing staff, subspecialty colleagues, and parents for appropriate sedative and analgesic care of a child are inappropriately high and can lead to frustration, stress, or outright panic on the part of the primary clinician. Unfortunately, these situations more commonly produce just the result one is trying to prevent— a frightened, uncooperative, and wholly unhappy child. The purpose of this chapter is to provide a brief overview of the indications for and safe provision of sedation and analgesia in children, including suggested pharmacologic

149

management guidelines that provide some specific medications and doses, but also, and more importantly, are applicable to a variety of practice conditions and institutional resources. For purposes of clarity, the review is divided into two sections—sedation and analgesia—although this distinction is somewhat artificial in clinical practice. For example, opioid analgesic–induced sedation is often a beneficial and desired side effect, although it can, at its extreme, be detrimental or even life-threatening. Finally, as the title implies, this review is focused on pharmacologic means of achieving sedation and analgesia in children; it does not address the critically important role of nonpharmacologic techniques (e.g., cognitive-behavioral interventions, hypnosis), which are described in detail elsewhere.[1,2]

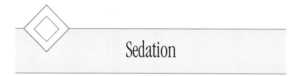

Sedation

Pharmacologic sedation is indicated for inpatient and outpatient procedures that do not require an operating room or general anesthesia. The most common procedures for which sedation is used include laceration repair, closed fracture reduction and casting, radiologic procedures [e.g., CT and magnetic resonance imaging (MRI)], and bone marrow aspiration. Pharmacologic sedation may also be indicated for agitated patients in an intensive care unit, particularly those requiring mechanical ventilation.

A variety of intellectual, emotional, and ethical reasons may be offered to rationalize the use of such sedative therapy: it makes the care team's job of diagnosis and treatment more efficient; it improves patient comfort and safety; it reduces parental stress; it reduces caregiver stress; it is what we, as parents, would want our children to receive. However, objective evidence for such rationalizations is hard to find. Although in some instances (e.g., an agitated

and thrashing toddler with a suspected cervical spine injury) sedation may arguably provide improved patient safety, sedation also potentially increases the risks for both minor (e.g., somnolence) and major (e.g., respiratory depression, airway obstruction, and pulmonary aspiration of gastric contents) complications, particularly in those who are very young (less than 1 year) or who have underlying medical conditions.[3] Thus, in the absence of data demonstrating improved patient outcome as a result of sedation, patient safety must always be the primary concern.

Targeting this issue of patient safety, both regulatory [e.g., Joint Commission on the Accreditation of Health Care Organizations (JCAHO)] and professional [e.g., American Academy of Pediatrics (AAP), American Society of Anesthesiologists (ASA)] organizations have published guidelines to help ensure the safety of children receiving pharmacologic sedation.[4–6] These guidelines address issues such as the child's current and past medical conditions, the availability of appropriate monitoring, the experience of immediate health care personnel, and the availability of emergency resuscitation personnel and equipment. The presence or absence of such personnel and equipment may dictate different sedation options from one institution to the next and from one patient to the next.

Choosing a Regimen

Owing to the inherent variabilities in patients' ages, medical issues, planned procedures, and institutional resources, it is clear that no single "cookbook" protocol for providing pediatric sedation will suffice for all, let alone a majority of cases. Thus, offered below is one approach—a "Five-Step Plan"—that makes five specific inquiries as to the patient and the planned procedure (Table 11-1), the answers to which will determine an appropriate pharmacologic sedative regimen that is tailored to the individual circumstance.

Table 11-1

The "Five-Step Plan" for Sedation Choice

1. Is "conscious" or "deep" sedation required/
   desired?
2. What monitoring equipment, personnel, and
   resuscitation tools are available?
3. Is the patient appropriately fasted to reduce
   volume of gastric contents?
4. Is the procedure painful or not painful?
5. Is intravenous access present?

1. *Is "conscious" or "deep" sedation required/
desired? Conscious sedation* is defined as a controlled state of depressed level of consciousness
that meets three criteria: The patient can maintain (a) protective airway reflexes (i.e., the gag
reflex), (b) appropriate response to physical
stimulation and verbal command, and (c) a
patent airway independently and continuously.
This level of sedation adequately guards against
apnea and pulmonary aspiration of gastric contents and thus is indicated for children who
have not been appropriately fasted (see below)
to reduce the volume of gastric contents (e.g.,
acutely injured or other emergent patients), as
well as for fasted children who only require
mild-moderate levels of sedation (that is, patient
wakefulness and movement will not interfere
with the planned procedure). Conscious sedation may be performed by properly trained,
nonanesthesia physician and nursing personnel with appropiate monitoring (see below).
Agents typically used for conscious sedation
include oral and intravenous opioid analgesics,
oral and intravenous benzodiazepines, chloral
hydrate, pentobarbital, and nitrous oxide (see
Table 11-2).

Deep sedation is defined as a controlled state
of depressed level of consciousness (usually
unconsciousness) in which the three requirements of conscious sedation listed above are not
met. Deep sedation can be performed without

an endotracheal tube if the patient is appropriately fasted to reduce the risk of pulmonary
aspiration of gastric contents (see below). Otherwise, the presence of an anesthesiologist (or
other individual trained to secure the pediatric
airway with an endotracheal tube) is mandatory.
Agents typically used for deep sedation include
intravenous propofol, sodium thiopental, ketamine, and benzodiazepines, or volatile (gas)
anesthetics (see Table 11-2).

2. *What monitoring equipment, personnel,
and resuscitation tools are available?* Because
the monitoring equipment and personnel required for conscious and deep sedation differ,
their availabilities will dictate sedation options.
During conscious sedation, the minimum
requirements established by the AAP and ASA[4,5]
to diagnose and treat the life-threatening complications of respiratory depression or airway
obstruction include: (a) continuous pulse oximetry; (b) support personnel *in addition to the
practitioner performing the procedure*, whose
sole responsibility is to monitor the patient's
physiologic status, vital signs, and level of consciousness, and to assist in any supportive/
resuscitative measures as needed; (c) immediately available resuscitation equipment necessary to secure the pediatric airway (i.e., high
flow oxygen, bag/mask device, suction appara-
tus, and full size range of intubation tools) and
reverse unwanted drug effects (e.g., naloxone
for opioid overdose, flumazenil for benzodiazepine overdose), as well as personnel who
know both where the equipment is kept and
how to use it; and (d) physiologic monitoring
and observation until the patient meets established discharge criteria (Table 11-3). The AAP
and ASA guidelines are clear that if these minimum requirements cannot be met, conscious
sedation should not be performed. During deep
sedation, the personnel requirements are for an
anesthesiologist (or other individual trained to
secure the pediatric airway with an endotracheal
tube), and the monitoring requirements are
those of the ASA for the provision of general
anesthesia.[7]

Table 11-2

Common Pharmacologic Agents for Sedation and Analgesia in Children

CLASS	DRUG	DOSE/ROUTE[a]
Benzodiazepine	Midazolam	0.5 mg/kg (PO, PR)
		0.05–0.15 mg/kg (IV)
	Diazepam	0.3 mg/kg (PO)
		0.1 mg/kg (IV)
Barbiturate	Thiopental	4–7 mg/kg (IV)
	Methohexital	30 mg/kg (PR)
		1 mg/kg (IV)
Other sedative-hypnotic	Propofol	2–4 mg/kg (IV)
		0.025–0.2 mg/kg/min (IV)
	Ketamine	5–10 mg/kg (PO, PR)
		2–5 mg/kg (IM)
		1 mg/kg (IV)
Opioid	Morphine	0.025–0.1 mg/kg (IV)
	Fentanyl	0.005–0.015 mg/kg (OT)
		0.001–0.003 mg/kg (IV)
	Codeine	1 mg/kg (PO)
Nonopioid analgesics	Acetaminophen	10–15 mg/kg (PO)
		20–40 mg/kg (PR)
	Ibuprofen	5–10 mg/kg (PO)
	Ketorolac	0.5 mg/kg (IV, IM)

KEY: PO, oral; PR, rectal; IV, intravenous; IM, intramuscular; OT, oral transmucosal
[a] *Note:* 1 mg = 1000 μg (i.e., 0.010 mg/kg = 10 μg/kg)

Table 11-3

Recommended Discharge Criteria after Conscious Sedation

1. Cardiovascular function and airway patency are satisfactory and stable.
2. The patient is easily arousable and protective reflexes are intact.
3. The patient can talk (if age-appropriate).
4. The patient can sit up unaided (if age-appropriate).
5. For a very young or handicapped child incapable of the usually expected responses, the presedation level of responsiveness or a level as close as possible to the normal level for that child should be achieved.
6. The state of hydration is adequate.

SOURCE: From the American Academy of Pediatrics,[4] by permission.

3. *Is the patient appropriately fasted to reduce the volume of gastric contents?* As pulmonary aspiration of gastric contents is a highly morbid yet preventable complication of pediatric sedation, all efforts should be made to minimize its occurrence. For this reason, the use of conscious rather than deep sedation is preferred, since the protective airway (gag) reflexes, which will prevent aspiration in the event of gastroesophageal reflux or vomiting, are retained. In addition, an appropriate period of fasting prior to sedation for an elective procedure (e.g., bone marrow aspiration, CT or MRI, colonoscopy) will reduce gastric volume, and hence the potential for aspiration of gastric contents. Absolute times for presedation fasting that guarantee an empty stomach are somewhat subject to debate.[8] In our local institutions, the guideline of 2 h fasting for clear liquids, 4 h fasting for breast milk, and 6 h fasting for solids and nonclear liquids is routinely employed. It is obvious that such fasting practices are impractical in the treatment of acutely injured children (they are rarely fasting upon emergency room arrival) as well as unreliable in children with underlying conditions that predispose to esophageal reflux and aspiration (e.g., gastroesophageal reflux disease, severe obesity, skeletal muscle weakness or myopathy, quadriplegia, static encephalopathy).

4. *Is the procedure painful or not painful?* Painful procedures (e.g., laceration suture, fracture reduction and casting, bone marrow aspiration) typically require both analgesia (systemic or local) and sedation. The combination of systemic opioid analgesics and benzodiazepines, however, carries an increased risk of synergistic respiratory depression.[9] Nonpainful procedures (e.g., CT or MRI) require only sedation, which should be provided without the use of systemic opioids to reduce the risk of synergistic respiratory depression. This is of particular importance in the context of CT for closed head injuries because hypoventilation-induced hypercapnea will elevate intracranial pressure (due to cerebral vascular dilation) and potentially aggravate underlying brain injury.

5. *Is intravenous access present?* The presence of a functioning intravenous line offers the practitioner both a wider choice of drugs for sedation and analgesia as well as the ability to more safely titrate these drugs to the desired effect compared with other routes of administration. Opioid (naloxone) and benzodiazepine (flumazenil) reversal agents can also be administered more expeditiously by the intravenous route in the event of unintentional overdose or unexpected sensitivity to the drugs.

Despite these strong arguments for placement of an intravenous line, it is acknowledged that obtaining intravenous access in children is not without difficulty; in the case of minor procedures, it may be more problematic than the scheduled procedure itself. In these cases, oral, rectal, or transmucosal drug administration is indicated (see Table 11-2), although these routes result in more variable and unpredictable drug effects, so that a higher index of suspicion for side effects (e.g., oversedation) must be maintained when drugs are administered by these routes.

Pharmacologic Choices

An abbreviated list of sedative agents and recommended doses is provided in Table 11-2. It should be noted that these (and other textbook) recommended doses must take into account the spectrum ("bell curve") of responses that any given drug and dose will elicit from a diverse group of individual patients. Furthermore, it is important to remember that as drug dose is increased, drug effects (both desired *and* undesired) will also increase. Because the expected effects from these agents are both widely variable and somewhat unpredictable, published dose recommendations are purposely low, so that if error occurs, it will occur on the side of safety. This helps explain the seemingly frequent frustration of administering a sedative agent and achieving a less-than-adequate response. This issue also argues strongly for the use of intravenous sedation (and analgesia) in children, because of its more rapid onset of action and safe titration "to desired effect" that cannot be provided when such agents are administered by other routes.

Complementing the information provided in Table 11-2, three arbitrary categories of sedation needs and indications are listed below, along with several "pearls" for each category:

1. *Mild/moderate sedation required, no intravenous access.* Clinical scenarios include painless diagnostic studies (e.g, CT and MRI), repair of simple lacerations, incision and drainage of small abscesses, and wound care/dressing changes. Systemic opioid analgesics are rarely indicated for these cases, although local anesthesia/analgesia (regional or field block) is frequently employed. Oral or rectal midazolam (0.5 mg/kg) is commonly used for such conscious sedation, having an onset time of 15 to 30 min, a duration of 1 to 3 h and the added benefit of producing limited anterograde amnesia. Midazolam is quite bitter to the taste and requires administration in fruit-flavored syrup or carbonated soda. It can also be delivered intranasally, although few children will sit quietly while several milliliters of liquid are squirted into their nares. In the event of either inadequate effect or "disinhibition" at 30 min, a second dose of 0.25 mg/kg will often be successful. Disinhibition (evidenced by agitation and a *worsening* of cooperation) often occurs at plasma midazolam levels just below those necessary for sedation; thus, the usual success of administering a second dose at 30 min. Alternatives to benzodiazepines are also available. These include chloral hydrate (25 to 75 mg/kg orally or rectally; onset time, about 60 min; duration, 4 to 6 h, which may limit rapid achievement of discharge criteria) and oral transmucosal fentanyl citrate (Oralet®, 5 to 15 μg/kg; onset time, about 30 min; duration 2 to 4 h; indicated for procedures that require both analgesia and sedation).

2. *Mild/moderate sedation, intravenous access present.* Clinical scenarios include repair of complex lacerations, closed reduction/casting of fractures, bone marrow aspiration, gastrointestinal endoscopy, and extended radiographic diagnostic procedures in a multiply-injured, but otherwise "stable" child (i.e., no major cardiovascular, respiratory, or neurologic injury). Intravenous administration is indicated for those cases where a more "profound" level of conscious sedation is required to achieve adequate patient cooperation.

These procedures often require concomitant systemic opioid analgesia and conscious sedation. Owing to the synergistic respiratory depression that occurs with combined opioid and benzodiazepine therapy, it is suggested that all starting drug doses be decreased by 50 percent and then titrated to their desired effect.[9]

Intravenous midazolam is a common choice, with an onset time of 2 to 5 min and a duration of 1 to 3 h. The starting dose is 50 μg/kg and can be repeated every 5 min, with the vast majority of patients achieving appropriate sedation with a total dose of 150 μg/kg or less. Alternatively, diazepam (100 μg/kg starting dose) may be used, its advantage being a longer duration (4 to 6 h), which may be of benefit for prolonged diagnostic or therapeutic procedures, particularly in children to be admitted to the hospital or who are already inpatients. Typical intravenous opioid analgesic choices are morphine and fentanyl (see below).

3. *Moderate/deep sedation, intravenous access present.* Clinical scenarios include bone marrow aspiration, intrathecal medication (e.g., chemotherapy) administration, gastrointestinal endoscopy, sedation on the intensive care unit, and acutely injured patients with significant cardiovascular, respiratory, or neurologic injuries who required prolonged diagnostic evaluation and/or invasive procedures (e.g., angiography, diagnostic peritoneal lavage). Intravenous access is obviously required for these cases.

For elective procedures in fasted and hemodynamically stable children, intravenous propofol (2 to 4 mg/kg bolus; 25 to 200 µg/kg/min continuous infusion) provides for rapid onset of sedation (<1 min) that resolves within 10 to 30 min upon its discontinuation. The primary drawback of propofol use (in its current formulation in intralipid) is pain on injection when delivered into small peripheral veins.

Ketamine is an intravenous alternative (1 mg/kg) with an onset time of less than 1 min and a duration of 10 to 30 min. Its primary drawback is the small (about 10 percent) incidence of aural and visual emergence hallucinations in children—an effect related to its structural similarity to the street drug phenylcyclidine (PCP).

With a critically injured child in whom muscle relaxation with paralytics is necessary for endotracheal intubation or to facilitate diagnostic or therapeutic maneuvers, it is important to recall that muscle relaxants have absolutely no central nervous system sedative properties, although they produce a very "sedated-appearing" (immobile!) child. Thus, in patients with hemodynamic stability (*not* in a multiply-injured child in hypovolemic shock), sedative agents (preferably benzodiazepines due to their associated amnesia) should be administered concurrently with muscle relaxants.

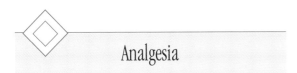

Analgesia

Analgesia can be provided for children with the use of systemic opioids, nonsteroidal antiinflammatory drugs (NSAIDs), acetaminophen, and/or local anesthetics administered topically or as a regional or field block. On the other hand, opioids are typically reserved for the treatment of moderate to severe pain, as they act in a dose-dependent fashion (with regard to both desired analgesic and undesired side effects) and are capable of controlling virtually all degrees of pain. At the extreme, opioids can even ablate intraoperative surgical pain, but at the price of

severe respiratory depression necessitating endotracheal intubation and mechanical ventilation. In contrast, NSAIDs and acetaminophen act in a dose-dependent manner but at some point reach a ceiling effect whereupon increasing dose results in additional side effects but no additional analgesia (Fig. 11-1). Thus, these agents are valuable analgesics but are typically used for mild pain complaints, with great care taken to avoid systemic toxicities of renal impairment (NSAIDs) and hepatic dysfunction (acetaminophen) by not exceeding established daily maximal doses. These nonopioid agents are also routinely used for more significant pain in combination with systemic opioids (e.g., acetaminophen-codeine formulations) because their "opioid-sparing" effects will result in improved analgesia at lower opioid doses (hence fewer opioid-related side effects).

Systemic opioid analgesia is mediated by the interaction of an administered opioid agonist with specific opiate receptors in the periaqueductal gray matter of the brainstem. Thus, it is important to appreciate that between the syringe of codeine elixir held in the nurse's hand and the eventual opiate receptor target lie a series of potential impediments to achieving the desired

Figure 11-1

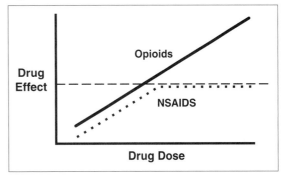

Opioid analgesics provide dose-dependent analgesia that can treat virtually all degrees of pain, although with dose-dependent side effects that limit clinical use. In contrast, nonsteroidal anti-inflammatory drugs (NSAIDs) provide dose-dependent analgesia to a certain point, then exhibit a "ceiling effect" that limits their analgesic efficacy.

analgesic effect: patient refusal to consume medication, nausea or vomiting, impaired intestinal absorption of drug (due to other gastric contents), poor bioavailability (e.g., due to hepatic metabolism of drug on the first pass through the portal circulation), impaired cerebral perfusion, altered blood-brain barrier, and abnormal receptor function due to long-term drug administration (i.e., tolerance). Given this chain of potential impediments, it is a wonder that opioid analgesia works as well as it does! Thus, one's expectation of analgesic effect should reflect these reasons for highly variable outcomes from child to child or even from one dose to the next.

Side Effects

Although analgesia can be mediated by both mu-1 and kappa opiate receptors, all currently available opioid analgesics are mu-1 agonists. This is important because in addition to being responsible for decreasing pain, mu-1 receptors also mediate a variety of undesirable side effects, including euphoria, sedation, apnea, miosis, nausea/vomiting, constipation, urinary retention, pruritus, and drug tolerance. Of these, several deserve special mention:

1. *Central nervous system.* Euphoria, dysphoria, apnea, sedation, and cough suppression result from opioid interaction with opiate receptors scattered in other portions of the brain stem and the limbus. Meperidine (Demerol) is metabolized into normeperidine, which reduces the seizure threshold; thus, meperidine is not recommended for chronic use.
2. *Gastrointestinal system.* Nausea and vomiting are frequent side effects of opioid therapy, although tolerance to these effects typically develops within 2 to 4 days. Often a change in opioid therapy is made during this time to prevent nausea. When the nausea subsides (often due to tolerance and unrelated to the medication change), the patient is inappropriately labeled as "allergic" to the initial opioid.

   Constipation is another frequent side effect, especially for chronic opioid users (e.g., oncology patients, cutaneous burn patients). Tolerance to the analgesic effects of opioid therapy develops after as little as 2 weeks of therapy, yet tolerance to its constipating effects may never occur. Because of the risk of progressive and problematic constipation, a regular bowel regimen of stool softeners and possibly peristaltic agents should be initiated promptly if chronic therapy is anticipated.
3. *Skin.* Opioid-induced pruritus is centrally mediated and not histamine-induced (except possibly with morphine use). However, the typical therapy given for opioid-induced pruritis is antihistamine administration that merely offers coincident relief through the unintended mechanism of sedation.
4. *Respiratory depression.* Opioids are powerful respiratory depressants but can be used safely owing to the counterbalance of pain as a potent respiratory stimulant. Clinically important respiratory depression occurs if too much opioid is given, opioid clearance is reduced, or pain is taken away (e.g., regional nerve block).

   Treatment of respiratory depression is with intravenous naloxone (1 μg/kg titrated carefully to a respiratory rate in the low-normal range in cases of non-life-threatening bradypnea; 5 μg/kg in cases of frank apnea). Care should be taken to avoid excessive opioid reversal that can result in an agitated, hypertensive, and tachycardic child in excruciating pain. Because the duration of naloxone effect (about 1 h) is significantly less than the duration of most commonly used opioids (3 to 6 h), these patients carry the risk for "renarcotization" when the initial naloxone effect dissipates. One preventive strategy against renarcotization is to administer, immediately following the initial therapeutic intravenous dose of naloxone, a second, identical dose intra-muscularly. This intramuscular dose acts as a depot for systemic uptake over several subsequent hours and better approximates the time course of previously administered opioids.

5. *Opioid tolerance and dependence.* Although not of concern when opioids are used for one-time treatment of pain-related to proce-dures, tolerance and dependency may occur with longer durations of treatment. Opioid *tolerance* is characterized by the develop-ment of decreasing analgesic (or other) effect with chronic therapy and develops at different rates for different effects (e.g., nau-sea/vomiting effect, 2 to 4 days; analgesic effect, about 2 weeks; constipating effect, little or no tolerance develops). Tolerance is a challenging issue with chronic analgesic use, particularly in pediatric oncology out-patients. Opioid tolerance presents with increasing pain complaints despite compli-ant analgesic use and necessitates an increase in opioid dosing, often to levels well above those recommended in standard texts (including this chapter). A significant hurdle to overcome by all caregivers at this point is to understand that as long as life-threatening complications of opioid use (e.g., respiratory depression, significant oversedation) are not present, opioid dosing can and should be increased—irrespective of the mg/kg dose—until the desired anal-gesic effect is obtained.

Physical dependence is characterized by the development of the abstinence syn-drome (yawning, lacrimation, agitation, tremors, insomnia, fever, and tachycardia) upon abrupt withdrawal of opioid therapy. It can be prevented by tapering opioid use by 10 to 20 percent per day in patients receiving opioids for greater than 2 weeks, or even more slowly (10 to 20 percent per week) in patients receiving longer periods (months) of therapy. If the opioid with-drawal symptoms occur, they are effectively treated with opioid administration at 20 to 40 percent of the previous daily dose. *Psy-chological dependence* is characterized by abnormal behavior that results in opioid use for reasons other than pain relief. Its inci-dence in children receiving opioids for med-ical conditions is unknown but likely very rare, as in adults it is estimated at 1:10,000 for non-substance-abusing patients receiv-ing postoperative opioid therapy.[10]

Routes of Administration and Dosing

Oral, oral transmucosal, intramuscular, and intravenous dosing can be used for opioid ther-apy. Each route offer both benefits and limita-tions. Oral administration of opioid elixirs in children allows accurate dosing in a relatively palatable formulation (e.g., fruit-flavored syrup), in contrast to tablets or capsules, which may be less acceptable to small children and also come in a limited, and usually inconvenient range of dose sizes. Oral therapy, however, requires a functioning intestinal tract and can be limited by nausea and/or vomiting. In addition, the "first pass" effect of hepatic metabolism on drugs absorbed by the portal circulation results in vari-able oral analgesic potency.

Oral transmucosal opioid administration is typically palatable (e.g., fruit-flavored lozenges) to children and results in a rapid onset of action owing to prompt plasma uptake of drug through the buccal mucosa. Some cooperation from the patient is required, however, to limit biting, chewing, or swallowing of the lozenge, all of which result in decreased potency associated with enteral rather than transmucosal absorp-tion. Intramuscular administration may have a rare indication (e.g., a child in severe pain and difficulty obtaining intravenous access), but it is otherwise mentioned only to be condemned. Patients will tend to associate requests for anal-gesic medication with the immediate pain of the intramuscular injection and not with the anal-gesic effect that occurs 30 to 45 min later, which can lead to fewer analgesic requests and an increase in overall pain levels. In addition, plasma absorption of intramuscularly delivered drugs is highly variable, resulting in unpredictable analgesic and side effects.

Choices for intravenous administration include bolus dosing, continuous infusion, and patient-controlled analgesia (PCA). As with intravenous sedation, the titration of incremental opioid doses to the desired analgesic effect is most efficacious and safe. Using morphine as an example, the typical textbook dose recommendation for intravenous bolus dosing is 0.1 mg/kg. However, administering incremental doses of 0.025 mg/kg every 5 to 10 min provides a mechanism for safely treating a wide spectrum of patients, including those more sensitive to opioid effects, with the vast majority of nontolerant patients experiencing appropriate analgesia with a total dose of 0.1 mg/kg or less.

Continuous opioid infusion is a superior method for obtaining analgesia by maintaining relatively constant plasma opioid levels, unlike the peaks and valleys associated with intermittent bolus dosing. Morphine is most commonly used for continuous intravenous analgesia, at infusion rates of 10 to 40 μg/kg/h. A simple method for calculating and performing such infusions is to measure the child's weight in kilograms and add that same number of milligrams of morphine to a 100-mL bag of crystalloid solution (lactated Ringer's, saline, etc.). Then using an electronic infusion pump, infu-

sion flow rates of 1 to 4 mL/h will correspond to 10 to 40 μg/kg/h.

PCA can typically be used (in consultation with an anesthesiologist or pain specialist) in most children over 10 years of age and occasionally in those as young as 7 to 8 years of age, depending on the child's cognitive development. The most important aspect of PCA use is convincing parents that PCA stands for "patient-controlled analgesia" and not "parent controlled analgesia." This point is a safeguard against opioid overdose with PCA, because when administered only by the patient, oversedation will limit the patient's ability to activate the dosing button, thereby preventing overdose. With parental activation of the dosing button, this safeguard is lost and serious complications such as apnea are more likely.

Offered below is a three-step framework for determining the appropriate opioid analgesic starting dose for a variety of commonly used oral and intravenous agents in children: First, commit to memory the incremental dosing regimen for morphine (0.025 mg/kg administered every 5 to 10 min until desired effect is reached, usually at a total dose of 0.1 mg/kg or less). Second, if an opioid other than morphine is desired, use Table 11-4 to convert the morphine dosing regimen to the appropriate regimen for the desired drug. For example, since the "equipotent intravenous dose" of meperidine is 10 times greater than that of morphine, the incremental dose of meperidine would be

Table 11-4

Commonly Used Opioid Analgesics

Drug	IV Dose (mg/kg)	Duration	Bioavailability
Morphine	0.1	3–4 h	20–40%
Meperidine	1.0	3–4 h	40–60%
Methadone	0.1	4–24 h	70–100%
Fentanyl	0.001	0.5–1 h	30–50%
Hydromorphone	0.04	3–4 h	80–100%

0.25 mg/kg administered every 5 to 10 min until desired effect is reached, usually at a total dose of 1.0 mg/kg or less.

Third, if oral dosing of the opioid is desired, increase the intravenous dose determined above to adjust for bioavailability (the "first pass" hepatic metabolism of drugs absorbed into the portal circulation). For example, if the bioavailability is 30 percent, then the equivalent oral dose is three times greater than the recommended intravenous dose.

Procedural versus Background Pain Relief

In children as in adults, pharmacologic analgesia is indicated for both procedural pain (e.g., fracture reduction/casting) and background pain (i.e., the relatively constant pain associated with conditions such as malignancy or surgical wounds). It is important to keep in mind the distinct therapeutic goals for addressing these two specific analgesic needs, as the pharmacologic agents and administration methods employed will differ depending on which analgesic need is being targeted (Table 11-5). For procedural analgesia, the presence of intravenous access provides improved analgesia by permitting the rapid titration of short-acting agents (e.g., fentanyl, alfentanil). For background analgesia, as for postoperative or significant wound pain, the presence of an intravenous catheter allows continuous infusion of longer-acting agents (e.g., morphine). In the absence of intravenous access, agents with a fast onset (e.g., transmucosal opioids, nitrous oxide) may be preferable for procedural analgesia. For background analgesia, oral agents with long durations of action (e.g., methadone) or sustained intestinal release and absorption [e.g., morphine (MSContin®) or oxycodone (Oxycontin®) tablets] are convenient because they provide relatively constant plasma opioid levels. Regularly scheduled (as opposed to "as needed") administration of standard oral opioid analgesics may also improve background analgesia by increasing the time which plasma levels are kept within the therapeutic range (Fig. 11-2).

Pain Assessment

Pain assessment in children is challenging due to their variable physical, psychological, and cognitive development, which depends on age, family and peer support, and environmental

Table 11-5
Targeting Analgesic Therapy

ISSUE	PROCEDURAL PAIN	BACKGROUND PAIN
Pain characteristics	Intermittent; moderate–severe intensity	Constant; mild–moderate intensity
Pharmacologic goal	Potent analgesia with rapid onset and short duration	Constant plasma analgesic levels in therapeutic range
Potential solutions	1. IV >> OT >> PO opioids 2. Nonopioid analgesics (e.g., nitrous oxide) 3. Nonpharmacologic opioids (e.g., behavioral) therapy	1. Continuous IV opioid infusion 2. "Long-acting" oral opioids 3. transdermal opioids 4. regularly scheduled analgesics (opioid and other)

KEY: PO, oral; IV, intravenous; OT, oral transmucosal.

Figure 11-2

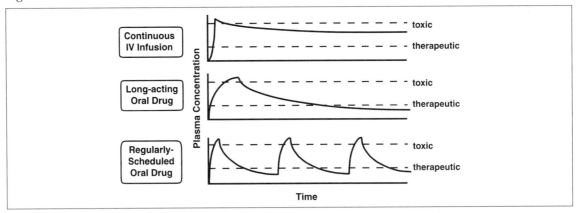

Background pain relief is improved when plasma opioid levels are maintained in the "therapeutic window" (above the therapeutic analgesic threshold but below the level that produces unwanted side effects). Three common strategies for maximizing the time–plasma opioid levels within the therapeutic window, depending on the presence of intravenous access and medication choice, are shown.

surroundings. This task is most difficult in the infant and toddler group, for whom reliable and valid pain assessment tools are difficult to find. Use of a pain assessment tool on a daily basis for patients with ongoing pain issues provides two tangible benefits to both patient and caregiver (see below). These benefits are maximized when pain assessment occurs regularly (i.e., on daily rounds or regularly scheduled clinic visits), when both background pain and procedural pain are assessed, and when results are recorded in the medical record or bedside chart so that all caregivers are aware of the level of pain, recent changes in pain, and the effects of recent analgesic interventions.

Pain assessment instruments include use of a standardized pain score (e.g., the verbal scale of 0 to 10 in adolescents and older children). In children 3 to 10 years of age, pictorial scales, like the Oucher[11] (Fig. 11-3) probably provide the most accurate assessment of the patient's pain and thus serve as the most reliable guide to analgesic needs. When obtainable, patient pain scores can be compared from day to day to determine whether (1) pain is changing or

(2) recent analgesic interventions have had the desired effect on pain reports. Further, by eliciting and recording a daily pain score, the communication of pain and analgesic needs between caregivers is simplified. Such a standardization of pain reports obviates the need for interpretation of patients' pain by nursing staff, particularly as nurses change from day to day or shift to shift. Similarly, pain management by "on-call" physicians or others not primarily responsible for a particular patient's care is simplified by the ability to refer to a chronologic record of patient-reported pain scores and medication records.

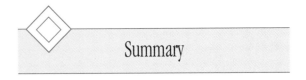

Summary

The assessment of pediatric pain and the provision of safe and effective sedation and analgesia in children are typical of valuable medical skills—they are challenging to perform effec-

Figure 11-3

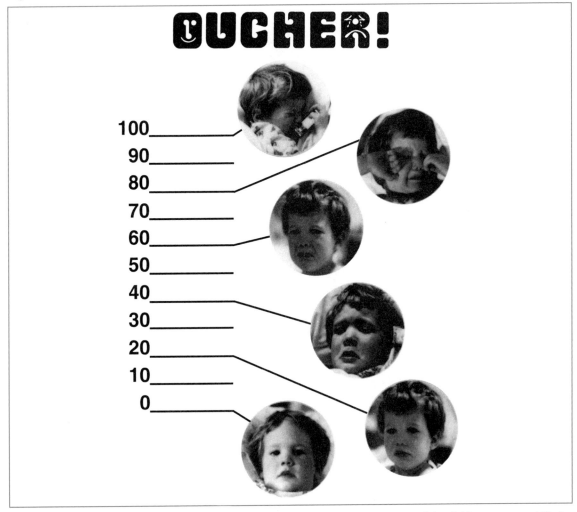

The "Oucher" pain scale is designed for pain assessment in children ages 3 to 15 years. If the child can count to 100, the numerical scale may be used to assess pain intensity. If not, it is explained to the child that the bottom picture (or 0) is "no hurt," whereas the top picture (or 100) is "the biggest hurt one could ever have." The child then selects the picture that best reflects the hurt being felt, and the corresponding numeric score is recorded. The Caucasian version of the scale is shown, with Hispanic, Asian, and African-American versions also available. (Reprinted with permission.)

tively yet provide generous reward to both patient and caregiver. To complement this brief review, the reader is referred to more detailed works[13,14] that may provide additional information or alternative approaches to the goal of safely and effectively managing the child who is anxious, frightened, or in pain.

References

1. Wagner AM: Pain control in the pediatric patient. *Dermatol Clin* 16:609–617, 1998.
2. Zeltzer LK, Jay SM, Fisher DM: The management of pain associated with pediatric procedures. *Pediatr Clin North Am* 36:941–964, 1989.

3. Malviya S, Voepel-Lewis T, Tait AR: Adverse events and risk factors associated with the sedation of children by nonanesthesiologists. *Anesth Analg* 85:1207–1213, 1997.

4. American Academy of Pediatrics, Committee on Drugs: Guidelines for monitoring and management of pediatric patients during and after sedation for diagnostic and therapeutic procedures. *Pediatrics* 89:1110–1115, 1992.

5. American Society of Anesthesiologists, Task Force on Sedation and Analgesia by Non-Anesthesiologists: Practice guidelines for sedation and analgesia by non-anesthesiologists. *Anesthesiology* 84:459–471, 1996.

6. *Comprehensive Accreditation Manual for Hospitals: The Official Handbook.* Oakbrook Terrace, IL, Joint Commission on the Accreditation of Health Care Organizations, 1998.

7. American Society of Anesthesiologists: Standards for basic intraoperative monitoring. *ASA Newsletter*, December 1986.

8. American Society of Anesthesiologists, Task Force on Preoperative Fasting: Practice guidelines for preoperative fasting and the use of pharmacologic agents to reduce the risk of pulmonary aspiration: application to healthy patients undergoing elective procedures. *Anesthesiology* 90:896-905, 1999.

9. Bailey PL, Pace NL, Ashburn MA, et al: Frequent hypoxemia and apnea after sedation with midazolam and fentanyl. *Anethesiology* 73:826–830, 1990.

10. Porter J, Jick H: Addiction rare in patients treated with narcotics. *N Engl J Med* 302:123–124, 1980.

11. Beyer JE, Denyes MJ, Vallarruel, AM: The creation, validation, and continuing development of the Oucher: a measure of pain intensity in children. *J Pediatr Nurs* 7:335–346, 1992.

12. Marvin JA: Pain assessment versus measurement. *J Burn Care Rehabil* 16:348–357, 1995.

13. Cote CJ: Sedation for the pediatric patient: a review. *Pediatr Clin North Am* 41:31–58, 1994.

14. *Acute Pain Management in Infants, Children, and Adolescents: Operative and Medical Procedures.* AHCPR publication #92-0020, US Department of Health and Human Services, Washington, DC, Pubic Health Service, 1992.

Chronic
Problems

Alan L. Goldbloom

Chronic Pain

Chronic pain in children challenges the wits of both parents and health care providers. Physicians usually find it easier and more satisfying to establish a specific cause (and treatment) for acute pain—whether due to injury such as a sprain or an illness such as appendicitis—than to determine etiologies for recurrent or chronic pain syndromes. While most chronic pain problems of childhood are not threats to overall health, they do trigger understandable distress and fear for parents and children and therefore merit thoughtful attention from the health care provider.

The late American pediatrician Dr. Harry Gordon astutely commented that "The physician's mission is to reduce anxiety—and all our knowledge, research, diagnosis and treatment are only means to that end." Indeed, this is the tradition of medicine. It is only recently that we have been able to reduce anxiety by actually curing disease, and even now, that outcome accounts for only a minority of physician-patient interactions. Most of the time, we reduce anxiety by helping people understand and cope with the situations they face. We rarely cure migraine headaches or recurrent abdominal pain, any more than we cure spina bifida, developmental delay, or diabetes. However, we help patients and families manage and deal with all these problems; the more effectively we do so, the more we have fulfilled the mission of the physician.

This chapter is not a diagnostic manual for the assessment of pain or determination of its etiology. Nor is it a guide to such relatively unusual and poorly understood pain syndromes as reflex sympathetic dystrophy. It is, instead, a guide to some office-based approaches to the most common pain syndromes in children. There will always be a group of children at one end of any spectrum whose pain problems defy the usual attempts at management and who may benefit from the focused expertise of pain management specialists or pain clinics. However, the majority of chronic pain problems are part of the bread-and-butter practice of those who look after children. They are the target of the advice provided in this chapter. The problems highlighted include recurrent stomachaches, growing pains, teething, headaches, and chest pain.

General Approach

Few situations are more distressing to parents than seeing their child in pain. Parents often consider pain to be the sign of a potentially serious problem that needs immediate attention. Understanding and acknowledging this fundamental concern is the key to a successful therapeutic relationship. Physicians may well understand, within the first few minutes of an encounter, that the problem causing the pain is relatively minor. Yet a dismissive approach ("There's nothing wrong, nothing to worry about. . .") may bring the office visit to a conclusion without resolving the fundamental concern of the parent. All parents want their issues, no matter how trivial, to be taken seriously. Key points to be used in assessment of recurrent pain are shown in Table 12-1.

Conveying Concern

A physician can convey concern by attitude, words, and action. A detailed history, allowing parent and child sufficient time to talk about the problem, will not only help piece together the story but also convey the physician's interest— an immediate therapeutic benefit. Equally important, a detailed and careful physical examination performed in front of the parents (when

Table 12-1

Key Points in Assessing Recurrent Pain

Nonjudgmental, interested approach.
Enough time for detailed history and physical examination.
Determine what the parents think is the cause of the underlying problem and what their worst fear is.
Ask about similar symptoms/illnesses in relatives.
Determine effect on school attendance, sports, and other activities.
Obtain relevant history of "life events" (births, deaths, separations, moves).
Ask about other consultations, referrals, tests, and results.

age-appropriate for the child), will also indicate the seriousness with which the problem is being addressed. Parents will not accept a physician's reassurances about the absence of physical disease if they do not believe that the problem was seriously considered in the first place. Laboratory investigations are no substitute for the physician's time and interest. While they may provide a convenient mechanism for dealing quickly with the issue and avoiding a prolonged office encounter, they are rarely useful in resolving the presenting problem in the absence of specific indications. In fact, laboratory tests often delay the inevitable—the session in which a thoughtful approach to the problem of a child's pain must be established.

After eliciting the full history of the pain problem, a little more digging into the underlying agenda can be helpful. Most parents have already wondered about a few frightening diagnostic possibilities but rarely voice them at the initial meeting. Make it easy for them to do so (e.g., "I don't know about you, but many parents whose children have recurrent headaches are already wondering about certain diseases or conditions. Have you had any such concerns?"). Getting the issues out on the table is the first step in addressing them and further assures the parents that you are at least considering the same possibilities that they are. Also, ask whether they are aware of any other family members or friends who have had similar or related problems. A relative who has just been diagnosed with colon cancer may heighten the concerns about any chronic abdominal complaint in a child (especially if the cancer was not diagnosed immediately after symptoms began).

The Psychobiological Perspective

Traditional categorization of pain as either organic or psychological is an outdated and limiting concept. Furthermore, to many parents (and some physicians), such categories have specific implications (e.g., *organic* means "real," while *psychological* means "fake"). Far more useful is the psychobiological perspective, which recognizes the complexity of pain as a phenomenon influenced by a multitude of factors. Not only do individuals have different thresholds for feeling or expressing pain but they are also subject do a variety of moderating factors including personality type, family issues, and external stresses. Exploration of family, school, and environmental issues is therefore an essential component of history taking in children with chronic pain. One must understand how the pain has affected the child and the family. How many days of school have been missed? Have the parents lost time at work? How has this affected the other children? Has the whole issue been stressful for the parents, and if so, how? What are other relatives and friends saying? When these questions are asked in a concerned manner and in the context of a thorough review of the problem, they are rarely viewed by families as intrusive. In fact, most families appreciate the time and interest being devoted to a difficult and long-standing problem.

Time Frame

Unlike the case with acute pain, the time frame for many types of chronic pain ranges from months to years. A child may not be obviously unwell but may have been complaining about the same symptoms for a very long time. Parents might be much more accepting of similar symptoms in themselves or another adult, but in the case of their children, they are particularly worried about missing something important. Sometimes, parents are convinced that there must be something wrong simply because the complaints have lasted so long. In fact, the reverse is often true; the shorter the duration, the more likely the pain will be due to some serious identifiable pathology or abnormality—although time alone is not a reliable way to tell whether pain is due to an illness. In dealing with a child who has had recurring pains over months or years, it is useful to point out that most of the "bad" diseases would have declared themselves by now.

Exploration of the frequency of pain can sometimes be turned to therapeutic advantage. If a parent is worried that a particular pain has been occurring approximately once a month and lasting 3 or 4 h, it can be helpful to point out that the child is *not* having pain for the remaining 29 days and 20 h of the month and that it is highly unlikely that any serious disease would cause symptoms so infrequently!

Parent-Child Relationship

Finally, an alert clinician must watch for any clues that the problem of chronic pain is simply the presenting symptom of more serious dysfunction in the parent-child relationship. In the vulnerable-child syndrome, the child becomes the unwitting victim of parental psychopathology. In other words, the presence of recurring symptoms or chronic illness in the child fulfills a parental need. In its most extreme form (Munchausen's syndrome by proxy), a parent may actually deceive clinicians and take a child from one facility to another, having repeated invasive investigations—or even surgery—based on a concocted history. While this end of the spectrum will be a rare occurrence for most practitioners, there are many well-meaning parents whose caregiving and nurturing needs are most rewarded when their children are ill. They seem incapable of seeing their child as healthy. For such parents, the concept of illness is not that of an occasional interruption in normal life activities; it is, instead, a full-time preoccupation. Sometimes, the problem is mild enough to be nothing more than an amusing character trait in the mother. (What clinician has not had the experience of being consulted about a vigorous, active, and well-grown 3-year-old whose mother's opening statement is "He's been sick since the day he was born!"?) For others, however, the implications are a little more serious, especially when they are interfering with schooling and making an otherwise healthy child a chronic patient. In sorting our this problem, be sure to elicit a clear history of previous consultations and investigations about the same issue. How many physicians have been involved? What tests were done, and what were the results? Has the child been hospitalized, and if so, why? Have other children in the family had similar problems? Be wary of answers that seem evasive or inconsistent. Ask permission to obtain prior records, and be suspicious if permission is denied.

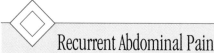

Recurrent Abdominal Pain

Recurrent abdominal pain (RAP) affects 5 to 10 percent of children at one time or another. It is frequently seen by pediatricians and has been a subject of study in the pediatric journals for decades, including a classic paper by Apley in which the characteristics of "little bellyachers" are well described. *Most textbooks list hundreds of causes of recurrent abdominal pain. However, those hundreds of causes usually account for about 5 percent of all the children who have these symptoms. For the remaining 95 percent, an obvious disease is rarely the cause.* Understandably, no parent wants his or her child to be part of the 5 percent and is usually concerned that nothing be missed.

Over the years, new theories about cause have emerged. Each idea rides a wave of popularity for a while. Some of the suggested causes that have appeared in both the medical and lay press in recent years are shown in Table 12-2.

Although each of these entities may occasionally be the problem, it is unlikely that any one accounts for a significant proportion of the many children with RAP. Food allergy in particular has always been a convenient "wastebasket" diagnosis for many conditions that elude specific etiology, and yet the evidence to support it as a widespread culprit is sadly lacking. Food restriction is a major burden to impose on child and family and should not be done in the absence of a fairly obvious cause-and-effect relationship to pain.

What is clear is that no single cause prevails and that the majority of children with RAP will never be diagnosed with a disease related to it. Nevertheless, there are several factors that may contribute to the situation, and each parent and caregiver should consider them.

Table 12-2

Popular Theories Regarding the Causes of RAP

Lactose intolerance
Gastroesophageal reflux
Helicobacter pylori infection
Food allergy
Irritable bowel syndrome

Description of the Pain

First is the question of language. Most children do not willingly describe the pain; instead, they usually say "My tummy hurts." Literal interpretation makes that a statement of pain. In fact, young children use the word *hurts* to describe *any* sensation different from their usual range of experience. It is helpful to point this out to parents, and indeed many will acknowledge that they often suggest that a child go to the bathroom as a first step toward relieving a "tummy-ache." The sensation that adults recognize as indicating a need to defecate may well be a "hurt" to a young child. Similarly, young children may use the term *hurt* to describe a variety of other sensations, including nausea, nervousness or "butterflies," hunger, a feeling of fullness after a meal, mild cramps, or the need to urinate. These are all sensations that the parents, as adults, will recognize and be familiar with. Making them aware of this analogy can help them develop a balanced perspective on their child's abdominal pain. Depending on the attention that has been paid to the matter, the child's descriptive pattern may become ingrained and may remain as part of an older child's vocabulary as well.

Sometimes, the physician can successfully elicit alternate descriptions of the pain while interviewing the child with the parents present. By using examples that the child recognizes, one may be able to narrow down the problem. ("When your tummy hurts, does it feel like you have to throw up . . . like you have to poop (or pee) . . . like you ate too much. . . etc.?"). From the parents, one can elicit the time pattern of recurrent pain (e.g., just before leaving for school, just before bedtime, or after meals) and determine how the child actually looks while he or she complains of pain. Some children relate the description in a very matter-of-fact manner and a few minutes later go out to play. Assess the degree to which the problem interferes with activities the child enjoys (playing with friends, etc.) and those he or she may not enjoy (such as school). Although all this information was always available to the parents, they may not clearly see the pattern until the physician draws it out during the interview. In other words, the history itself can be a useful exercise in helping parents to develop insight into their child's problem.

Stool Patterns

RAP can be associated with constipation. Sometimes the problem is evident because the child simply does not have a bowel movement very often. Yet there are also children whose constipation may not be so obvious because they seem to move their bowels daily. Such children may still have a lot of stool backed up in the bowel, causing frequent cramps, yet pass only a small amount of the total backlog. Many of these children get pain relief when fiber is added to their diets, even though they never complained of constipation. Occasionally, children will develop characteristic patterns of stool-withholding that may be difficult for them to change on their own. These children with full-fledged encopresis may have a large accumulation of stool in the colon and rectum, and may pass a bowel movement in the toilet only once every few days. Although the management of encopresis is beyond the scope of this chapter, every physician should be aware that recurrent abdominal pain may be the presenting symptom at the office visit, and the parent may not mention the bowel difficulties unless specifically asked.

Home Environment

An awareness of events in the child's environment (home, family, and school) is helpful in understanding recurrent abdominal pain. Children are creatures of habit, and major changes in their world can be quite disruptive. Some children express their upset or anxiety in words, but others show it in the development of a variety of physical symptoms, including abdominal pain. Moving—resulting in a change of city, home, or school—is disturbing to many children. The death of a relative or even a pet is difficult for children to understand and may trigger problems. The birth of a baby brother or sister is almost guaranteed to produce some degree of sibling rivalry (in other words, such reactions are normal), but may have a particular impact on some children. Finally, tensions within the home, especially marital difficulties, virtually always affect children to some degree.

Secondary Gain

Physicians can also help parents understand the pattern of secondary gain or positive reinforcement that develops in some children with RAP. Being ill usually attracts the concern and attention of one's parents. Children may not plan it this way, but the attention does reinforce a pattern of behavior that may have started quite innocently. Thus, some parents can track the onset of abdominal pain to an episode of gastroenteritis, which may have caused some cramps and discomfort. Yet the pain pattern persists well beyond the illness. Finally, in children whose parents are separated, being ill may be the one thing that brings the parents together in a mutual interest around the child.

Parental Issues

In approaching RAP, it can be illuminating to ask parents to take a close look at themselves. Parents who have chronic abdominal problems are more likely to have children with RAP. Some adults do indeed have intestinal symptoms on a regular basis without necessarily having a disease. Eliciting such a history is another way to help them develop insight into their child's problem. ("Do you have irritable bowel syndrome? Do you get diarrhea whenever you are

nervous or upset? Do you have a sensitive stomach? Do you vomit more easily than most people? Do you have problems with chronic constipation?") A "yes" answer to any of these question may indicate that the pattern is familial. Remind them that the apple does not usually fall far from the tree! The situation may be aggravated by the fact that adults who have these problems tend to focus on them more and may talk about them in front of their children, so that children have considerable exposure to these issues during their formative years.

Parents should also take a close look at their own concerns and anxiety. If a relative has recently been diagnosed with Crohn's disease, a parent may be particularly worried about stomach pain in a child. By recognizing the source of the concern, a parent may be able to keep it in perspective and avoid unduly increasing the child's anxiety. Also, by sharing the fear with the physician, a parent provides an opportunity to deal with the matter specifically, and thereby be reassured.

Tests

Many parents feel that some tests should be done to rule out serious disease. Testing for the sake of "ruling out," in the absence of evidence to suggest a particular diagnosis, is rarely helpful. Often, it may do more harm than good by subjecting the child to procedures that make him or her feel even more ill and vulnerable. Parents (and physicians) may be doing the child an even greater favor by ensuring that no unnecessary testing is done. It is far more valuable to spend the time reviewing some of the issues listed above than to go on a blind "fishing expedition" of laboratory tests and x-rays. In the end, each child's problems must be carefully considered on their own merits.

Management

Once you determine that a child belongs to the 95 percent whose pain cannot be easily related to a specific disease, share with the parents a sense of relief; this is *good* news. This conclusion may be difficult for parents to accept because of their fear that something has been overlooked, so make sure that they have an opportunity to have all their questions answered. This is the time when it is crucial that the parents feel that their concerns have not been dismissed. Booking a follow-up visit in a month or two is a good way to assure them that you have not lost interest and that you are available should the situation change. Be positive, but let them know that your door is always open. Some guidelines for the physician dealing with parents of children with RAP are shown in Table 12-3.

In explaining RAP, help parents understand that the child is not "making up" the symptoms. Explain that pain is a very subjective sensation, and we all learn different thresholds for pain as we grow up. The abdominal discomfort may be very real to the child, even when no disease is involved. Again, use an example with which adults can identify. An adult who develops diarrhea when nervous or who becomes nauseated at the sight of blood is not "making up" these symptoms, yet such reactions are very much linked to the brain and emotions—in both adults and in children.

Although most of this chapter focuses on the 95 percent of children with no underlying dis-

Table 12-3

General Guidelines for Parents of Children with Recurrent Abdominal Pain

Never ask child about pain. (If it hurts enough, he or she will tell you.)

Encourage child to deal with pain independently when it occurs

Emphasize need to address clearly identified psychosocial issues, and refer if necessary

Empathetic but firm insistence on return to school and normal activities

ease, recurrent abdominal pain that is associated with weight loss, recurrent fevers, chronic diarrhea, blood in the stools, pain or difficulty with urination, or frequent vomiting will require a different approach. The location of the pain may also be noteworthy. Usually, children will point to their navel as the site of the pain; if the pain is persistently on one side or if it is felt in the back, then further assessment is usually appropriate. Always be open to reviewing the clinical situation if new signs or symptoms appear.

In the absence of a serious illness requiring specific treatment, the physician is left wondering what to advise the parent. Specific advice must obviously be customized for each situation. Nevertheless, here are some general tips that may be helpful and can provide the parent with some concrete steps to follow:

1. Do not ask your child about pain if he or she has not brought it up and never ask if he or she had any pain today. If you ask the question, most children will say "yes"; if you don't ask, the child may not mention it. You can be sure that if the pain is significant, the child will bring it up. If the subject is not discussed, it is less likely to be inadvertently reinforced and may ultimately disappear. In other words, even talking about a child's pain can sometimes be "rewarding" for the child because it makes him or her the center of attention. This does not mean that the child is doing anything on purpose; but we do know that any behavior that is rewarded is usually repeated.

2. Teach the child ways to deal with the discomfort on his or her own, without disrupting routines for the rest of the household. The child may want to go to the bathroom and then perhaps lie down in the bedroom for a little while until the feeling passes. (Similarly, in school, it is preferable that the child lies down for a few minutes in the nurse's office rather than come home.)

3. If there are some obvious psychological or social stresses that may be playing a role

(death of a relative, recent move, marital problems), they must be dealt with openly. Professional counseling may be appropriate in this situation. Note that the counseling need not focus on the abdominal pain but may rather look at the stresses that underlie it.

4. Display an attitude of understanding and empathy while simultaneously encouraging your child to participate in normal routines to the greatest extent possible. School attendance is particularly important. Remember that when adults are ill or disabled, a major focus of treatment and rehabilitation is to enable a return to the workplace. School is, in fact, the child's workplace. Some parents feel that a child somehow needs to be protected from such real-world situations during any time of discomfort, but this approach may send the wrong message to the child and to others. It can be helpful to remind parents that one of the goals of the treatment of children with very serious ailments, such as cancer, is to get them back to school on a regular basis as quickly as possible. Indeed, parents of children with a variety of lifelong disabilities often become powerful advocates for the right of their children to attend school despite their significant difficulties. We should do no less for the child with chronic or recurrent abdominal pain.

5. Avoid extremes in dietary habit and try to maintain regular mealtimes. Although most recurrent abdominal pain is not due to food allergy or food intolerance, some children may be sensitive to excesses in their diet. For example, children who consume huge amounts of fruit juices each day, especially apple juice, may have abdominal discomfort. By the same token, adding a little fiber to the diet—in the form of whole wheat bread, popcorn, fiber cereals or high fiber cookies—may reduce symptoms in children with RAP.

Growing Pains

The common term *growing pains* usually refers to pains in the legs in young children. How growing pains got their name is a mystery. There is no real evidence that they have anything to do with growing except that they occur in childhood, when growth is admittedly occurring on an ongoing basis. Although there is no real explanation for them, they are indeed very real. Furthermore, they have some characteristics that are so common as to be very helpful in establishing a diagnosis.

Typically, these pains occur in children between the ages of 3 and 10 years, with a predilection for the younger end of the spectrum. They usually occur at night, often after the child is in bed, and seem to affect mainly the lower legs, especially the knees and shins. Because they occur at night, they frequently attract the attention of both parents and can become a fairly persistent pattern of disruption. In most cases, it is not difficult to differentiate growing pains from other, potentially serious problems in the legs. Here are some hints that can be shared with parents:

• Growing pains generally affect both legs. An injury or abnormality other than growing pains is more likely to involve only one leg.
• With growing pains, the problem often occurs when the child is motionless and not bearing weight. In almost any other problem of bone, joint, or muscle, the pain is worse when the affected part is in use or is at least bearing weight. Children with growing pains do not limp and are able to participate in their usual activities, including sports.
• Children with growing pains get relief from someone rubbing or massaging of the affected area. A child with a sore joint or a bruise does not like to have the area touched.

- Once asleep, children with growing pains rarely awaken until morning, and at that time are usually fine. More serious problems are unlikely to resolve that quickly.
- This problem often runs in families. Ask whether either parent was similarly affected (they may need to check with the grandparents). A positive response can be reassuring and helpful in understanding this as a common but transient childhood condition.

Like most problems in childhood, there is a wide spectrum of severity. Most children will have a pattern that is easily recognizable. Those with atypical or unilateral problems may need more focused assessment and investigation. These children may benefit from a referral to a physician experienced with such problems and may require some tests before a diagnosis can be made. There is no test for typical growing pains, however. It is a diagnosis made by observing a classic pattern and by being assured that there is no evidence to suggest any other cause for the pain.

Treatment tends to be simple. A simple pain reliever such as acetaminophen, ibuprofen, or aspirin (when not contraindicated) may provide relief at bedtime. Massage of the area or application of heat may also be helpful.

Teething Pain

Does teething cause pain? Generations of parents are absolutely convinced that it does. Teething has also been alleged to cause fever, rash, diarrhea, and vomiting in young infants. Historically, teething was considered a far more ominous malady; in 1839, over 5000 deaths among infants and children in England and Wales were officially attributed to teething. Despite centuries of concern about this universal phenomenon, there is not a shred of reliable evidence to support its role in any of these common childhood problems!

The many beliefs about teething are not unique to European or North American culture. In many cultures, teething is also seen as a disease requiring specific intervention and treatment. Is it conceivable that millions of parents, grandparents, and great-grandparents could be wrong? Let us consider some facts.

From the time they are born, infants are continually exposed to a variety of common viruses in their environments. The most common signs of illness when infants are infected with such viruses are fever, rash, and diarrhea—the same signs attributed to teething. Why then, does teething get the blame? The usual sequence of events is as follows: A parent notes that the infant is warm, has a rash, or has diarrhea; the parent then looks in the baby's mouth, specifically at the gums. From about 3 to 4 months until 2 1/2 years of age, there is virtually *always* a tooth about to erupt or erupting. As soon as the parent sees the swollen gum, he or she assumes that a diagnosis has been confirmed. The fact is that if the parent looked at the gums on a day when the baby had no symptoms, he or she would probably see a very similar picture!

It may be reasonable to assume that the little bit of swelling and redness observed over the gum just before the tooth breaks through might cause slight discomfort, but there is no logical way to connect the other symptoms described above. Even when babies drool and put things in their mouths, it is not clear whether they do this because of gum pain or is simply as part of normal development. After all, some normal infants do not have a tooth erupt until 12 months of age, but they still start putting things into their mouths at 4 to 5 months. The danger in blaming illnesses on teething is, of course, that it may provide false reassurance in the presence of a more serious problem.

If teething is not a disease, does it require treatment? A stroll through any drugstore reveals a wide array of preparations sold for the purpose of treating teething pain. In general, it is wise to avoid them. Most are fairly benign when used appropriately, but there have been rare instances of children suffering serious side effects, such as methemoglobinemia, when such medicines were improperly used (as when a 2-year-old ate an entire tube of teething gel containing local anesthetic). Unlikely as this may be, it hardly seems worth any risk if one is treating a "nondisease." After all, what could possibly be more normal than the eruption of teeth through the gums in a healthy baby? Simply stated, it is a part of normal human growth, and we should treat it as such.

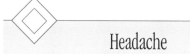

Headache

Like abdominal pain, headache tends to be a recurrent phenomenon in some children. Although some parents feel that headache should not occur in children, it is in fact quite common, especially in school-age and adolescent children. Headache may be a part of the symptom complex of any viral illness; however, this section focuses more on chronic or recurrent headaches.

The underlying fear of every parent whose child has headaches is the potential of an ominous underlying problem. The worst fear is that of a brain tumor, and although parents rarely mention it, they usually acknowledge having thought about it. All clinicians must obviously be alert to the possibility of intracranial disease in any child with unrelenting headache, early morning headache and vomiting, seizures, difficulty with speech or movement, or a change in consciousness. However, in a given practice, such children would be a fraction of a percentage of all those who may complain of occasional headaches.

Simply put, some children are headache-prone. They often take after at least one of their parents. The pattern of recurrent headache may develop at a fairly young age, but it is more likely to start after they are in school. These are children who are otherwise healthy and function normally in every way, but periodically they develop a bad headache. A frequent cause is migraine.

Migraine

Fortunately, migraine is something most parents have heard of. They are less likely to know that it can occur in childhood. Making them aware of this fact and that it occurs commonly is an important first step in helping them cope with it. Help them understand that there is no single cause of migraine, but that it does run in families (it is often comforting to parents to recognize that they are dealing with a condition that others in the family have). This is another situation in which parent education is a worthwhile investment. Clear explanations are appreciated and reinforce parents' confidence in the provider. For example, "Migraine is triggered by a change in size of the blood vessels that carry blood to the brain. Arteries, being lined by muscle, have the ability to become narrow or wider. In migraine headache, the arteries first constrict (become tighter), sometimes causing symptoms such as visual disturbances or 'funny feelings', and then dilate (become wider). When they dilate, the headache usually begins."

When a physician can knowledgeably and calmly elicit the classic signs and symptoms, he or she can paint a familiar picture and use this as the basis for explanation and reassurance. Children with migraine often feel nauseated and may even vomit. They frequently want to avoid bright light and loud noises and may be most comfortable when they lie down in a dark room and go to sleep. The fact that the physician is so familiar with the problem is in itself reassuring for concerned parents.

Once a child is known to be prone to migraine, there may be certain triggers that will set it off. Even if parents are not immediately aware of any pattern, it may be helpful for them to keep a prospective migraine diary. This has the added advantage of making them active partners in the therapeutic strategy and provides them with a sense of understanding and control that is very important. Sometimes fatigue, exercise, or long periods in the sun can trigger the headache. Also, food triggers can sometimes be identified; it may be valuable to keep a record of what was eaten just prior to a headache to see if a consistent pattern emerges. Common culprits include nuts, caffeine (as in cola drinks), spiced meats, etc. With time, parents (and children) become the real experts in identifying their patterns of migraine. They can usually tell when an episode is beginning and know what to do.

Most children with migraine can be treated with the simple measures listed above and with acetaminophen or ibuprofen. Ergotamine tartrate (usual dose is 1 mg) is used with some success in older children. In using medication, it is important to give it as early as possible and in sufficient initial dosage to be effective. Parents are generally loath to use pain medication unless absolute necessary—a practice which, in most situations, makes good sense. However, with migraine, the longer it has been present, the more difficult it is to get rid of. Therefore, once parents are familiar with a child's migraine pattern, they should be encouraged to treat early rather than late. In fact, analgesia and rest in a quiet room, if initiated at the very first sign of a headache, may be effective in aborting the episode. It is wise to ensure that the school staff is also instructed as to how to proceed.

Some migraine is particularly troublesome and may not respond to these simple measures. Sumatriptan, a specific and selective 5-HT receptor agonist, has been an effective drug for treating migraines in adults. It is not presently licensed for children under age 18. Biofeedback and self-hypnosis are used in some centers with children over 8 years of age.

Tension Headaches

Tension headaches are the other major cause of head pain in children. While more common in adolescents, they can occur in preteens as well. These headaches produce a sense of tightness around the head, especially over the temples. There may also be tightness of the neck muscles.

Typically, tension headaches are responses to stress. Most of us have experienced them at one time or another—after a particularly difficult day at work or an emotionally draining event at home. Children and teens are no different in their responses to stress; the challenge may be to find out just what the stress is. Indeed, the children themselves may not recognize the triggers. Just as events in a child's environment (family, school, and home) may be factors in recurrent abdominal pain, they can also be at the root of tension headaches.

If children are unwilling to talk openly about these issues with their parents (and parents may be part of the problem), further help may be necessary. Sometimes a referral to a psychologist, psychiatrist, or other professional counselor may be valuable. With such expert help, it may be possible to better understand the underlying issues; also, many psychologists can effectively teach the child some relaxation techniques to help relieve the headaches when they first occur. Thus, the child gains more control over what happens to his or her body and becomes less vulnerable.

Chest Pain

In children, chest pain is less common than some of the other problems mentioned in this chapter. Nevertheless, it always frightens parents, probably because it has a very different implication in adults. We are trained to think of chest pain in adults as one of the first signs of a possible myocardial infarction. In children, heart problems are extremely rare causes of chest pain.

In most cases, tests are not very helpful in determining a cause for chest pain. The story of the pain is far more useful, and by asking the right questions, an experienced clinician can often decide whether or not further investigation is needed.

The commonest cause of chest pain is a musculoskeletal problem. Given that the entire thoracic cage is lined with muscles, a cramp or spasm in any one of the muscles can cause a sharp pain, especially when the child is taking a deep breath. Such pain is sometimes referred to as a "stitch." Some children and adolescents are particularly prone to this. Both parent and child need to understand that, just as muscles in the leg can get sore or pulled from overuse, so can the muscles in the chest. Thus, a child with a bad cough may eventually develop chest pain from all the coughing, although this usually improves as the cough gets better.

Esophageal pain may be typical from its location, timing, and symptoms. Most adults have heard of "heartburn" as a cause of chest pain, but they do not always realize that it has nothing to do with the heart. Again, the physician can explain the mechanism of irritation from acid that the stomach regurgitates upward into the chest. This is less common in children but can occur, causing a burning pain in the center of the chest.

Parents should not feel that they have to figure out chest pain on their own. A visit to a physician will often help to sort out whether or not a significant problem exists. Parents should know, however, that most causes are minor and that the problem will improve with time. Even anxiety and depression can cause chest pain, and in these situations it is more important to find the cause of the problem than to provide

pain medication. Chest pain that is severe and persistent, is associated with fever, or causes shortness of breath needs medical assessment.

Conclusion

What conclusions can be drawn from all this? First, no single rule can apply to many different situations, and each child's problem needs to be considered individually. Second, the majority of chronic pain problems in childhood are not due to serious underlying disease. Third, even when disease is not present, children do not usually "make up" their pain.

No primary physician can be an expert on every kind of pain. Yet he or she can bring enormous comfort to families by reducing the anxiety that is associated with many kinds of chronic pain in children. Avoid the pitfalls of "diagnosis by exclusion," a chain of events that can lead to never-ending investigations of increasing invasiveness. Diagnoses are made by positive findings, not negative ones. And always remember the old adage that the definition of a normal person is someone who has not been adequately investigated!

Bibliography

Pediatric Pain—General

Apley J, MacKeith R, Meadow R: Recurrent pain, in *The Child and His Symptoms*. Oxford, UK, Blackwell, 1978, pp 58–76.

Dolgin MJ, Phipps S: Pediatric pain: the parents' role. *Pediatrician* 16:03–109, 1989.

McGrath PJ, Craig KD: Developmental and psychological factors in children's pain. *Pediatr Clin North Am* 36:823–836, 1989.

Siegel LJ, Smith KE: Children's strategies for coping with pain. *Pediatrician* 16:110–118, 1989.

Smith MS, Tyler DC, Womack WM, et al: Assessment and management of recurrent pain in adolescence. *Pediatrician* 16:85–93, 1989.

Zeltzer LK, Barr RG, McGrath PA, et al: Pediatric pain: interacting behavioral and physical factors. *Pediatrics* 90:816–821, 1992.

Zeltzer L, Bursch B, Walco G: Pain responsiveness and chronic pain: a psychobilogical perspective. *J Dev Behav Pediatr* 18:413–422, 1997.

Recurrent Abdominal Pain

Apley J: *The Child with Abdominal Pains*, 2nd ed. Oxford, UK, Blackwell, 1975.

Coleman WL, Levine MD: Recurrent abdominal pain: the cost of the aches and the aches of the cost. *Pediatr Rev* 8:143–151, 1986.

Hyams JS: Recurrent abdominal pain in children (commentary). *Curr Opin Pediatr* 7:529–532, 1995.

Hyams JS, Hyman PE: Recurrent abdominal pain and the biopsychosocial model of medical practice. *J Pediatr* 133:473–478, 1998.

Levine MD, Rappaport LA: Recurrent abdominal pain in school children: the loneliness of the long-distance physician. *Pediatr Clin North Am* 31:969–991, 1984.

Limb Pain

Bowyer SL, Hollister JR: Limb pain in childhood. *Pediatr Clin North Am* 31:1053–1080, 1984.

Sherry DD: Limb pain in childhood. *Pediatr Rev* 12:39–46, 1990.

Teething Pain

Bennett HJ, Brudno DS: The teething virus. *Pediatr Infect Dis* 5:399–401, 1986.

Swann IL: Teething complications, a persisting misconception. *Postgrad Med J* 55:24–25, 1979.

Headache

Holden EW, Levy JD, Deichmann MM, et al: Recurrent pediatric headaches: assessment and intervention. *Dev Behav Pediatr* 19:109–116, 1998.

McGrath PJ, Humphreys P: Recurrent headaches in children and adolescents: diagnosis and treatment. *Pediatrician* 16:71–77, 1989.

Smith MS: Comprehensive evaluation and treatment of recurrent pediatric headache. *Pediatr Ann* 24:450–466, 1995.

Chest Pain

Kocis KC: Chest pain in pediatrics. *Pediatr Clin North Am* 46:189–203, 1999.

Jeffrey A. Wright

Enuresis and Constipation

Elimination of waste products is a basic biological function. Nearly all parents at one time or another have questions or concerns about this function in their child. Questions range from those dealing with normal developmental stages, such as toilet training, to concerns about failure to achieve those stages or other specific disorders such as constipation, bedwetting, and urinary or fecal "accidents." It is either too much or too little or it occurs at the wrong time or place! This chapter considers the child in a developmental context to give an approach to analysis and management of some of the most common concerns about elimination.

Elimination problems can be classified under the general rubrics of defecation dysfunction and urinary dysfunction. Dysfunctional defecation includes constipation and encopresis.

Urinary dysfunction includes the dysfunctional voiding syndrome and enuresis. While related, motility disorders such as irritable bowel syndrome, chronic abdominal pain, and recurrent urinary tract infections are not discussed here but are reviewed in other chapters.

These conditions are model biobehavioral conditions, having both emotional and biological origins and consequences. Sorting these various components is intellectually challenging and well-suited for generalists who like to think broadly about their patients. Patients do well with providers who can respond to both biological and behavioral components. Most patients with elimination disorders can be managed within the care domain of the generalist.

As many as 10 percent of first graders have nocturnal enuresis and up to 2 percent have encopresis.[1] About 4 percent of visits to pediatricians are for constipation and 16 percent of 2-year-olds are said to be constipated by parental report.[2,3] These conditions are treatable and largely preventable. With resolution, the deep appreciation felt by patients and family make these problems rewarding to manage.

Despite the frequency of defecation disorders, there is a relative lack of research, especially clinical trials, to date. For example, there is no population-based study of encopresis prevalence reported in United States children. Despite the increasing average age of toilet training through the generations, there does not appear to be a decline in the rate of failure or complication. It is difficult to make clear recommendations to parents about ideal toilet training without some basic epidemiologic information.

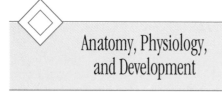

Anatomy, Physiology, and Development

The sphincters controlling elimination intrinsically link the anatomy of the urinary and intestinal tracts. Both urinary and anal sphincters are composed of the muscles in the puborectalis sling. The sphincters are made up of layers of muscles that share innervation and work as a syncytium. It is not possible to independently regulate the sphincters, and it is common for dysfunction in one area to be associated with dysfunction in the other. In short, dysfunction results from either high or low resting tone of the sphincters, or the inability to either constrict or relax the sphincters at will. The urinary and gastrointestinal systems are similar in that emotional state affects the functioning of the sphincters. Having an intestinal nervous system that controls motility and consequently bowel transit time further complicates fecal elimination. The power of these small muscular sphincters over the lives of children and their families is impressive.

There is a "dance," of sorts, between the brain, the internal anal sphincter (IAS), and the external anal sphincter (EAS). Continence is maintained by involuntary tonus of the IAS and somewhat by reflex constriction of the EAS. The internal sphincter is autonomic and responds differently depending on whether the rectum is filled slowly or quickly. If the rectum is acutely distended, as when feces descend into the rectum, the IAS relaxes and the EAS constricts reflexively. Relaxation of the EAS requires voluntary cortical overriding of the reflex constriction to allow defecation to proceed. A bowel movement occurs when the constriction is consciously released or is overwhelmed by pressure within the rectum. Many children with constipation have a high resting tone of their EAS and seem unable to relax it through cortical control. Some children paradoxically constrict the EAS with efforts to expel feces. The harder they push, the tighter the sphincter becomes. There are a variety of terms—including *rectal dyssynergy*, *anismus*, and *paradoxical anal constriction*—that describe the situation when the "dancer stumbles" in this manner.

The urinary system is similarly afflicted in the case of dysfunctional voiding. The process is the same, with inability to cortically control the external urethral sphincter. The bladder accommodates a gradual increase in urine volume until a critical volume is achieved. Until then, there is no real urge to urinate. Once the critical volume is reached, the detrusor muscle constricts, causing a sudden increase in pressure. Sudden gushes of urine may occur when the detrusor muscle contracts, overwhelming the ability of the sphincter to withhold urinary flow (causing urgency and accidents). In dysfunctional voiding, there is residual urine after voiding because of incomplete emptying due to high external sphincter tone. The bladder's critical volume is achieved more readily (causing frequent urination). Various terms describe this condition, including *frequency-urgency syndrome, overactive bladder*, and *dysfunctional voiding.*

As with all motor skills, some children are "naturals"; others only accomplish the skill with maturation and repeated practice. Using an analogy with sports skill development may help parents understand that their child is not a "gifted athlete" when it comes to the skill of urinary or fecal control. Children with urinary and/or defecation dysfunction develop maladapted behaviors in response to their ineffective elimination. This destroys their confidence and further compounds their anxiety about elimination, making the problems worse.

Defecation Dysfunction

Defecation dysfunction occurs when any one system—the central nervous system (CNS, or cortex), the autonomic and gut nervous system, or the motor neuronal system—fails to operate in concert with the others. The cortex is under the influence of innate factors such temperament and learned responses (a painful bowel movement) and emotional state (stress, generalized anxiety, etc.). The gastrointestinal nervous system responds to a host of gut hormones, dietary content, and emotional influences. The neuromotor unit has a physiologic resting state that determines sphincter tone, and motility coordination also changes with development.

Cortical and emotional influence have long been blamed as the origin of encopresis. This is only part of the picture. There are both afferent (gut to brain) and efferent (brain to gut) interconnections; the "gut-brain highway." Children with constipation and encopresis have defects in the afferent system. Rectal stimulation fails to produce normal cortical evoked potentials; it is not "all in their head." The concept of the "gut-brain highway" can be explained to parents, using, as example, people who experience diarrhea, cramps, or "butterflies in the stomach" when they are under emotional stress (brain to gut) and by citing how terribly intestinal cramps and nausea can make people feel (gut to brain).

Initially all children are incontinent. Newborn elimination patterns are chaotic. There is a high sensitivity to stimuli from eating. Often, a newborn will have a bowel movement with each meal. At 3 to 4 months of age, at the same time the infant is developing diurnal rhythm in sleep, the intestinal nervous system (INS) stabilizes and the number of bowel movements may suddenly decrease. This is the first of several critical periods for the development of constipation. If the peristalsis slows a fraction too much, feces will become larger and drier, making them more difficult to pass. Parents often mention, at the 4-month health supervision visit, their observation of their infant turning red in the face and straining to defecate. This has been termed "the grunting baby" and may represent early learning about the coordination of defecation.[4] Breast-fed infants tend to pass more frequent and softer feces than their formula-fed peers, and they seem to have fewer problems with constipation in infancy. Adding solids to the diet may slow bowel transit time and increase intraluminal bulk, causing constipation.

The colon's sole function is to extract water from feces and hold the feces until an appropriate time for elimination. The stomach empties about 1 h after a meal and small bowel transit is completed about 4 h later. The feces then enter the cecum. The time from entry into the cecum until defecation varies between 12 and 72 h. The ascending colon has a predominantly retrograde peristalsis, back toward the cecum. The ascending colon and cecum are saccular and easily distended. The transverse colon has a to-an-fro motion, moving feces forward and then backward. The motion of the descending colon is predominantly directed toward the sigmoid. Several times each day, often after meals, there is a strong forward propulsive wave from the cecum to the sigmoid. This moves the bolus of feces from the ascending to the transverse and from the transverse to the descending colon, and sigmoid, and rectum. This stimulates the urge to defecate. Upon defecation, some people empty only the rectum while others empty the contents of their bowel to the splenic flexure, depending on the power of the forward propulsive motion.

During early toddlerhood, a new spinal reflex develops. When feces enter the rectum, they stimulate local relaxation of the internal anal sphincter. A signal is sent, via a spinal arc, causing reflex constriction of the external anal sphincter. Prior to development of this reflex, there would be relaxation of the external sphincter and spontaneous elimination. Now, the external sphincter constricts and pressure builds within the rectum. A parent, noting his or her child's awareness of the urge to defecate, might use this opportunity to capture the product in the preferred location. For most children this is not a problem and they are eager to please their parents. However, the sensitive or anxious child may react to these attempts at toilet training by associating the "defecation urge anxiety" with the toilet. Such a child may withhold and display behaviors of leg crossing or hiding until the sensation abates. This results in further accumulation of feces in the rectum, initiating a cycle of retention and progressive colorectal enlargement.

Another common time for children to develop difficulties with defecation is when they venture from their usual surroundings to more public facilities such as day care, school, or other places of travel. Here the sensitive, poorly adaptive child may react negatively to unfamiliar odors, feelings of lack of privacy, or even to facilities that are cold to touch. Many parents note that their school age child will admit to withholding their bowel movement all day, waiting until they come home to use their more familiar bathroom.

In summary, the INS is highly balanced with the CNS. The abilities and state of one affect those of the other. This can be thought of as similar to a thermostatic control—a basic autonomic set point responds to cortical input and affects gastrointestinal motility. Reciprocally, there are cortical responses sending signals to the gut. If the child is "all put together," the systems work smoothly, but if anything goes awry, a prolonged period of dysfunctional defecation may follow.

The development of elimination skills can be explained to parents by comparing it with other areas of development. Just as a toddler often understands more than he or she can say, children may have cognitive understanding of the goals of toilet training before they are neurodevelopmentally able to perform the task. For most children, time is all that is required for maturation to occur. As in the case of most biological phenomena, there is a bell-shaped distribution to acquiring these skills, with some predictable minority destined to be the last.

There is a cluster of comorbidities with encopresis including attention deficit hyperactivity disorder, learning disorders, oppositional defiant disorder, and motor dysfunction. This highlights the fact that children with mild neurologic dysfunction have higher rates of elimination disorders. One might postulate that because there are higher rates of all these conditions among males, males tend to experience a neurologic delay in maturation and/or integration compared to females.

Children with more severe neurologic impairment—such as those with mental retardation, cerebral palsy, meningomyelocele, or other spinal cord disorders—frequently have associated bowel and bladder dysfunction. Soiling with these conditions is specifically excluded from the diagnosis of encopresis in the American Psychiatric Association's *Diagnostic and Statistical Manual of Mental Disorders*, 4th ed. (DSM-IV) and is more correctly is termed *incontinence*. Similarly, any bowel disorder resulting in diarrhea with "accidents" is not called encopresis by definition.

Evaluation

It is incumbent on the health care provider dealing with children to ask about elimination. Owing to its sensitive nature, many patients or parents will not volunteer that there is a problem. It is the story obtained during the course of health supervision visits that gives clues to such problems. Remember that children are usually cleaned and dressed for their visit to the doctor, so soiled underpants may be a hidden fact unless specifically asked about. Parents may not know about normal defecation behavior, fecal quality, or frequency of elimination. In brief, bowel movements should occur about daily, and feces should be soft and painless to pass. Their consistency should be like that of toothpaste, with no scybala (the small balls that can look like "rabbit raisins"). Using this definition of normal, constipation is a deviation from that either because of decreased fecal frequency, hardness, pain with defecation, or difficulty in passing feces, as indicated by straining.

A general caveat: the earlier the constipation is diagnosed and the more aggressively it is treated until resolved, the shorter will be the duration of problem with fewer secondary consequences. Identifying the constipated toddler and making sure that constipation does not persist can prevent many cases of encopresis. The constipated toddler persages most cases of encopresis.

With this background, the origins of constipation can be divided into the causes outlined in Table 13-1.

The medical history is usually sufficient to make a diagnosis of constipation and to understand its etiology. The average number of bowel movements after infancy is about six (plus or minus two) per week. The cause of constipation is either slow gut motility or obstruction of elimination. Obstruction can occur because of anatomic disorders or disorders involving the process of defecation. Possible anatomic disorders include anal stenosis, anterior dislocation of the anus, or outlet obstruction due to mass. Anal abnormalities are present from birth and should be diagnosed early, but it is amazing how often these are overlooked.

Anorectal incoordination or poor motility leads to accumulation of feces in the rectum and a large fecal diameter. Scybalous feces are characteristic of slow motility or low dietary fiber content. If there is a clear history of regularly passing large-diameter feces, there is no need to test further for Hirschsprung's disease.

Irritable bowel syndrome usually presents as diarrhea, but in toddlers and some older children there may be a history of diarrhea alternating with constipation. These children may have gushes of liquid stool, often confused with retentive encopresis with overflow incontinence or with nonretentive encopresis (see below).

There is a controversial condition that has been called *intestinal neuronal dysplasia*. It is controversial because it is not clear whether the condition really exists. Symptoms are intractable idiopathic constipation. Some have found changes in the bowel wall on microscopic examination. It remains for pediatric gastroenterologists to define this condition more clearly, but at present there is no specific treatment other than that for constipation.

ARE RECTAL EXAMS NECESSARY?

Rectal examinations are usually touted as an essential step in the evaluation of the child with

Table 13-1

Causes and Typical Clinical History of Constipation

CAUSE	TYPICAL CLINICAL HISTORY
Infantile incoordination of peristalsis	A 4 month-old with sudden onset of impaction, distention, and abdominal pain.
Dietary factors	Chronic hard small feces noted to have onset with change in diet.
Change from breast to formula	
Change from formula to cow's milk	
Cow's milk protein intolerance	
Initiation of solids	
Low fiber intake	
Slow transit time	Relapses after laxatives discontinued.
Intrinsic low motility	
Hypothyroidism	
Secondary to medication or medical disorder	
Anxiety	A toddler who will only defecate in a diaper, the "pull-up pooper." May use the toilet for urination.
About passing feces	
About using toilet	
Fear of falling in	
Fear of monsters	
Secondary to painful event	
Anal fissure	
Sexual abuse	
Secondary to overcoersion	
Oppositional disorder	Preschool–age child who runs from parents or has a tantrum in response to efforts to encourage use of the toilet.
Heightened emotional state	Parents are unaware of the elimination pattern, disagree on management, or accuse the other parent of contributing to the problem.
Dysfunctional family	
Divorce	
Abuse	
Anatomic disorders	History of constipation dating to the newborn period and persisting.
Anterior anus	
Anal stenosis	
Short-segment Hirschsprung's	
Mixed	Inappropriate parental response to the other causes with secondary emotional state or anxiety.

constipation. Although this simple examination may yield valuable information, it does have some risks. All children should have external inspection of the anus, which can provide information about anatomy, location, and resting sphincter tone. A gaping anus can be the result of either long-standing constipation or repeated anal sexual abuse. The presence of anal fissures, tags, hemorrhoids, or prolapse can be due to long-standing constipation, anal sexual abuse, or chronic malabsorption. The rectal digital exam can help to identify sphincter weakness due to neurologic disorders and the presence of a prominent posterior shelf, found in anterior dislocation of the anus. The rectal exam can serve as a "poor man's anal manometry." A simple maneuver can be performed by asking the patient to constrict and then relax the anal sphincter. Then the patient is asked to attempt to push the examiner's finger out of the rectum. Paradoxical anal constriction may be diagnosed if an increased sphincter tone is noted on attempts to expel the finger and poor ability to relax voluntarily. Some of these children also have a high resting anal tone with the ability to neither relax nor constrict, but this is usually not apparent on rectal exam. Inspect the lower back looking for dimples, hair tufts, or mass; these may lead to discovery of spinal dysraphism or presacral teratoma.

The risk in performing a rectal exam is that the child may have been sensitized by prior invasive experiences, perhaps because of anal sexual abuse or either prescribed or parent-initiated treatment. Parents who have used enemas, suppositories, or anal stimulation may have created a vicious cycle of pain, personal invasion, and further fecal withholding. There are horrific stories of parents chasing children about the house, capturing and holding them down with legs spread, to insert well-meaning therapy into the rectum. This is abusive, and we do not recommend this approach. If the child is unable to cooperate or permit a rectal exam or there is a known history of anal abuse, the exam should be deferred to a later time. Rarely, exam under general anesthesia may need to be done.

A careful history is usually sufficient to make the diagnosis of constipation, fecal withholding, or incontinence. The rectal exam helps identify the rare organic cause of these problems. For completeness, it should be done, but failure to obtain the exam need not postpone initiation treatment in the fearful child. If treatment fails, then the evaluation should be completed, looking for rare causes.

ARE ABDOMINAL ROENTGENOGRAMS HELPFUL?

Often abdominal flat-plate roentgenograms are obtained to evaluate the degree of fecal impaction. The advantage of the radiograph is that this shows parents physical evidence of a biological disorder. Parents who had been angry with their child may become compassionate in view of a now obvious medical disorder. This can be a powerful tool to initiate a new beginning in the parent-child relationship. That aside, the radiograph is often overinterpreted, with presence of any feces read as impaction. The radiograph has poor inter- and intraobserver reliability and poor correlation with motility and outcome. Some use the radiograph to scale the aggressiveness of laxative therapy. There are no randomized controlled trials to show that radiographs guide therapy better than history or examination. Roentgenograms do not need to be done unless the physician determines that this tool is needed to ensure a therapeutic relationship. The value of such a relationship exceeds the cost and risk of the test, and a few more minutes of communication may save that money and radiation exposure.

Treatment of Constipation

The main concept for treating constipation is that treatment should be intensified until resolution occurs. The earlier and more effective the treatment, the less likely will be the long-standing problems or complications.

Increasing fiber in the diet is the mainstay of treating constipation in adults, but children just do not like to eat fibrous foods. Sneaky ways to increase fiber include switching from white to whole wheat or other whole-grain breads, adding bran to cookies or muffins, increasing the amount of fresh fruit and vegetables in the daily menu, and by making drinks (fruit smoothies, Ultra Slim Fast) with added fiber. Eating a cup of popcorn and an apple a day will add 2 to 4 g of fiber. Increasing fiber is a gradual process and goal. It really involves changes in the whole family's eating pattern and acceptance of new foods into the child's regimen. This takes time and repeated exposures. Also, children may rebel against the parents' attempts to get them to eat "what is good for you." Children should learn to feed themselves and regulate their energy intake. This means that parents may need to compromise and use medicine to treat constipation rather than food.

However, there is another dietary modification that can benefit the child—namely, the reduction of cow's milk in the diet. A number of studies show that cow's milk intake is associated with constipation. Theories about cause range from calcium fatty acid soaps to milk protein allergy.[5] Whatever the cause, if the child is a large cow's milk or cheese consumer, a reduction in this intake may improve the constipation.

Assuming that there are no organic causes of constipation, treatment is geared toward softening the stool or increasing colon motility. A wide variety of laxatives are available (see Table 13-2 for examples). Laxatives can be divided into stimulant, lubricant, surfactant, osmotic, and bulk-forming agents. They all work, but individuals have preferences for one form over another because of palatability or side effects. Most laxatives are derived from natural substances, but patients who prefer a "natural" remedy can choose from a variety of herbal teas, bulking agents, or fruit mixture concoctions. Chewing sugar-free gum or eating dietetic candy provides an alternative source of sorbitol. Fruit juices such as pear or prune also have high sorbitol content. A caution: "natural" laxatives are often as strong or stronger than traditional pharmaceutical laxatives. They often contain senna, cascara, aloe, or other stimulants in amounts greater than those in over-the-counter preparations.

Colon motility is increased with most laxatives. In addition, a number of other prokinetic medicines are used to increase bowel motility. Drugs such as metoclopramide, cisapride, and other drugs stimulating contraction—including erythromycin or parasympathomimetics such as neostigmine or bethanechol—have been used. Cisapride has been the most studied in children and appears to be effective in idiopathic constipation. However, cisapride has been recently cited as causing heart condition changes and is no longer recommended. Because these medications are more expensive than laxatives and diagnostic tests for bowel motility disorders are expensive and often unavailable (requiring an experienced pediatric gastroenterologist or surgeon), it seems prudent to try laxatives before turning to prokinetic agents.

Laxative abuse and dependency are overrated concerns. Laxative abusers share common features with those diagnosed with anorexia nervosa and bulimia; treatment of constipation does not cause these conditions. There is really no evidence of dependency on laxatives in children in the existing medical literature.

Other components of treatment include ensuring adequate fluid intake, regular exercise, and general bowel hygiene, including response to urges to defecate. See the discussion below of maintenance therapy for retentive encopresis to obtain additional management tips.

Encopresis

The definition of encopresis is fecal soiling after the expected age of toilet training in the absence of medical disorders (see Fig. 13-1, an algorithm for the evaluation and treatment of fecal soiling).

In the United States, the current age expected for completed toilet training is a mental age of 4 years. Fecal soiling occurs when there is too much pressure from within the gut so that it overwhelms a normal anal sphincter or when normal peristalsis encounters a sphincter that does not work properly. The evaluation of soiling involves looking for those physical disorders that increase intraluminal pressure or alter sphincter function. It becomes somewhat of a semantic conundrum when one considers that retentive encopresis leads to sphincter dysfunc-

Table 13-2

Common Laxatives and Dosages

Category Generic (Brand)	Adverse Effects	Usual Maintenance (Constipation) Dosage for Children 6–12 Years of Age	Cleanout Dosage
Stimulants Bisacodyl (Dulcolax) Senna (Senokot)	Cramps	5–10 mg/day 5–10 mL qhs or 0.5–1 tsp granules qhs	
Bulk-producing Psyllium (Metamucil) Polycarbophil	Implication if inadequate fluid intake.	2.5–5 g qd–qid	
Surfactant Docusate (Colace)	Not recommended for use with mineral oil.	40–120 mg/day	
Lubricant Mineral Oil	Aspiration risk.	1–3 tbsp/day	9–12 tbsp/day
Osmotics Sugars Lactulose Sorbitol	Gas, bloating, cramps.	1–2 mL/kg/day in 2–3 divided doses	
Salts Magnesium (hydroxide in milk of magnesia, citrate in magnesium citrate)	Watch use of magnesium in patients with renal dysfunction.		
Polyethylene glycol electrolyte solution (GoLYTELY, CoLyte, MiraLax)	Nausea, bloating, vomiting, cramps	2 mL/kg/day in 1–2 divided doses 1 tbsp/8 oz water per day	500–1800 mL/h; usually requires nasogastric tube.

tion, as discussed previously. I believe that, as understanding increases, more cases of encopresis will be considered "organic" and that the term will then have outlived its usefulness. In current usage, the organic disorders excluded are those from the presently labeled gastrointestinal or neurologic disorders.

The principal gastrointestinal disorder to consider is irritable bowel syndrome. Children with this condition have periods of constipation or diarrhea. Sometimes there is a rush of peristalsis with a sudden increase in rectal pressure. The child may be surprised by a quick spurt of feces that is usually liquid. Diagnosis is reinforced by a positive family history of irritable bowel or spastic colon. It is also reinforced by a patient's past history of colic or nonspecific diarrhea as a toddler. These children have abdominal cramps

Figure 13-1

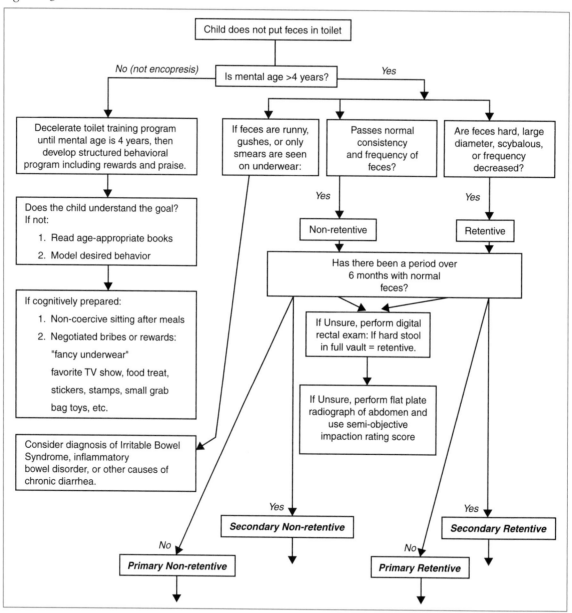

Algorithm for evaluation and treatment of fecal soiling.

Figure 13-1(cont.)

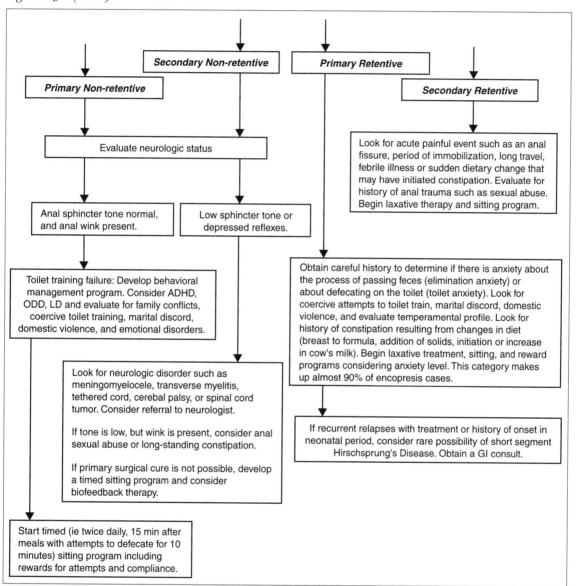

or nonspecific chronic abdominal pain. Because they have loose feces more often than constipation, the differentiation between the impacted retentive encopretic with overflow incontinence and the child with an irritable bowel depends on a careful history and exam that excludes fecal impaction.

Neurologic disorders include transverse myelitis, myelomeningocele, lipoma of the cord, tethered cord, aganglionosis, and a variety of peripheral neuropathies. As described previously, the central neurologic system affects elimination control by cortical influences on the external anal sphincter.

It is usually easy to determine by history the difference between these causes. Spinal cord lesions usually lead to incontinence. Outlet obstruction or aganglionosis results in small-diameter feces.

WHEN SHOULD MANOMETRY AND RECTAL BIOPSY BE DONE?

If the child has a history that dates the onset of fecal retention to the neonatal period and the anal exam is normal, then the only clear way to exclude Hirschsprung's disease is by rectal biopsy. This does not need to be done if the child is passing large-diameter feces. There is a minute possibility of missing ultra-short-segment aganglionosis, but many with that condition have been effectively managed by conservative laxative therapy. Another indication for biopsy then is repeated failures of laxative therapy despite good compliance; this means sincere efforts for a long period (months or years). A third population in which to consider biopsy is in children with Down syndrome, who have a much higher risk of Hirschsprung's disease. Many gastroenterologists perform manometry as part of their evaluation. Other than in research, it is not clear that manometry gives more information than by proceeding directly to biopsy, as biopsy is the definitive test for Hirschsprung's disease.

WHEN SHOULD THYROID FUNCTIONS BE MEASURED?

Hypothyroidism can cause constipation. Although there are anecdotal reports of cases of hypothyroidism presenting with constipation, it is very unlikely that a child with hypothyroidism will have no other stigmata of the disease. Constipation is common and hypothyroidism is rare. Most children with enough thyroid dysfunction to cause constipation also have coarse hair, poor growth, increased weight for height, cold intolerance, declining cognitive performance, bradycardia, etc. Our local experience with over 1000 encopretic children has yielded no case of hypothyroidism, so the tests do not need to be done unless other stigmata are present. Again, children with Down syndrome are an exception because they have a cumulative lifetime prevalence of 15 percent who become hypothyroid. They should be tested regularly.

Treatment of Encopresis

The current standard treatment of encopresis consists of three general phases, a cleanout phase, a maintenance phase, and a weaning phase. Patient education helps to develop a working partnership with the family and also increases the rate and speed of recovery. Psychosocial management is needed throughout all phases.

Cleanout empties the colon and rectum. Rectal distention blunts the normal sensation. The rectum receptors are stimulated by tension in the wall of the rectum. With chronic dilatation, the diameter of the rectum is enlarged, with consequent reduction in tension in the wall. It is important to start treatment with a clean rectum and attempt to keep the diameter reduced. Theoretically, since the urge to defecate is caused by stimulation of the rectal tension receptors and since tension increases relative to the radius of a tube to the fourth power, keeping the diameter small would greatly increase receptor stimulation. Also, a dilated rectum and colon may have decreased muscular propulsive effectiveness because the muscle fibers may be stretched beyond their effective contractile range.

The maintenance phase is longer than most want or expect. It usually takes 6 to 12 months of sustained compliance to achieve benefits. Loss of enthusiasm for the program may lead to relapse, requiring a restart of the whole process. The physician becomes the coach and cheerleader for the family to help them stay with the program. Nurse clinicians, social workers, and psychologists all offer additional encouragement and can take a leading role to direct the program. *The essential ingredients are involvement and follow-up. This is not a prescription to dispense but a team process requiring involvement.*

The weaning phase is based on individual response. Children with mild problems or problems of short duration may be weaned over several months, while those with an intrinsic predisposition to constipation or long-standing problems may need some vigilance to bowel hygiene for their entire lives.

THE CLEANOUT PHASE

Cleanout can be accomplished by using oral laxatives, enemas, or suppositories. If there is no acute abdominal pain, there is no clear advantage to cleanout from below. There may be potential adverse effects, as discussed previously. Some believe that rectal stimulation helps the child associate bowel movements with local sensations, but there is no experimental evidence to support this. Since stimulants may cause cramps in an impacted bowel, it is usually more successful to use high-dosage oral mineral oil (up to 9 to 12 tablespoonfuls per day). To improve palatability and reduce the risk of aspiration, it is best to give it in a food that is cold and creamy (ice cream, frozen yogurt, pudding, etc.), or oily (peanut butter, chocolate, poured on pancakes with syrup, or in salads with dress-

ing, etc.). Mineral oil does not cause vitamin deficiency in normally nourished children, and it can be used for months to years. Mineral oil aspiration may occur when used in infants (under 12 months) or in children with neurologic impairment; the oil should be avoided in these groups.

Children with megarectum, a grossly distended rectum with severe impaction, or those who are unable to comply with high-dose oral laxatives may require an inpatient bowel flush. This is usually done using a nasogastric polyglycolate solution. This solution does not appear to cause electrolyte imbalance, even when given at rates as high as several liters per hour. The insertion of a nasogastric tube can be traumatic, so a small, soft feeding tube is usually preferable. Sedation may be needed in some children. Although this technique is effective in clearing the bowel, it is a more expensive and invasive method to use, especially on a repeated basis. It should be used only if compliance with the maintenance phase is likely. Do not let parents or children rely on periodic bowel flush to avoid the longer, more difficult maintenance phase.

Rarely, manual disimpaction under general anesthesia is required. This is reserved for the greatly impacted or very anxious patient who is unable to comply with high-dose oral therapy or a nasogastric tube. Some children with past traumatic experiences or sexual abuse will do better if they do not add the trauma of a bowel cleanout to their concerns. As with the bowel flush, there is no reason, other than acute abdominal pain, to use this method of cleanout if there is little likelihood of compliance with a maintenance program immediately afterwards.

A few brief words on enemas and suppositories: do not use them unless there is acute abdominal pain and urgent relief is needed. They are unpleasant for the parent, child, and provider and no more effective than an oral cleanout. Phosphate enemas may cause electrolyte abnormalities. There is no scientific rationale supporting the use of foodstuffs in the rectum, such as molasses or milk as an enema.

The exceptions for enemas include use of self-administered enemas or suppositories in an older child with chronic bowel disorder (e.g., postoperative complication or meningomyelocele). Likewise, children who are profoundly neurologically impaired may require a bowel management program, including periodic enemas.

The use of an appendiceal cecostomy to give antegrade colonic enemas (ACE) provides direct access to the bowel for periodic flushing. This procedure is rapidly gaining in popularity, but there are no studies showing use of this technique in treating encopresis. It has been used to treat idiopathic chronic constipation. Generally, these procedures are reserved for children in the same categories as those mentioned above requiring chronic enemas, as a way to improve their lifestyle.

Cleanout should be accomplished within the first week of therapy. It is preferable to start on a Friday so that the weekend is available to manage the copious amounts of feces often eliminated. This warrants keeping children home from school if needed to avoid embarrassing accidents.

THE MAINTENANCE PHASE

The maintenance phase includes several components: (1) continued softening of feces, (2) a toilet-sitting program, (3) a behavioral management program, and (4) dietary management.

Fecal Softening

The goal of ongoing fecal softening is to provide experience with passing soft feces (anxiety reduction, rectal sensation enhancement, and propulsive muscle strengthening). It is better to err toward the supraphysiologic range of two to three bowel movements per day. Children with encopresis should never go more than 2 days without a bowel movement because they are at risk of reaccumulating an impaction, requiring another cleanout phase.

Any tolerated laxative is acceptable. The range of choices is broad, including mostly dietary treatment with fiber, tea or fruit paste, or medicinal treatment with lubricants, stimulants, or osmotic or surfactant laxatives. See Table 13-2 for a list of laxatives and dosages that may be used. The important goal is to find one that the child is willing to take on a regular and prolonged basis without creating conflict with the parent. Like defecation, eating is an activity governed by the child, not the parent. The parent's job is to create an environment conducive to compliance with the regimen. This means reducing the adverse effects of the medication (taste, side effects) and rewarding willingness to take it. The child's job is to take the medication. Sometimes children tolerate smaller dosages of two types of laxatives rather than a larger dosage of one. There may be some advantage to using a lubricant and mild stimulant together, but this treatment is empiric with no supporting studies.

Toilet Program

The toilet-sitting program should be designed considering any toilet or defecation anxiety and the developmental status of the child. Also, this should not be punitive, and parents with anger or frustration are not ready to do this. The child should take responsibility, but the parent should express the intention and reward attempts approximating the desired outcome. In young children it may be best to revert to using diapers for a period of 3 to 6 months. The "toilet phobic" child should participate in selecting the seat to use (and perhaps decorating it with stickers or colors; there are fuzzy seat covers, or cushioned rims with reduced ring size and cartoon characters that may reduce anxiety). A small stool on the floor is often less threatening than an adult-sized toilet. The child's feet should rest on a surface to aid in the Valsalva maneuver. If the child is unable to tolerate entering the bathroom because of anxiety, additional counseling will be needed before the encopresis program can succeed.

To take advantage of the gastrocolic reflex (increase in peristalsis after meals), a good time to sit is about 15 minutes after eating. This means the family may need to restructure their morning routine, because the strongest propulsive waves often occur the morning. Today's frenetic lifestyle of waking children at the last minute so they can rapidly ingest their cereal and dash off to school leaves inadequate time for this normal bowel response. Parents unwilling to adjust their schedule are making a statement about the priority of this issue in their lives. When the child sits, he or she can blow bubbles, a horn, or balloons to help increase intraabdominal pressure. Hopefully, the laxative therapy has made the feces soft enough to pass easily. The child should attempt to push out feces for about 5 or 10 min. If there is elimination of feces, the parent should celebrate, reward, and praise. If there is no product, the parent should maintain a supportive but neutral attitude and encourage another try later.

The child should be told to respond to any urges to defecate. This may need to be coordinated with the school. Teachers often feel that children are trying to avoid classwork by running to the bathroom (and indeed some are), but these children need specific support and exceptions to rules. It may require development of a special hand signal, hall pass, and use of the private (lounge) restroom to give privacy and reduce anxiety about the use of public facilities.

The child is trying to figure out how to defecate by a trial-and-error process. Children can be told that this is like trying to learn how to wiggle their ears. They have to explore their muscles and try to coordinate their action. This is a crude treatment methodology, but no superior method is known.

Behavior Management

Rather than focusing on the product of elimination, parents should reward their child for compliance with the process, specifically for taking laxatives and making attempts to defecate. Before therapy, the parents had been focused on the product, with resultant anxiety, frustration, and anger. Redirecting their efforts to provide positive encouragement of the process gives an opportunity for a fresh start with their child.

Children may participate in creating a token reward system. The rewards should be small and reproducible, frequent and meaningful for the child. Younger children will work for stickers, stamps, or candy. Older children can work for electronic game time, baseball cards, money, or extra time with a parent. A calendar can be used to log compliance. Praise should be coupled with the token reward because most children prefer parental affection to tokens, and it will aid in reducing the tokens during the weaning phase.

Dietary Management

In contrast to treating constipation, diet is not the most important part of the treatment plan. As mentioned previously, children do not particularly care for foods with increased fiber content. Asking parents to increase their child's intake of fiber is likely to create another area of conflict. Eating and elimination are physiologic events under the control of the child, not the parent. There is no way to "get" a child to eat just as there is no way to "get" a child to defecate or urinate on parental command. It is wise not to push this issue, though diet will be the eventual treatment for children with innately slow colonic motility. There is time to develop a diet later.

A reduction in cow's milk intake may reduce the firmness of feces, as discussed above, under the treatment of constipation.

The Weaning Phase

Treatment takes longer than would be desired. It wears on the patience of parents, teachers, and the children to comply with a complex daily regimen involving medications, a sitting program, and a reward system. *One of the main causes of treatment failure is insufficient duration of therapy. Most patients require 6 to 12 months of laxative therapy.*

The desired outcome is placement of feces into the toilet, no soiling of underwear, and no discomfort with defecation. There is no need to repeat roentgenograms or other tests; the out-come is obvious from the parent and child reports.

Attempts to gradually wean and discontinue laxatives will likely be successful after the child has not had soiling for about 3 months. Some children have periods of relapse that require a resumption of previous laxative dosages. Some children seem to require a small dose of laxative for many years. A general bowel hygiene plan would include a modest increase in dietary fiber, regular exercise, and awareness of bowel activity. The child should be encouraged to take time to respond to defecation urges and try to expel some feces on a daily basis. A structured daily routine, such as sitting on the toilet for 15 min after breakfast each day, may prevent a relapse.

There is no evidence-based approach to weaning. Gradually reduce the amount of laxative and monitor the number of bowel movements in the toilet per week. If the child begins to skip days with fecal output, then the laxatives should be increased. A common technique is to have the child record the sessions of sitting on the toilet and note whether or not feces are expelled. The child can be rewarded for completing the chart, sitting, and taking the laxative. The focus should be on the desired outcome rather than on the number of soiling accidents. Should these occur, they should be noted but not punished. The child should be taught to focus on his or her body signals. He or she should respond to any urges to defecate and be told to try to expel feces every day.

Parent and Patient Education

Parents need to understand that this condition is not a result of their parenting. Here the explanation of encopresis as a biopsychosocial disorder is helpful. Some parents really believe that this is a physical disorder and expect a quick medical treatment to cure it. They may push for additional tests. Some parents feel their child is soiling as an act of disobedience. Most parents have some degree of guilt about their failure as parents to train their child. Some also have guilt about the anger and abuse they may have committed during episodes of frustration in dealing with their child's accidents and lack of progress. Some parents are really angry with their child and show dislike.

Parents can be told that this is a physical disorder, with incoordination and dysfunction of the defecation process. The colon is stretched and will not contract normally. The rectal urge sensation is blunted. Explain that this is a developmental disorder requiring help, analogous to a learning problem, attention deficit, clumsiness, cerebral palsy, or even a need to wear eyeglasses. This instills hope that the condition will improve with maturation, which it often does. They can be told about the cortical influences on the sphincter, and that stress and anxiety may make the condition worse. Parents need to become their child's advocates and coaches. This may be difficult for the frustrated and angry parent; additional family counseling may be needed. This is especially important if the family is otherwise dysfunctional or disrupted by divorce. If the parents are fighting with each other over custody, money, or parenting style, the encopresis is less likely to resolve.

The child must have a conceptual understanding of the goals. If the child is young, books about "pooping" (*Everyone Poops*, by

Taro Gomi), the toilet process (*Once Upon a Potty: His or Hers*, by Alona Frankel, or *Going to the Potty*, by Fred Rogers) can help establish the expectations. Use of peer pressure by exposure to other children in preschool, role modeling by other family members, or bribes of fancy underwear are all appropriate tools that may work for individual children. Older children may benefit from play therapy (modeling clay) or group sessions.

PSYCHOSOCIAL MANAGEMENT

As alluded to above, support of the family and resolution of family strife are important to the recovery process. Parents unable to provide encouragement or with competing emotional issues will not be successful. Children bring a complex array of innate factors and issues to the relationship too. Each child has behavioral style and developmental status that may or may not fit with parental expectations. Children with learning or sensory integration disorders, attention deficit, or oppositional defiant disorder require extra patience. Even bright, sensitive children do not always respond rationally to their internal distress and lack of control over their bodies; they seem prone to these problems. For these reasons, it is important to consider the psychosocial aspects of the family and possibly building a team to help with the issues identified. A child does better when there is stability and structure in its life, where the parents are nurturing and emotionally stable, and when there is a broader network of social support.

Many have evaluated whether the rate of emotional or behavioral problems is higher in children with encopresis, and they have found inconsistent results. It is generally accepted that much of the behavioral morbidity is a consequence of the condition, with its ostracism, ridicule, exclusion, and emotional abuse. Most likely there are some vulnerable children who have underlying associated neurodevelopmental disorders and some children who suffer sec-ondary emotional trauma. The condition is associated with primary and secondary emotional issues. There should be a low threshold for referral to mental health services.

Children who soil often have poor self-esteem. They come to their doctor visits with their baseball caps pulled down over their faces. They sit cross-legged in the corner and do not speak. They may draw violent or death-riddled images. Their parents have "tried everything," from scolding and ridicule to physical punishment. Their peers call them "stinky." They are at higher risk of comorbidities like learning disorders, attentional deficit, oppositional defiant disorder, conduct disorder, and childhood schizophrenia. It is simplifying to state that a complete psychosocial screen must be done as part of the evaluation and treatment of encopresis. A majority of the treatment time is spent addressing the emotional milieu of the family and the behavioral consequences of this problem. The clinician with some training in family counseling or solution-oriented therapy can make vast improvements within a few visits. *The first goal is to "demystify" the condition by explaining how the bowel works, how the sphincter can be influenced by emotions, and that this condition is common.* It is not a topic brought up at family get-togethers and is suppressed as a failure of parenting. The parents and child often do not know of any other person who has experienced this problem. Just telling them that they are not alone is therapeutic.

All of the treatment should include acknowledging that this is a sensitive area, and the emotional state of the child should be monitored. All protection should be given to the child's sense of control over his or her body and the child should participate in treatment choices. The physician and parents should work with the school to protect the child from exposing the problem to peers and from any public humiliation.

If the physician does not personally have interest or skills in this area, it is appropriate to refer the child to family counseling with a social worker, psychologist, or psychiatrist.

Sadly, few controlled studies have been conducted that support any one particular treatment plan over another or comparing various types or regimens of laxatives. It is not known if encopresis is increasing or even how commonly it occurs. Clearly there is a need for further research.

What about outcome? In one study, data were available on 110 of 127 children treated for 1 year. With initial bowel cleanout, counseling, education, and a supportive maintenance program, 51 percent did not have accidents after 6 months. About 8 percent showed no improvement during the year.[6]

Nonretentive Encopresis and Fecal Incontinence

Whereas 90 percent of encopretics are retentive, the remaining minority are nonretentive. This group is more challenging and less likely to be effectively treated.

Besides retentive versus nonretentive, encopresis has been further categorized into cases that are either primary or secondary. It is called primary encopresis when the child never had a period of 6 to 12 months of successful toileting.

Secondary cases are those who were using the toilet for at least 6 to 12 months and then began to soil. Table 13-3 shows common causes of encopresis using this categorization system. With a new onset of soiling, one must consider whether it is due to an acquired neurologic disorder. This is easily checked by an exam of gait, rectal sphincter tone, and distal reflexes (ankle deep tendon reflexes test L3-4 and anal wink tests S4-5). If these are intact, the spinal cord is not the cause of the soiling. If sphincter tone is low or reflexes are suspect, then consultation with a neurologist is indicated. MRI of the spinal cord should be considered.

A troublesome group comprises the secondary onset, nonretentive encopretic, especially those presenting after 10 years of age. These children most likely have significant emotional disorders that are not amenable to simple behavioral modification regimens. They should be evaluated and comanaged with a child psychologist or child psychiatrist. Outcome from this group is worse than that from the retentive children.

Treatment of children with nonretentive soiling is directed toward catching feces in the toilet instead of the pants. A structured sitting program with attempts to defecate on the toilet twice each day is presented with a positive reinforcement strategy. If the child is able to place

Table 13-3

Categorization of Encopresis and Examples of Causes

	RETENTIVE	NON-RETENTIVE
Primary	Constipation	Meningomyelocele
	Dysfunctional defecation	
	Anatomic—anal stenosis	
	Anterior anus	
Secondary	Constipation	Transverse myelitis
	Postoperative	Cord tumor
	Anal fissure	Sexual abuse
	Sexual abuse	Emotional disorder

feces in the toilet, there is less risk of a soiling accident at other times during the day. Some add a mild laxative to the regimen to facilitate daily elimination, but this need should be evaluated on an individual basis.

The primary focus of treatment is to address the underlying psychosocial disorder. The principal etiology is stress or a heightened emotional state. Children with nonretentive encopresis are often found in families in chaos and in those with severe marital discord, domestic violence, and physical or sexual abuse. Some children or their parents have diagnosable mental illness as well.

Urinary Dysfunction

The development of bladder control parallels that of bowel control. The bladder of the neonate empties automatically with filling. The awareness of a full bladder appears to develop between 1 and 2 years of age. The bladder is interesting in that it gives signals only when full, not when partially full. The amount of fullness needed to stimulate emptying or the urge to empty depends on a number of factors, including biological, genetic, developmental, and emotional ones. Analogous to the rectal external anal sphincter, the external urethral sphincter is under cortical influence. Many children who become excited or who are under stress develop increased urges to urinate. They dance on their toes trying to postpone their urge.

Urinary disorders are divided into urinary accidents that occur only at night (after age 4), and accidents that occur during the day or both day and night. Daytime accidents are due either to developmental problems or dysfunctional voiding. Boys and girls are seen with different types of urinary disorders. Boys are more commonly slow to become dry at night. Girls are seen more frequently with urinary infections and urgency-frequency disorders.

Like constipation, most causes of urinary dysfunction are not organic. Most organic causes can be discovered through history, physical examination, and urinalysis. As with encopresis, enuresis is a symptom, not a disease. Most urgent medical disorders can easily be excluded by a urinalysis. The most common cause of new-onset urinary incontinence is a urinary tract infection (see Chap. 7). Urinary tract infections are a major cause of urinary urgency and frequency. A urinary tract infection can be suspected by microscopic examination of the urine or by a dipstick test that shows a positive leukocyte esterase, nitrate, or hematuria.

It helps to differentiate pollakiuria from polyuria, urinary urgency, urinary incontinence, and dysuria. *Pollakiuria* refers to extraordinary urinary frequency. *Polyuria* implies a large amount of urine. *Urgency* is the urge to urinate regardless of the volume. *Urinary incontinence* exists when there is an inability to withhold dribbling of urine. Many reserve this term for neurologically caused disorders. *Dysuria* is pain with urination. *Enuresis* is incontinence of urine where voiding is normal. It may be voluntary or accidental, primary or secondary. Dysfunctional voiding, also called the *frequency-urgency syndrome*, is characterized by pollakiuria and urinary urgency, but urine volume is normal. Polyuria is worrisome for inability to concentrate due to antidiuretic hormone dysfunction, renal tubular defects, psychogenic water drinking, or from extra solute in the urine, as in diabetes mellitus. Failure to concentrate the urine, as indicated by a very low specific gravity, is a sign of diabetes insipidus. If the specific gravity is above 1.010 to 1.015 in a morning-voided specimen, diabetes insipidus would be very unlikely. The presence of glucose in urine would diagnose diabetes mellitus.

To distinguish dysfunction from normal functioning, it is interesting to review the secular trends and cultural differences in toilet training.

Brazelton, in 1962, showed that about 40 percent of children were toilet trained by the age of 18 to 24 months and over 90 percent were trained by 24 to 30 months.[7] Taubman, in 1997, reported that 50 percent of boys were not trained until 30 to 36 months and that this figure reached 90 percent after 42 months of age.[8] In contrast, the East African Digo use "nurturant conditioning" to achieve continence by 5 to 6 months of age.[9] It appears that an attentive and involved parent can induce early continence, but this is not something easily prescribed. The reality is that in the United States the current general expectation is that a child will be out of diapers before starting school at 4 or 5 years of age. Sparing the discussion of what is right or wrong with society, any child with bedwetting or daytime wetting after 4 years of age needs an evaluation and discussion with parents. (Figure 13-2 provides an algorithm for the evaluation and treatment of urinary wetting.)

Nocturnal Enuresis

There is a normal developmental progression to achieving urinary continence at night. About 10 percent of 1-year-olds remain dry at night; this number increases by 15 percent of the remainder for each year of age. So, about 50 percent of 2-year-olds are dry at night, and there is then a slow, long taper, with 10 percent of 6-year-olds and 1 to 5 percent of adolescents who still have nighttime wetting.[10]

There are various etiologic theories and associations with regard to nighttime wetting, including association of wetting with certain sleep cycles, increased rates of enuresis with learning problems, socioeconomic status, familial genetic patterns, small bladder size, and central control of urine concentration. One or more of these potential etiologies can be found in an individual patient. It is not clear that determining this makes any difference in treatment. It helps to use these theories to explain to parents that this problem is neither their, nor their child's fault. If a familial pattern is found, it can be used to encourage understanding and compassion.

The dominant etiology is usually developmental immaturity. There are two important facts to remember when explaining this to parents. First, children will mature at their own rate; no way to make children mature more rapidly has been found. Children do need to know what is expected, and parents need to provide an environment supportive of the process. Second, with time and patience, the problem is likely to resolve without any specific intervention. With that in mind, the parents can only make things worse by using punishment, scolding, or humiliation in an attempt to hurry things along.

TREATMENT

There are many treatment options. First, it may be that no treatment is the best treatment. This means the child is given permission to mature at his or her own rate and that the family will provide ways to deal with the urinary accidents. This is the treatment of choice in children under 6 or 7 years of age. Parents should protect the bed by covering it with plastic and allowing the child to use absorbent diapers at night. The issue should be defined as one for the child and not the family. The child can place soiled bedclothes in a hamper or washing machine by the mental age of 4 or 5 years. This should be taught using positive reinforcement, thus removing the family from having to be angered by this issue.

As the child ages, he or she may express a desire to spend nights with friends. This creates the wish for additional treatment. Any of the options discussed below work in some children. It should be the goal of the physician to discuss the hassles and benefits of each choice and to determine with the family which to try. Here are the choices:

SIMPLE REWARD PROGRAM Give the child a token (stamp, sticker, baseball card, candy, money,

Figure 13-2

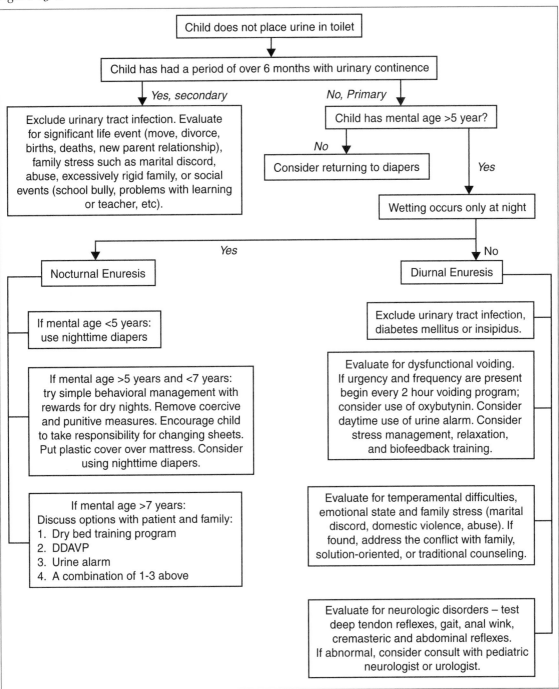

Algorithm for evaluation and treatment of urine wetting.

extra game time, etc.) for each night of dryness. Such rewards should be frequent and small but of a kind the child finds desirable. The use of rare rewards (e.g., a bicycle) does not allow periodic reinforcement. A simple calendar can be used to record the success. The rewards can be tiered—for example, giving a bonus award for three consecutive dry nights. *Hassles:* There may not be a dry night, so reinforcement is not possible. This is best used if there is an occasional dry night. The child will tire of this program unless new and novel awards are periodically introduced. In addition, the parent must maintain involvement with praise and encouragement. If the parent forgets the reward, the program will degenerate. *Benefit:* This is not invasive, it is inexpensive, and it is a good starting point for the younger child. It can teach parents how to give praise and positive reinforcement that can be used in other circumstances.

DRY BED TRAINING   A more complex behavioral management program can be developed that may include bladder stretching exercises, visualization and imagery training, and night waking by the parent in addition to simple rewards. *Hassles:* This is an intensive program that may create anxiety in children and parents if not applied with understanding and calm. It may be too intensive for disorganized families. *Benefits:* This program is very structured, which may appeal to certain parents. It has the tone of parental control without being too rigid.

URINE ALARM SYSTEMS   These have been available for many years and have become very sophisticated in the last decade. A small moisture-sensitive sensor that can be comfortably attached to underwear has replaced the original bed pad that rings an alarm when moistened. This sensor may be hard-wired to a buzzer attached at the shoulder of the nightshirt or remotely signal a pager to vibrate or alarm when triggered by a few drops of urine. They are effective in the motivated child over 7 years of age. Parents can

be told that there is a success rate of 85 percent with this technique. The alarms can be ordered over the Internet and cost about $50. http://www.palcolabs.com/pediatrics; http://www.pottypager.com. They take about 3 to 5 months of use to reach maximum effectiveness. *Hassles:* Some children do not wake with the alarm, but the whole family does! This is not a system that is easily taken on overnight trips to friends. It must be used at home well in advance of the travel time. *Benefits:* This is a nonmedicinal approach that uses the lure of technology and gadgets that appeals to many boys. It is very effective.

DESMOPRESSIN   Some children have been shown to lack the normal nocturnal rhythmicity of vasopressin, so dilute urine continues to be produced during sleep. Once the bladder fills, it empties. Desmopressin, or DDAVP, replaces the antidiuretic hormone and causes urine concentration. *Hassles:* This medicine costs about $90 per month and the condition tends to relapse once the medicine is stopped. *Benefits:* This is a good choice for children who have never had a dry night. It proves they can stay dry. It is a good choice, if it works, to use before an overnight visit with a friend.

IMIPRAMINE   This tricyclic antidepressant probably acts both centrally and, with anticholinergic effects, directly on the sphincter. It was used for many years as a primary therapy for nocturnal enuresis with fair success. Nearly 50 percent of children appear to respond. *Hassles:* Recent concerns about cardiovascular toxic effects have created a loss of interest in its use. The drug should not be around young children because of the potential for poisoning. There is a significant relapse rate after the medicine is stopped. *Benefits:* This medication may work when other treatments have failed. It may also work in the child who has never had a dry night. It may be a good choice for the 1-week camp if given with supervision.

HYPNOTHERAPY This is another way of developing understanding of bladder function and uses mental imagery and relaxation techniques. *Hassles:* Most providers do not feel comfortable providing this treatment without specific training in hypnotherapy. It may be costly for parents because it requires several professional visits. *Benefits:* This is another nontoxic way to treat the condition, with about a 67 percent chance of cure.

Daytime Enuresis

Urinary accidents that occur only during the day are either due to stress and emotional factors or to dysfunctional voiding (see below). A careful inventory of family or social stresses usually reveals a potential source of anxiety. For some children, their innate temperament manifests as high sensitivity to the world around them. Normal amounts of stimulation may cause an exaggerated response. The source of the stress must be dealt with, or the child must be taught coping skills such as imagery, relaxation, or thought blocking.

Most children with daytime enuresis also have nighttime enuresis. Some approach this condition by using alarms during the day in addition to the night.[11] Some advocate the use of bladder exercises by having the child withhold urine as long as possible after the urge to void is detected, but this technique has not been subjected to controlled trials.

Dysfunctional Voiding

Symptoms of voiding dysfunction are due to the incomplete emptying of the bladder. It may seem that the child has a small bladder capacity because there is often increased urinary frequency and occasionally a dramatic urge to void. Two events occur: the bladder does not empty and the sphincter closes too soon. The bladder does not send signals of the urge to void until it reaches a certain volume. In this disorder, the child does not empty with a void. This reduces the bladder volume below the threshold for urge, but with a small amount of refilling, the threshold is soon regained. This occurs in a cyclic pattern. The second event involves the urethral sphincter. The sphincter closes prematurely or does not relax. This seems to be related to anxiety and general emotional level, but there is a cycle of urinary accidents leading to anxiety, so it is not clear whether the stress is primary or secondary.

Dysfunctional voiding can place the kidney at high risk when vesicoureteral reflux is present. The high pressure during detrusor contraction can cause direct damage to the kidney. In addition, there is a heightened risk for urinary tract infections that can cause renal scarring.

EVALUATION

Extensive testing including cystourethrogram, electromyographic (EMG) testing of pelvic floor muscles, sonography, and cystoscopy are all expensive and invasive procedures that have been recommended as part of the evaluation. Generally, an initial attempt to treat using behavioral management can be applied without doing these tests. Children should be evaluated for possible urinary infection with a simple urinalysis. Further testing should be reserved for recalcitrant cases.

Usually the diagnosis can be made by history. The classic features are urinary frequency and urge with inability to withhold urine. Urine is often released in a sudden gush or is staccato. Then the stream may stop abruptly, giving the impression that there was little urine present. Some girls develop a stereotypic "curtsy"; with urge to urinate, they drop to one knee placing the heel of one foot onto the perineum to withhold urine.

History should explore for past incidents of urinary infection, constipation, and the possibility of sexual abuse. Any or all of these may also be present and contribute to the origin of this condition.

TREATMENT

The best results have been reported with behavioral management using voiding training and biofeedback.[12] Anticholinergics (such as oxybutynin chloride, 5 mg two to three times per day) are often used but have not been shown to be superior to biofeedback training. There is no role for urethral dilatation as a treatment.

Simple behavioral training can begin with a timed voiding schedule—for example, every 2 h during the day. The use of a countdown timer or alarm may be helpful. Girls should be told to sit on the toilet backward, because some will obstruct urinary outflow by clamping their thighs together. Seeing the urinary stream also provides visual reinforcement that may help improve its quality. Compliance with the sitting program can be reinforced with a positive reward system and praise. Children should be told to void even though they "don't feel like they have to go." It usually takes several weeks to see any improvement. The main component of this program is an enthusiastic cheerleader and coach to maintain enthusiasm and consistency. A parent, teacher, physician, or nurse can provide this.

The use of portable sonography to measure postvoid residual bladder volume can provide objective data showing improvement in bladder emptying efficiency. The program can be made more sophisticated by using periurethral EMG to provide direct visualization of sphincter muscle relaxation. Surface perineum or leg EMG is probably not as effective but is commonly done. Biofeedback and behavioral management is cited as over 80 percent curative of this condition.

Summary

Elimination is as natural as eating. Yet there is an innate revulsion with the products of elimination. This normal response protects the individual from exposure to the harmful infectious agents found in feces. But this revulsion may be transferred to the producer of elimination, especially in the case of children with defecation dysfunction.

Both urinary and fecal elimination disorders are biobehavioral problems that share common features, including the tendency to resolve with maturation. However, the emotional morbidity of these conditions warrants immediate attention rather than waiting for maturation to occur. Treatment may range from simple reassurance to a complex regimen including family counseling and a structured behavioral management program, depending on the needs of the child and family.

References

1. Bellman M: Studies on encopresis. *Acta Paediatr Scand* 1966.
2. Fleisher DR: Diagnosis and treatment of disorders of defecation in children. *Pediatr Ann* 5: 700–722, 1976.
3. Issenman RM, Hewson S, Pirhonen D, et al: Are chronic digestive complaints the result of abnormal dietary patterns? Diet and digestive complaints in children at 22 and 40 months of age. *Am J Dis Child* 141:679–682, 1987.
4. Levine MD: Encopresis: its potentiation, evaluation, and alleviation. *Pediatr Clin North Am* 29: 315–330, 1982.
5. Iacono G, Cavataio F, Montalto G, et al: Intolerance of cow's milk and chronic constipation in children (see comments). *N Engl J Med* 339:1100–1104, 1998.

6. Levine MD, Bakow H: Children with encopresis: a study of treatment outcome. *Pediatrics* 58:845–852, 1976.
7. Brazelton, TB: A child-oriented approach to toilet training. *Pediatrics* 29:121–128, 1962.
8. Taubman B: Toilet training and toileting refusal for stool only: a prospective study. *Pediatrics* 99:54–58, 1997.
9. deVries MW, deVries MR: Cultural relativity of toilet training readiness: a perspective from East Africa. *Pediatrics* 60:170–177, 1977.
10. Forsythe WI, Redmond A: Enuresis and spontaneous cure rate: study of 1129 enuretis. *Arch Dis Child* 49:259–263, 1974.
11. Halliday S, Meadow SR, Berg I: Successful management of daytime enuresis using alarm procedures: a randomly controlled trial. *Arch Dis Child* 62:132–137, 1987.
12. Schulman SL, Quinn CK, Plachter N, Kodman-Jones C: Comprehensive management of dysfunctional voiding. *Pediatrics* 103:E31, 1999.

F. Estelle R. Simons

Chapter

14

Asthma

Asthma—a persistent inflammatory disorder of the airways (Table 14-1)—is the most common chronic respiratory disorder in the pediatric population. The prevalence of asthma is increasing in many industrialized countries; it now affects 2 out of every 10 children.[1]

Asthma is nearly always associated with sensitization to environmental allergens in young patients, many of whom have other allergic disorders, such as rhinitis, rhinoconjunctivitis, and atopic dermatitis. The worldwide increase in asthma has been associated with an increase in these other allergic disorders and is therefore likely due to an actual increase in the number of people with the disease rather than to increased recognition of asthma or to "lumping" of various disorders involving wheezing under the diagnostic label of asthma.

Although there are many risk factors for asthma—with complex interactions among genetic, environmental, microbiologic, and age-related anatomic and physiologic factors—the increase in asthma and allergic disorders is attributed primarily to lifestyle and environmental changes during the past century. In some populations, for example, asthma prevalence is inversely related to microbial infections.

The pathophysiology of asthma is summarized in Fig. 14-1. The chief characteristic feature is inflammation throughout the airways. Smooth muscle spasm (bronchoconstriction) of the airways, although present, is no longer considered to be the most important aspect of asthma pathophysiology.[2]

This chapter focuses on the diagnosis and management of chronic persistent asthma, which is an important practical concern for primary care clinicians. The assessment and management of acute asthma in children seen in the emergency department or hospital is discussed briefly.

Table 14-1
Characteristics of Asthma

Airway inflammation is associated with bronchoconstriction due to mucous plugging, airway wall edema and remodeling, and increased airways hyperresponsiveness ("twitchy" airways).

Individual children and adolescents have their own unique trigger factors and symptom patterns.

Severity ranges from mild-intermittent to mild-, moderate-, or severe-persistent.

Prognosis is variable; although many children with asthma improve during adolescence, only those with the mildest disease actually "outgrow" it.

Asthma is associated with atopy (genetic predisposition for development of IgE-mediated responses to common allergens), and with disorders such as allergic rhinitis and atopic dermatitis.

Figure 14-1

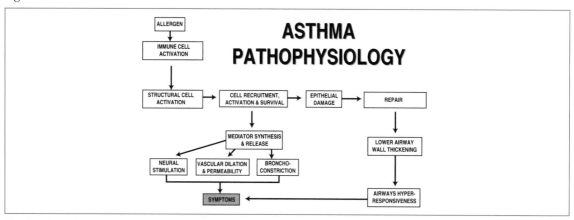

This flowchart illustrates how allergen exposure may result in asthma symptoms. Immune cells include T lymphocytes, B lymphocytes, and Langerhans (allergen-presenting) cells. Denervation and disruption of the epithelium occur, and other structural cells such as endothelial cells are activated. The cells recruited and activated are mast cells, eosinophils, and basophils. Airways remodeling, a repair process, involves mucous gland hyperplasia, smooth muscle hypertrophy and hyperplasia, and vascular proliferation as well as loss of elastic fibers, fibroblast proliferation, and collagen deposition beneath the basement membrane. The chemical mediators of inflammation synthesized and released include histamine and leukotrienes. Bronchoconstriction is placed in context as only one of many aspects of the pathophysiology of asthma. (Adapted by permission from Howarth.[2])

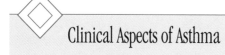 Clinical Aspects of Asthma

Airway inflammation in asthma is associated with intermittent episodes of coughing, wheezing, shortness of breath, and chest tightness or discomfort that may interfere with daily activities and sleep. Asthma is classified as "mild intermit-tent" or "mild moderate," or "severe persistent" based on the severity, frequency, and duration of symptoms, the level of airflow obstruction, and the extent to which the asthma interferes with daily activities. Although fewer than 10 percent of affected children and adolescents have severe-persistent disease with frequent intermittent acute episodes, most asthma fatalities and nearly 80 percent of all hospital inpatient days for asthma occur among individuals in this group. The morbidity caused by asthma, even by mild or moderate disease, is widely underestimated (Table 14-2). Asthma severity as assessed by symptoms, lung function, and airways hyperresponsiveness is influenced by asthma duration; therefore early diagnosis and intervention are crucial.

Until adolescence, asthma is found more commonly in boys than in girls, but the reverse is true after puberty. Although asthma improves or even disappears during adolescence in many children, only rarely is it truly outgrown. Risk factors at age 7 years that independently predict current asthma in an adult include female gender, atopy (for example, a history of atopic dermatitis), presence of low midexpiratory flow rates on spirometry, history of asthma in the mother or father, early onset (before 5 years) and having more than 10 acute asthma episodes, or having severe or prolonged exacerbations.[3,4]

Disease patterns vary greatly. Although airway inflammation is present all the time, regardless of asthma severity, symptoms are generally intermittent rather than continual or progressive.

They may be seasonal or may occur year round. Patients generally have typical patterns of symptoms: for example, acute episodic wheezing, coughing, and shortness of breath during viral upper respiratory tract infections; coughing and subclinical wheezing for weeks after viral infections; symptoms in a specific setting, such as a school classroom; or symptoms at specific times of day, as at night or in the early morning and/or following specific forms of exercise.

Asthma symptoms can also be triggered by a variety of inhaled substances and varying circumstances (Table 14-3). Exposure to allergens such as dust mites, cat and dog danders, and cockroaches may occur not only in the child's home but also in day care, school, and other public places. Any change in the home, day care, or school environment and any disruption

Table 14-2

Asthma Morbidity: Impact on Child and Caregivers

Limitation of activities, especially participation in sports
Nocturnal or early morning awakening(s), loss of sleep, and consequent adverse effects on behavior or school performance
School absences due to physician's office visits, urgent care visits, emergency department visits, hospitalizations
Adverse effects on growth or development due to the asthma itself or to the medications used to treat it
Interference with family routines and recreation; effect on the family dynamics
Economic impact (parents have to take time off from work)

Table 14-3

Triggers of Asthma Symptoms

Airborne allergens[a]
Viral upper respiratory tract infections[b]
Exercise[c]
Tobacco smoke and other irritants (strong odors, air pollutants, dust particles, vapors, gases, and aerosols)
Exposure to cold, dry air (also other changes in air temperature or humidity or in the weather)
Emotions (laughing, crying, anger, fear)
Concomitant gastroesophageal reflux
Endocrine factors (menstrual cycle, thyroid disease)
Medications (aspirin and other nonsteroidal anti-inflammatory drugs, β_2-adrenergic blockers)

[a] Indoor allergens (e.g., cats, dogs, house dust mites, cockroaches, and molds) and outdoor allergens (e.g., tree, grass, and weed pollens and molds).
[b] May trigger severe acute asthma exacerbations that last for weeks.
[c] Triggers brief transient episodes lasting less than 1 to 2 h; less likely to be triggered by some forms of exercise such as swimming than by others such as running or skating.

in usual activities (for example, sleepovers, field trips, camping, vacations, or moving) may cause an exacerbation of symptoms. There is now incontrovertible evidence that passive exposure to tobacco smoke leads not only to asthma symptoms and exacerbations but also to deteriorating lung function over time.[5]

Diagnosis of Asthma

There is no specific immunologic, biological, or physiologic marker for asthma. Instead, the diagnosis is based on the symptoms and signs of asthma and associated atopic disorders and on response to treatment. It can be confirmed only when obstruction to airflow has been documented to be reversible and other disorders involving coughing and wheezing have been excluded. The differential diagnosis for common asthma symptoms such as cough is extensive (Table 14-4).

History

Tipoffs in the history that the diagnosis is *not* asthma include neonatal onset, failure to thrive, recurrent bacterial respiratory tract infections, and history of choking or vomiting with wheezing. The most common masquerader of asthma in infants and young children is bronchiolitis. The viral upper respiratory tract infections that trigger wheezing in infants and young children with asthma also trigger transient wheezing in infants without asthma due to the small diameter of the airways, with a disproportionately large effect of edema and mucus secretion and smooth muscle constriction on airway patency. In infants and preschool children with virus-induced wheezing, longitudinal follow-up may be necessary to confirm or rule out the diagnosis of asthma with certainty.

Table 14-4

Differential Diagnosis of Asthma (Cough and/or Abnormal Expiratory or Inspiratory Sounds and/or Shortness of Breath)

Upper and middle respiratory tract
Allergic rhinitis[a]
Upper respiratory tract infections[a]
Sinusitis[a]
Foreign body
Croup
Pertussis
Epiglottitis
Hypertrophy of adenoids or tonsils
Structural abnormalities of the upper
    and middle respiratory tract[b]
Vascular rings
Space-occupying lesions (e.g., tumor)
Vocal cord dysfunction
Enlarged lymph nodes
Toxic inhalation
Lower respiratory tract
Bronchiolitis (viral)
Chronic lung disease[c]
Cystic fibrosis
Foreign body
Tuberculosis
Gastroesophageal reflux[a]/chronic aspiration
Alpha₁ antitrypsin deficiency
Bronchiectasis
Hypersensitivity lung diseases
Pulmonary eosinophilia
Pulmonary edema
Mitral valve prolapse
Tumor
Hyperventilation syndrome
Toxic inhalation
Loffler's syndrome
Churg-Strauss syndrome
Hemosiderosis

[a]Allergic rhinitis usually coexists with asthma; other disorders such as upper respiratory tract infections, sinusitis, or gastroesophageal reflux may also coexist with asthma.
[b]Choanal atresia, laryngeal webs, laryngomalacia, tracheomalacia, tracheoesophageal fistula, tracheostenosis, bronchostenosis.
[c]Also called bronchopulmonary dysplasia; occurs in children with a history of prematurity and mechanical ventilation.

Physical Examination

On physical examination, typically, a child with asthma may have evidence of allergic rhinitis (allergic "shiners" with discolored, swollen eyelids; transverse nasal "crease" because of constant nose-rubbing, mouth-breathing, and edema of the nasal mucosa), and/or sinusitis (malodorous breath), and/or atopic dermatitis (erythematous, scaly excoriated skin). Tipoffs in the physical examination that the diagnosis is *not* asthma include unilateral wheezing, monophonic wheezing, focal lung signs, cardiovascular signs, digital clubbing, or failure to thrive.

Ancillary Tests

A wide variety of tests are available for investigating and monitoring asthma in children (Table 14-5). Some are suitable for use in a primary care setting, such as an office practice, and others are available only in subspecialist clinics or at children's hospitals. In asthma, the chronic inflammation of the airways is associated with obstruction to airflow, which by definition is reversible either spontaneously or by at least 15 percent after inhalation of albuterol or similar short-acting bronchodilators. The obstruction to airflow can be objectively measured using peak

Table 14-5

Investigations in Asthma

Primary care
  Pulmonary function tests[a] (e.g., peak expiratory flow, forced expiratory volume in 1 s (FEV_1) and other spirometric tests)
  Bronchoprovocation test (free-range running)
  Eosinophils (peripheral blood, nasal secretions)
  Chest radiograph
  Serum immunoglobulins G, M, and A
  Sweat chloride test
  CT scan or radiographs (e.g., occipitomental, anteroposterior, or lateral) for diagnosis of sinusitis
  Height measurement[a] (using wall-mounted stadiometer)
  PPD skin test (purified protein derivatives) (5TU intermediate strength)
Subspecialist care/children's hospital
  Pulmonary function tests[a] (flow volume loops, plethysmography, lung volumes, airway resistance, forced oscillation, infant/preschooler pulmonary function testing, pulse oximetry)
  Bronchoscopy
  Bronchoprovocation test (treadmill exercise, cold dry air, methacholine, histamine)
  Allergy tests for sensitization to specific airborne allergens (epicutaneous tests, RASTs, ELISAs)
  Gastroesophageal reflux disease evaluation (barium esophagram, esophageal pH monitoring, esophageal manometry, radionucleotide studies, esophagoscopy with biopsy)
  Ciliary structure and function evaluation
  Serum eosinophilic cationic protein[b]
  Hypertonic saline-induced sputum examination (for eosinophils, other inflammatory cells, and mediators of inflammation)[b]
  Nitric oxide[b]

KEY: RAST, radioallergosorbent test; ELISA, enzyme-linked immunosorbent assay; PPD, purified protein derivative; TU, tuberculin unit.
[a] Pulmonary function tests and height measurements are also used for regular monitoring
[b] Used in asthma research

expiratory flow meters or spirometry. For children under 5 years of age, who are too young to perform forced expiratory maneuvers, age-appropriate pulmonary function tests are available in the respiratory clinics and allergy clinics of most children's hospitals.

The inflammation in the airways is also associated with an increase in airway hyperresponsiveness to natural stimuli such as exercise or cold, dry air, and, in the pulmonary function test laboratory, to inhaled chemicals such as methacholine or histamine. Tests for airway hyperresponsiveness are useful in the diagnosis of mild asthma—for example, in children who cough after exercise. A challenge test can be performed only if a child is symptom-free and has an FEV_1 in the normal or near-normal range; the aim of the challenge is to produce a 20 percent decrease in FEV_1, not to produce asthma symptoms.

Specialized tests for gastroesophageal reflux may be indicated for children who vomit in association with wheezing, who have persistent nocturnal symptoms, or who do not respond to optimal pharmacologic treatment for asthma.

Allergy skin tests, although not useful for the diagnosis of asthma per se, are helpful in young asthmatics in order to identify sensitization to common airborne allergens, which are potential trigger factors for asthma symptoms.[6]

Management of Chronic Persistent Asthma

Current optimal approaches to management of persistent asthma are summarized in Tables 14-6, 14-7, and 14-8. The goals of therapy are to prevent the symptoms of coughing, wheezing, or breathlessness at all times and to minimize the need for urgent-care visits, emergency department visits, and hospitalizations. In addition to prevention of symptoms, other important

Table 14-6

Asthma Education: Objectives

Improve child's and parent's or caregiver's understanding of asthma (as a persistent disorder with intermittent symptoms of variable severity).

Improve ability to recognize and manage "breakthrough" symptoms and an acute asthma episode.

Discuss treatment goals, especially the goal of freedom from asthma symptoms.

Discuss the importance of avoiding trigger factors such as cigarette smoke and airborne allergens.

Improve ability to differentiate between preventer (anti-inflammatory) and reliever (bronchodilator) medications.

Discuss concerns over potential side effects of medications (including long-term effects).

Identify practical economic resources for the family (medications, transport to health care facilities).

Provide emotional support for the family.

Discuss potential barriers to meeting treatment goals (lack of faith in conventional medical treatment, "different" sociocultural beliefs, having close relatives with sub-optimally managed asthma).

goals are to improve pulmonary function as much as possible while avoiding adverse effects from treatment and meeting patients' and families' expectations. Delay in asthma treatment may be associated with a poorer prognosis.

Education

Asthma education is most successful when targeted to children of specific age groups and their families, e.g., preschoolers, school-age children, and adolescents. Ideally, it is based on the following principles: anticipation of asthma exacerbations, determination of an appropriate response, and rehearsal of solutions (e.g., when, why, and how to take or increase medications, and, if age- or disease severity–appropriate, when, why, and how to monitor peak expiratory flows).

The key objectives in asthma education are listed in Table 14-6. The importance of a written asthma action plan [a mutual agreement by the child or adolescent, the family, and the physician(s)] cannot be overemphasized. Having a self-management plan and increasing medications promptly at the onset of "colds" are associated with reduced likelihood of hospitalization or emergency department visits.

Avoidance of Environmental Allergens and Respiratory Irritants

Specific measures, such as washing bed sheets in hot water at least twice monthly to get rid of house dust mites (in house dust mite–sensitive children), are associated with significantly reduced hospitalization rates for asthma.[7] Avoidance of respiratory irritants, especially cigarette smoke, is a major barrier to successful asthma treatment in many children. Control of environmental allergens and respiratory irritants is easier said than done, and easier done than maintained over many years (Table 14-7).

Table 14-7

Avoidance and Control of Animal Dander and House Dust Mite Allergens in the Home

Cats, dogs, and other animals
If a child is allergic to animal dander, do not have an animal in the home.
If it is impossible to remove the animal, keep it outside as much as possible and bathe it weekly.
Never allow the animal into the child's bedroom. (Keep the door closed!). Seal off or cover the room's heating vent with a filter. Use a portable heater if necessary. A portable HEPA filter[a] may help to clean the room air.
House dust mites
Avoid carpets, rugs, and upholstered furniture in the bedroom, as one-third to one-half of a child's time is spent in this room.
Encase the mattress and box spring with airtight, dustproof covers or construction plastic. Seal zippers and seams completely with 2 in. duct tape.
Use new dust mite–free pillows. Dry on the hot cycle for 45 min every two weeks, and replace every few years.
Use cotton or synthetic bedding and mattress cover; wash weekly in hot water (130°F) and dry on the hot cycle.
Treat stuffed animals as for pillows or bedding.
Use washable window coverings.
Use a central vacuum system or a vacuum with a HEPA filter (e.g., Nilfisk). An upright vacuum or one with a double-bag is also satisfactory. Damp-dust all surfaces weekly.
Use a dehumidifier if the humidity in the home is >60%; mites (and molds!) thrive when humidity is high.
Do not use a humidifier.
Air cleaners are ***not*** helpful in removing dust mites or dust mite fecal pellets.

[a] The HEPA filter must have a high airflow (250 cu ft/min or more).

Table 14-8
Medications for Chronic Asthma Treatment[a]

Generic (Brand Name)	Comments
Inhaled glucocorticoids[b] Beclomethasone dipropionate (Beclovent, Vanceril, Vanceril-DS) Budesonide (Pulmicort Turbuhaler; Pulmicort Respules) Triamcinolone acetonide (Azmacort) Flunisolide (AeroBid, AeroBid-M) Fluticasone propionate (Flovent) Mometasone furoate (Asmanex)	Medications of choice for long-term control of moderate-severe persistent asthma; significantly more effective than any nonsteroidal medications on all outcome measures of asthma treatment: (↓ frequency of symptoms; ↓ need for "rescue" bronchodilator medication; ↑ airway patency and ↓ airway hyperresponsiveness). Risk of adverse effects on growth is significantly less than it is during oral glucocorticoid treatment or during severe uncontrolled asthma.
Inhaled cromolyn sodium/nedocromil sodium[b] Cromolyn sodium (Intal) Nedocromil sodium (Tilade)	Less effective than inhaled glucocorticoids for moderate or severe persistent asthma. Safe. Nedocromil may taste unpleasant to some patients.
Leukotriene modifiers Montelukast (Singulair) Zafirlukast (Accolate)	New oral medications. Effective for mild persistent asthma and for exercise-induced asthma. Steroid-sparing effects in moderate and severe asthma, and long-term safety are still being investigated. Zafirlukast may have potential for drug interactions at high doses.
Inhaled long-acting β₂-adrenergic agonists[b] Salmeterol (Serevent); salmeterol combined with fluticasone (Advair) Formoterol (Foradil)	Preferably used as a steroid-sparing agent with an inhaled glucocorticoid in patients with moderate-severe persistent asthma. Fixed-dose combinations with inhaled glucocorticoids are still being studied in children. Bronchoprotective effect may decrease over time. May cause tachycardia, tremor, and headaches.
Slow-release theophylline (Theo-Dur, Uniphyl, and others)	Preferably used as steroid-sparing agents. Serum concentrations should be monitored and should be kept in the range of 5–15 µg/mL (55–110 µmol/mL, lower than formerly recommended). Theophylline does not have a favorable benefit-to-risk ratio. Potential side effects include insomnia, restlessness, headaches, seizures, abdominal pain, nausea, vomiting, tachycardia, and diarrhea. Drug interactions, for example, when erythromycin is administered concurrently, may contribute to theophylline toxicity.

Table 14-8 (cont.)
Medications for Chronic Asthma Treatment[a]

Generic (Brand Name)	Comments
Inhaled short-acting β2-adrenergic agonists[b] Albuterol (Airet, Proventil, Ventolin, Airomir, Proventil-HFA, Ventolin Rotacaps) Terbutaline (Bricanyl) Bitolterol (Tornalate), Pirbuterol (Maxair)	Not recommended for regular daily use, but only for prevention of exercise-induced asthma and for relief of asthma symptoms. Increasing use of a short-acting β2-agonist or lack of effect of a short-acting β2-agonist indicates inadequate asthma control and the need for a regular preventer medication such as an inhaled glucocorticoid, or if patient is already taking a preventer medication, the need for a dose increase. All short-acting β2-agonist potentially cause tremor, tachycardia, and headache. Risk-to-benefit ratio of inhaled β2-agonists is superior to that of oral β2-agonists.
Oral glucocorticoids methylprednisolone (Medrol) prednisolone (Prelone, Pediapred) prednisone (Prednisone, Deltasone, Orasone, Liquid Pred, Prednisone Intensol)	For short-term treatment (usually 5–7 days) until acute asthma symptoms resolve) and peak expiratory flow returns to 75–80% of child's personal best value; there is no need to taper the dose. Rarely, used on a long-term alternate-day basis for management of severe persistent asthma; such patients require close monitoring in order to keep the dose as low as possible and to prevent systemic adverse effects.

[a] For correct doses and dose regimens, see Ref 8 and product monographs.
[b] Inhaled medications require assessment of a child's ability to use a particular inhalation device (metered-dose inhaler with spacer or metered-dose inhaler with spacer and face mask) or wet nebulization. Repeat assessment and coaching with regard to optimal use of inhaler device is fundamental for optimal prevention and control of asthma symptoms.

One trigger factor for asthma that should not be avoided is exercise; indeed, the adequacy of asthma control can often be assessed by a child's ability to keep up with his or her peers at recess, in physical education class, or while participating in organized sports.

Medications

A wide variety of medications is available for the prevention and control of asthma symptoms, and new medications are continually being introduced (Table 14-8). A stepwise approach to treatment is recommended.[8] For mild intermittent asthma (step 1), use of a short-acting β_2-adrenergic agonist bronchodilator a few times weekly is appropriate. In all other children, those with mild-persistent (step 2), moderate-persistent (step 3), or severe-persistent (step 4) asthma, regular daily use of an anti-inflammatory medication, usually an inhaled glucocorticoid, is the fundamental step in management.

The key to successful pharmacotherapy of asthma is to use each medication in the lowest dose that will prevent and control symptoms. Every physician caring for children with asthma should understand the benefits and risks of a few selected medications from each class and should also be able to demonstrate the optimal use of selected inhalation devices to children and their caregivers.

Polypharmacy should be avoided. Many children with mild-intermittent asthma require only one medication: a short-acting β_2-adrenergic agonist to relieve exercise-induced symptoms and to use for occasional relief of breakthrough wheezing. Most children with mild- or moderate-persistent asthma require only two medications: an anti-inflammatory drug to prevent or control symptoms and a bronchodilator reliever medication to use when symptoms occur. Even patients with severe persistent asthma require no more than two controller medications: an inhaled glucocorticoid and a steroid-sparing medication, and no more than two reliever medications for treatment of breakthrough symptoms (a short-acting inhaled β_2-adrenergic agonist, which will suffice in most children for most breakthrough symptoms, and an oral glucocorticoid for backup use when the breakthrough symptoms cannot be controlled with the β_2-adrenergic agonist).

B2 AGONISTS

β_2-adrenergic agonists, potent and rapidly acting bronchodilators, are no longer used on a regular basis several times daily in persistent asthma treatment. These drugs remain valuable when used intermittently to prevent exercise-induced asthma and for "rescue" treatment of acute asthma symptoms. They should be given by inhalation from metered-dose inhaler or dry-powder inhaler wherever possible, rather than by the oral route.

INHALED STEROIDS

Glucocorticoids inhaled once or twice daily regularly, although not a cure for asthma, are more effective than any other anti-inflammatory medications available for the prevention of wheezing and treatment of persistent symptoms.[9] There are clinically relevant differences among the inhaled glucocorticoids available, the devices used for inhalation, and the propellants used in metered-dose inhalers. Steroid-resistant asthma is fortunately rare; the most common reason for failure of response to inhaled glucocorticoids is lack of adherence to a treatment regimen of regular inhalations.

MAST CELL INHIBITORS

Antiallergic medications such as cromolyn or nedocromil are worth a try with mild persistent asthma[8] but are less effective than inhaled glucocorticoids and are no longer in common use.

THEOPHYLLINE

The role of sustained-release theophylline has also diminished during the past decade. Theophylline has a glucocorticoid-sparing effect in moderate-severe asthma.[8]

LONG-ACTING β2 AGONISTS

The long-acting β_2-adrenergic agonists salmeterol and formoterol, used as monotherapy, have a bronchodilator effect but otherwise are less effective than inhaled glucocorticoids.[8,9] Their role as steroid-sparing agents, especially in fixed-dose combination medications involving an inhaled glucocorticoid, appears to be promising, but this has not yet been adequately assessed in children.

LEUKOTRIENE MODIFIERS

Leukotriene modifiers are the first new class of medications to be introduced for persistent asthma treatment in 25 years. Their main role is likely to be for mild asthma[8] and for exercise-induced asthma; in children, their role as steroid-sparing agents for moderate-severe asthma is currently still being investigated.

ANTIHISTAMINES

Antihistamines (H_1-receptor antagonists) are not used primarily for asthma treatment; but when needed for the management of other allergic disorders such as allergic rhinoconjunctivitis, they do no harm in asthma and may actually contribute to symptom relief. The role of H_1-antagonists in prevention of asthma symptoms in atopic children who have not yet developed wheezing is unclear but is of considerable interest.

OTHER MEDICATIONS

The anticholinergic/antimuscarinic medication ipratropium bromide has no role in the out-patient management of persistent asthma in children. Also, antibiotics have no role in asthma treatment as the upper respiratory tract infections that trigger asthma episodes are viral rather than bacterial. For optimal improvement in asthma symptoms, associated upper airway disorders, including allergic rhinitis and sinusitis, should also be optimally treated.

Immunotherapy

Immunotherapy for asthma associated with allergy to airborne substances—such as house dust mites or tree, grass, and weed pollens, which are difficult to avoid in the environment—remains more controversial in the treatment of asthma than in other allergic disorders such as rhinoconjunctivitis. Immunotherapy is not recommended for preschool children with asthma.[6] Improvement in asthma after immunotherapy is related to the allergen dose that can be administered during a defined time frame and is thus easier to achieve when only one allergen, (e.g., house dust mite) is being injected. Long-term, low-dose, multiple-antigen immunotherapy is reported to add little to optimal treatment using control of environmental allergens and optimal pharmacotherapy, including inhaled glucocorticoids.[10]

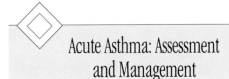

Acute Asthma: Assessment and Management

Asthma exacerbations are most likely to occur during viral upper respiratory infections, allergen exposure, or withdrawal of medication, particularly glucocorticoids. As any severe acute exacerbation is potentially life-threatening, assessment of the severity of the episode is important. Some patients are at particularly high

Table 14-9

Risk Factors for Near-Fatal or Fatal Episodes of Asthma

Previous near-fatal episode(s) (e.g., intensive care unit admission, intubation, and/or mechanical ventilation)[a]

Hospitalization(s), emergency department or urgent-care visit(s) for asthma during previous year

Excessive use of short-acting β_2-adrenergic agonists (e.g., two canisters per month or equivalent)

Concurrent use of or withdrawal from oral glucocorticoids

Poor perception of asthma symptoms and delay in treatment

History of noncompliance with asthma medications

History of psychosocial problems or psychiatric disease

Sensitization to *Alternaria* (mold)

Passive smoke exposure

Reduced access to health care, including medications, due to poor socioeconomic status

Poor formal education, language barrier, low-income or overcrowded housing

[a]*Note:* Patients with asthma who have concomitant anaphylactic sensitivity to foods are at increased risk for death during anaphylaxis.

risk for fatal or near-fatal episodes (Table 14-9). Subspecialist involvement may provide helpful support for such children and their primary care physicians.

For hospitalized patients with severe episodes of asthma, the initial assessment consists of a history and physical examination, particularly with regard to breathlessness, use of accessory muscles, respiratory rate, oxygen saturation, and, if feasible, peak flow or FEV_1; arterial blood gases may be needed in some patients (Table 14-10).[8] Frequent repeat assessments are necessary.

Treatment should be started promptly and should consist of oxygen, an inhaled short-acting β_2-adrenergic agonist, ipratropium bromide, and systemic glucocorticoids. Oral prednisone within 4 h of administration reduces the need

for hospitalization among children treated in the emergency department for acute asthma.[11] Sedation in any form is contraindicated in the treatment of any asthma exacerbation. Patients not responding to initial treatment should be transferred to and monitored in hospital units where staff are skilled in the management of acute respiratory disorders in children and where appropriate facilities for intubation and mechanical ventilation are available.

Every child discharged from an urgent care facility, emergency department, or hospital after an asthma exacerbation should receive instruction about the oral and inhaled glucocorticoid treatment regimen (dose, number of days of treatment) and an appointment for a follow-up visit with his or her personal physician during the next 7 to 10 days.

Table 14-10

Assessing the Severity of Asthma Exacerbations

	SEVERITY OF ASTHMA EXACERBATIONS		
CHARACTERISTIC	MILD[a]	MODERATE[b]	SEVERE
Breathless	Walking	Talking (for infants, softer, short cry; difficulty feeding)	At rest
Position	Can lie down	Prefers sitting	Hunched forward
Talks in . . .	Sentences	Phrases	Words
Alertness	May be agitated	Usually agitated	Usually agitated[c]
Accessory muscles and suprasternal retractions	Not noted	Usually	Usually[c]
Wheeze	Moderate, often only end-expiratory	Loud	Usually loud[c]
Pulsus paradoxus	Absent; <10 mmHg	May be present; 10–25 mmHg	Often present, >25 mmHg (adult); 20–40 mmHg (child)[c]
Peak expiratory flow after initial bronchodilator; % predicted or % personal best	>80	≈60–80	<60 predicted of personal best (<100 L/min in adolescents if response lasts <2 h)
Sa_{O_2} (on air), %	>95	91–95	<90
Pa_{O_2} and Pa_{CO_2} on room air	Test not necessary	>60 mmHg and <45 mmHg	<60 mmHg (often cyanotic) and >45 mmHg (impending respiratory failure)

[a] Patients can be managed in a primary care setting.

[b] Patients should be assessed and managed in a hospital.

[c] The presence of one or more of the following suggests that respiratory arrest may be imminent: drowsiness or confusion, paradoxical thoraco-abdominal movement, quiet chest (no wheezing), and bradycardia; in infants, a respiratory rate of >60 and an SaO_2 of <91 are danger signs.

Summary

Asthma is a common chronic disease that remains underdiagnosed and undertreated. The condition is not only a global health concern but also a practical concern for many physicians. Diagnosing asthma depends largely on the history, physical examination, and reversibility of symptoms with a short-acting bronchodilator, preferably confirmed using peak expiratory flow or spirometry before and after bronchodilator treatment.

The main goal in management, a symptom-free patient, is readily achievable in most children and adolescents by using a combination of avoidance of environmental trigger factors, pharmacologic treatment, and asthma education. Each young person with asthma needs an asthma action plan detailing how to avoid his or her trigger factors, how to prevent symptoms, and what to do if symptoms break through despite regular preventive measures.

References

1. Centers for Disease Control and Prevention: Asthma mortality and hospitalization among children and young adults—United States, 1990–1993. *MMWR* 45:350–353, 1996.

2. Howarth PH: Pathogenic mechanisms: a rational basis for treatment. *BMJ* 316:758–761, 1998.

3. Jenkins MA, Hopper JL, Bowes G, et al: Factors in childhood asthma as predictors of asthma in adult life. *BMJ* 309:90–93, 1994.

4. Godden DJ, Ross S, Abdalla M, et al: Outcome of wheeze in childhood: symptoms and pulmonary function 25 years later. *Am J Respir Crit Care Med* 149:106–112, 1994.

5. DiFranza JR, Lew RA: Morbidity and mortality in children associated with the use of tobacco products by other people. *Pediatrics* 97:560–568, 1996.

6. Ownby DR, Adinoff AD: The appropriate use of skin testing and allergen immunotherapy in young children. *J Allergy Clin Immunol* 94:662–665, 1994.

7. Lieu TA, Quesenberry CP Jr, Capra AM, et al: Outpatient management practices associated with reduced risk of pediatric asthma hospitalization and emergency department visits. *Pediatrics* 100:334–341, 1997.

8. Lemanske RF Jr, Busse WW: Asthma. *JAMA* 278:1855–1873, 1997.

9. Simons FER and the Canadian Beclomethasone Dipropionate-Salmeterol Xinafoate Study Group. A comparison of beclomethasone, salmeterol, and placebo in children with asthma. *N Engl J Med* 337:1659–1665, 1997.

10. Adkinson NF Jr, Eggleston PA, Eney D, et al: A controlled trial of immunotherapy for asthma in allergic children. *N Engl J Med* 336:324–331, 1997.

11. Scarfone RJ, Fuchs SM, Nager AL, et al: Controlled trial of oral prednisone in the emergency department treatment of children with acute asthma. *Pediatrics* 92:513–518, 1993.

Alexander K. C. Leung
Thomas J. Bowen

Seasonal Allergic Rhinitis and Food Allergy

Seasonal Allergic Rhinitis

Seasonal allergic rhinitis (or rhinoconjunctivitis), seasonal pollinosis, and hay fever all describe a symptom complex typically characterized by rhinorrhea, nasal congestion, sneezing, and itching of the nose, eyes, eustachian tubes, and pharynx. These symptoms are periodic in nature and occur during the pollinating season of the plants to which the patient is sensitive.

Epidemiology

The prevalence of seasonal allergic rhinitis in the general population has been estimated to be 5 to 22 percent, increasing during childhood from less than 1 percent during infancy, to 4 to 5 percent from 5 to 9 years of age, to 9 percent during adolescence, and to 15 to 16 percent after adolescence. Typically, seasonal allergic rhinitis does not develop until the patient has been sensitized by two or more pollen seasons. Both sexes are equally affected. Seasonal allergic rhinitis has a genetic predisposition. Most investigators believe that the mechanisms permitting the development of allergic rhinitis, asthma, and eczema are governed by multiple genes, often autosomal dominant with incomplete penetrance.

Pathogenesis

Seasonal allergic rhinitis is a type I immediate hypersensitivity reaction mediated by specific IgE antibody to a seasonal allergen. An aeroallergen, which enters the body through inhalation, interacts with antigen-presenting cells, T-cell and B-cell lymphocytes, and, if the patient is T-helper 2 (TH2) atopic–predisposed, these processes may result in the production of IgE antibodies. The IgE antibodies so formed bind to high-affinity receptors on mast cells and basophils and to low-affinity receptors on eosinophils.

On nasal reexposure to the same antigen, the antigen bridges two adjacent IgE molecules attached to the surface of these cells with resultant release of preformed chemical mediators such as histamine and chemotactic factors. These mediators cause immediate-phase symptoms that typically subside within 30 to 60 min. Other mediators such as leukotrienes and prostaglandins are synthesized through the metabolism of arachidonic acid in the cell membrane.

Late-phase reactions follow, with an influx of various inflammatory cells, including eosinophils, over a period of 30 min to 24 h. These late-phase reactions result in the release of more chemical mediators.

Seasonal allergic rhinitis is commonly caused by the pollens from nonflowering wind-pollinated plants, usually from the pollens one cannot see rather than those that are easily visible. In general, tree pollens cause symptoms in the early spring, grass pollens cause symptoms in the late spring and early summer, and ragweed and other weed pollens cause symptoms in the late summer and autumn until frost. Seasonal allergic rhinitis may also be caused by wind-borne mold spores. Insect-pollinated flowers or plants rarely cause allergic rhinitis because these pollens are too heavy to be airborne. Ingested foods do not usually cause allergic rhinitis, but patients with ragweed, birch, or alder allergies may experience oral allergy syndrome, as described later in this chapter.

Clinical Manifestations

SYMPTOMATOLOGY

The characteristic symptoms of allergic rhinitis include seasonal rhinorrhea, nasal congestion, nasal and ocular pruritus, and paroxysmal sneezing. The nasal discharge is usually clear and watery and results from a combined effect of increased secretory activity and plasma exudation. The watery rhinorrhea may cause patients to sniffle and blow their noses often. Posterior pharyngeal drainage gives rise to frequent clearing of the throat and coughing. Nasal congestion usually results from an allergic inflammatory edema of the nasal mucosa. Chronic and severe nasal congestion may lead to habitual mouth-breathing, nasal speech, snoring, and headache. Pruritus usually affects the nose, eyes, and eustachian tubes. Itching of the nose may cause children to rub the tip of the nose with the palm in an upward fashion (the so-called allergic salute), as shown in Fig. 15-1. Itching of the palate, throat, and ears is a less common but very suggestive symptom. Sneezing is caused by stimulation of irritant receptors supplied by trigeminal nerve endings, which initiates a central reflex. Paroxysmal repetitive sneezing, often 10 to 15 times in a row, is a classic symptom of allergic rhinitis.

PHYSICAL FINDINGS

The nasal mucosa usually appears pale, bluish, and edematous. The nasal turbinates are often enlarged. Nasal polyps are present in a small percentage of affected individuals. If nasal polyps develop before the age of 20 years, cystic fibrosis should be considered as a diagnostic possibility. Mouth breathing is common. The child may wrinkle the nose (rabbit nose or facial grimace) and rub it in characteristic ways (allergic salute). Constant rubbing of the nose in an upward direction may lead to a horizontal crease at the junction of the bulbous tip of the nose and the more rigid bridge (allergic crease). Dark circles under the eyes (allergic shiners) (Fig. 15-2, see Color Plate 24) have been attributed to infraorbital venous stasis resulting from swollen nasal and paranasal mucous membranes, which compress the veins that drain that area. Double folds of the lower eyelids (Dennie's lines or allergic lines) are also common. Conjunctival injection and edema are frequent findings in patients with associated allergic conjunctivitis. There may also be excessive lacrimation and chemosis.

Children may also develop elongated facies, narrowed maxillae, flattened malar eminences, and high arched palates (adenoidal facies) due to chronic nasal obstruction. The tympanic membranes may show evidence of secretory otitis media, immobility, or tympanosclerosis due to chronic inflammation with recurrent infections. Eczema and intermittent bronchospasm may also be evident.

Diagnostic Studies

NASAL CYTOLOGY

The nasal secretions may be examined by having the patient blow the nasal secretions onto a piece of plastic wrap or nonporous paper. After transfer to a glass slide, the secretions are heat-fixed and stained with Hansel stain. The presence of more than 5 percent eosinophils suggests allergic rhinitis. However, the test is not diagnostic, as nasal eosinophilia is also found in the nonallergic rhinitis with eosinophilia syndrome (NARES). The presence

Figure 15-1

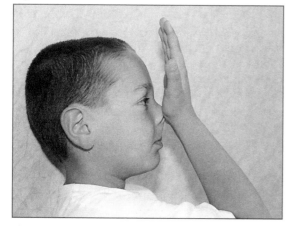

Children with allergic rhinitis tend to rub the tip of the nose with the palm in an upward fashion (the so called "allergic salute").

of neutrophils, on the other hand, suggests infection rather than allergy. Overlap between clinical conditions limits the utility of this test.

Skin Tests

Skin testing using high-potency standardized extracts is the diagnostic method of choice to demonstrate IgE antibodies and to identify sensitivities to allergens. Skin testing is rapid, specific, sensitive, and cost-effective. The common allergens used for testing include grasses, trees, cats, dogs, and house dust mites.

Skin testing is usually done by percutaneous or epicutaneous prick or puncture technique on the forearm or back and the result is examined in 10 to 20 min. Intradermal testing for inhalant antigens (not food antigens) may be done if the prick test is negative. Intradermal tests are more sensitive but may cause more false-positive reactions. Positive (histamine) and negative (saline) controls are applied by the same prick or puncture technique. A wheal (not including erythema) of 3 mm or larger in comparison with a negative control is considered positive. To avoid false-negative results, antihistamines and some antidepressants should be withheld for various periods prior to the skin testing.

In Vitro Tests for Total and Specific IgE

rast Radioallergosorbent tests (RASTs) and enzyme-linked immunosorbent assays (ELISAs) are often used to measure allergen-specific IgE in vitro. The clinical importance of measuring total serum IgE for allergic rhinitis is limited with overlap of serum IgE levels between normal subjects and patients with allergic rhinitis. Moreover, an elevated total serum IgE can be found in other allergic diseases (asthma, eczema), fungal infections (allergic bronchopulmonary aspergillosis, systemic candidiasis), viral infections (infectious mononucleosis, cytomegalic inclusion disease), parasitic infestations (visceral larva migrans, filariasis, schistosomiasis), immunodeficiency syndromes (hyperimmuno-

globulinemia E syndrome, Wiskott-Aldrich syndrome), and collagen vascular disorders (infantile polyarteritis nodosa and rheumatoid arthritis).

In the RAST, the patient's serum is incubated with various antigens. Antigen-specific IgE, if present in the serum, attaches to the antigen. RASTs are used mainly in patients with severe eczema or dermographism, in those who must keep taking antihistamines, and in those with risk of severe anaphylaxis. The advantages of the RAST are convenience and safety. The tests are not affected by medications or skin condition and the patient's serum can be tested for multiple different IgE molecules at one time. Disadvantages include high cost, limited number of antigens available, delay in obtaining results, detection of circulating IgE rather than cell-bound IgE, interference with the test result by circulating IgG antibody, and the use of radiation in the laboratory with attendant precautions. Also, RASTs may be less sensitive than skin testing.

elisa In the ELISA, an enzyme such as alkaline phosphatase or horseradish peroxidase is attached to the antigen-specific IgE rather than a radioisotope, and the enzymatic activity is then determined. The activity of the bound enzyme is proportional to the amount of anti-IgE bound to antigen-specific IgE. The ELISA has similar advantages and disadvantages as the RAST in the identification of antigen-specific IgE. For both the RAST and the ELISA, physicians ordering these tests must be concerned about quality control. Many laboratories do not perform these tests well.

Finally, although clinicians often like to use in vitro tests in children with extensive atopic dermatitis, these children often have markedly elevated serum IgE levels. A markedly elevated serum IgE concentration can interfere with the RAST and ELISA and give falsely elevated results. A comparison of skin tests and in vitro tests for specific IgE is shown in Table 15-1.

Table 15-1

Comparison of Skin Tests and in Vitro Tests for Specific IgE

SKIN TESTS	IN VITRO TESTS FOR SPECIFIC IgE
Results rapidly available	No risk to patient
Greater sensitivity	Irradiation hazard to technician
Less costly	Convenience
Wide allergen selection	Not affected by medications
Can detect non-IgE–mediated allergic reactions	Not affected by skin conditions
	Patient's serum can be tested for multiple different IgE molecules at one time
	Limited number of antigens available
	Detection of circulating IgE rather than cell-bound IgE

Management

ENVIRONMENTAL MODIFICATION

Patients with seasonal allergic rhinitis may benefit from keeping windows closed, using air conditioning or high efficiency particulate air (HEPA) air filters to filter allergens, limiting time spent outdoors when pollen counts are high, keeping windows closed while riding in cars, and avoiding contact with compost piles, barns, and hay. Mowing of grass, raking of leaves, and direct contact with pollinating plants should be avoided. A mask worn during such activities that cannot be avoided helps reduce the allergen exposure.

PHARMACOTHERAPY

Because it is difficult to completely avoid exposure to aeroallergens, most patients resort to drug therapy to prevent or alleviate the symptoms of seasonal allergic rhinitis (Table 15-2).

ANTIHISTAMINES Antihistamines are generally used as first-line treatment for seasonal allergic rhinitis. Antihistamines function by competing with histamine, through their ethylamine core, for receptors on sensory nerves, endothelial cells, and smooth muscle cells. Antihistamines, particularly those of the tricyclic class, may reduce the release of histamine from mast cells

Table 15-2

Effects of Different Drugs on Nasal Symptoms

DRUGS	NASAL ITCHING AND SNEEZING	RHINORRHEA	NASAL OBSTRUCTION	IMPAIRED SMELL
Antihistamines	+++	++	+/−	−
Oral decongestants	−	−	+++	+
Nasal decongestants	−	−	+++	+
Topical corticosteroids	+++	+++	++	+
Oral corticosteroids	+++	+++	+++	++
Mast cell stablizers	++	+	+	−
Ipratropium bromide	−	++	−	−

and basophils and may also curtail production of leukotrienes and kinins.

Antihistamines block both the vasodilation that results from stimulation of blood vessels by H_1 receptors and the mucous gland hypersecretion and sneezing that result from the reflex irritation. Antihistamines are highly effective in controlling sneezing, rhinorrhea, and itching, but they are less effective for relieving nasal congestion. They are also effective in reducing associated ocular symptoms. Because of their rapid onset of action, they are especially useful for symptoms of intermittent allergic rhinitis. They yield the best result, however, if given prior to an anticipated antigen exposure.

The first-generation antihistamines, such as diphenhydramine and chlorpheniramine, are lipophilic and penetrate the central nervous system easily. As such, they may cause sedation. A number of first-generation antihistamines also block muscarinic cholinergic receptors, with resultant undesirable effects such as dry mouth, blurred vision, urinary retention, and constipation.

In second-generation antihistamines such as astemizole, cetirizine, loratadine, fexofenadine, and terfenadine, alterations have been made such that these compounds are lipophobic and penetrate poorly into the central nervous system, thereby minimizing their sedative effect and anticholinergic action. In general, second-generation antihistamines are safe, effective, and well tolerated. Astemizole and terfenadine can cause serious cardiovascular events, including QT prolongation, torsades de pointes, and other cardiac arrhythmias in patients with cardiac disease or serious hepatic impairment as well as in patients who are concurrently taking agents or drugs that undergo significant metabolism in the liver (e.g., clarithromycin, erythromycin, cyclosporine, ketoconazole, itraconazole, cimetidine, and a long list of prescription and nonprescription agents). Astemizole may also cause increased appetite, with resultant weight gain. Ophthalmic and nasal preparations of antihistamines—such as antazoline, levocabastine, and olopatadine—are effective in the treatment of ocular and nasal symptoms. These medications not only relieve the itching but also treat the symptoms of allergic rhinoconjunctivitis.

DECONGESTANTS When nasal obstruction is a prominent symptom, an oral decongestant such as phenylephrine, pseudoephedrine, or phenylpropanolamine may be used alone or in combination with an antihistamine. These alpha-adrenergic agents constrict blood vessels and reduce blood supply to the nasal mucosa, thereby decreasing the volume of blood in the sinusoids and the amount of mucosal edema. Systemic adverse effects include restlessness, insomnia, headache, tachycardia, palpitations, and hypertension in susceptible individuals.

Nasal decongestant sprays and drops such as xylometazoline and phenylephrine have a more rapid onset of action and are more efficacious than systemic administration of alpha-adrenergic decongestants. Nasal decongestants may, however, cause rebound congestion, and with prolonged use, rhinitis medicamentosa.

CORTICOSTEROIDS Intranasal corticosteroids are the most effective agents for the treatment of seasonal allergic rhinitis. These agents act by modifying gene expression. When glucocorticoids combine with intracellular steroid receptors, the resulting complex interacts with DNA to form cell-regulating proteins. These proteins inhibit leukocyte priming, limit the secretion of cytokines and other mediators, and modulate enzyme systems. They also inhibit the migration of mast cells into the nasal mucosa and induce eosinopenia. As such, intranasal corticosteroids reduce inflammation, suppress neutrophil chemotaxis, decrease nasal vasodilation and edema, and decrease late responses to nasal allergen challenge.

The potency of intranasal corticosteroids exceeds that of antihistamines, decongestants, and mast-cell stabilizers. However, intranasal corticosteroids do not relieve palatal or ocular itching as effectively; therefore, if these symptoms are present, an antihistamine is often added to the regimen. Because of the delayed onset of action, intranasal corticosteroids are particularly effective when used prophylactically to affect both the early and late phases of the allergic response.

A variety of nasal steroid sprays are available: beclomethasone diproprionate, budesonide, flunisolide, fluticasone, mometasone, and triamcinolone. In general, the aqueous suspensions of intranasal corticosteroids are less irritating and better tolerated than sprays with a freon propellant and other nonaqueous media. Budesonide taken by nasal inhaler does not have a smell or taste and does not trickle down the throat and is therefore preferred by some patients.

Local side effects consist of nasal irritation, stinging, burning, and epistaxis. Some adverse effects may be due to the drug delivery device or to the local effect of the spray rather than being a side effect of the drug per se. Occasionally, temporary use of corticosteroid eyedrops is necessary in the child with severe allergic conjunctivitis. Rarely, short-term oral steroids may be required to settle severe ocular and nasal symptoms while other medications start to take effect and to break the allergic cycle.

MAST-CELL STABILIZERS Mast-cell stabilizers, such as sodium cromoglycate, nedocromil sodium, and olopatadine, act by inhibiting calcium transmembrane flux, thereby preventing antigeninduced degranulation. They are effective in reducing sneezing, rhinorrhea, and nasal pruritus. They are not very effective, however, in preventing nasal congestion. In general, the effectiveness of mast-cell stabilizers is less than that of intranasal corticosteroids. They are most effective if started early and used prophylactically. Because of the delayed onset of effect, concurrent antihistamine therapy may be necessary. The major disadvantage of sodium cromoglycate and nedocromil sodium is the frequent dosing requirement (four to six times daily), which reduces compliance. Adverse effects are uncommon and include sneezing, nasal stinging and burning, and, rarely, epistaxis.

Ophthalmic preparations of sodium cromoglycate, nedocromil, olopatadine, and lodoxamide have been found to be effective in the treatment of allergic conjunctivitis. The last two agents have a less frequent dosing requirement.

IPRATROPIUM BROMIDE Ipratropium bromide (Atrovent) is an anticholinergic agent. By blocking acetylcholine-mediated responses, ipratropium decreases tissue concentrations of cyclic guanosine monophosphate, thus reducing the volume of nasal secretion and providing some minor degree of vasoconstriction. As such, intranasal ipratropium is helpful in patients with excessive rhinorrhea or postnasal drip who have been unresponsive to other treatments. It does not, however, relieve sneezing, itching, or nasal congestion. Side effects include excessive nasal dryness, dry mouth, dizziness, nausea, blurred vision, constipation, and urinary retention.

IMMUNOTHERAPY

Allergen immunotherapy consists of a series of injections of allergen extract(s) or high dose sublingual administration with the aim of reducing the patient's sensitivity to the allergen(s). Allergy shots are administered subcutaneously in minute doses at weekly, biweekly, or monthly intervals; the dose is gradually increased as tolerated to the appropriate maintenance dose determined by the specialist supervising the immunotherapy. Immunotherapy is usually discontinued after 3 to 5 years of maintenance therapy. In general, immunotherapy should be considered for patients who have unacceptable symptoms that fail to respond to environmental modification or pharmacotherapy. Patients who require medications for more than 6 months per year, two or more seasons of unacceptable pollinosis, or have intolerable side effects from pharmacotherapy are candidates for immunotherapy. Immunotherapy has been shown in double-blind studies to be effective in reducing the symptoms of seasonal allergic rhinitis with therapy starting as early as age 5. Immunotherapy produces a number of immunologic changes that include an increase in serum allergen-specific IgG-blocking antibodies; reduction of allergen-specific IgE production; blunting of the usual seasonal increase in IgE levels; reduction in mast-cell, basophil, and lymphocyte responsiveness to antigens; generation of antigen-specific suppressor T cells; and reduced production of some lymphokines.

Side effects of immunotherapy consists mainly of local reaction at the injection site. Preloading with nonsedating antihistamine may modify this problem. Systemic reaction, including anaphylaxis, may rarely occur but are less frequent with sublingual therapy. Appropriate facility precautions are warranted, such as having the patient wait for 30 min in the facility after the injection has been administered.

Emerging Concepts

Other immune therapies under clinical trial include chemokine and antichemokine therapy, humanized monoclonal anti-IgE antibody therapy, and intranasal vaccines, DNA vaccines, and gene therapy.

Food Allergy

Food allergy is an abnormal immunologic response resulting from the ingestion of food or food additives. It is unrelated to any physiologic effect of the food. The term *food allergy* is used interchangeably with *food hypersensitivity*.

Prevalence

The incidence of food allergy in children has been variously estimated to be between 0.3 and 7.5 percent; it decreases with age, with only 1 to 2 percent of the pediatric population affected by their fourth birthday. The incidence of food allergy is significantly increased in children with atopic disease.

Pathophysiology

Although any food can be allergenic, certain foods are responsible for the majority of food-related allergic events. The most frequently implicated foods include eggs, cow's milk, tree nuts, peanuts, soy, wheat, seafoods, citrus fruits, and chocolate (Table 15-3).

Under normal circumstances, exposure to food antigen via the gastrointestinal tract results in a local IgA response and preferential suppression of systemic IgM, IgG, and IgE antibody production as well as cell-mediated immune responses to the food antigen.

The most common immunologic reaction that leads to classic food allergy is the type I anaphylactic, IgE-mediated, or immediate hypersensitivity reaction. Oral tolerance fails to develop in genetically susceptible individuals, and exposure to a specific antigen stimulates the production of antigen-specific IgE. A type II cytotoxic reaction occurs when an antigen present on a cell surface combines with an antibody, either IgG or IgM, with resulting complement activa-

Table 15-3

Foods Most Commonly Implicated as Causing Allergic Reactions

Eggs
Cow's milk
Tree nuts/peanuts
Soy/soy products
Wheat/flour
Seafoods (fish/shellfish/mollusks/crustacea)
Citrus fruits
Chocolate

tion and cytolysis. A type III or antigen–antibody complex reaction occurs when antigen and antibody (IgG, IgM, IgA) combine to form immune complexes to which complement is fixed. Tissue damage may result if there are high concentrations of the immune complexes. Serum-sickness reaction may result if there is an antigen excess; an Arthus-type reaction may result if there is an antibody excess. A type IV or delayed hypersensitivity reaction occurs when antigen reacts with sensitized T lymphocytes and results in the production of cytotoxic cells and cells that release lymphokines. Thus far, there is very little evidence to support "pure" type II, III, or IV mechanism in the production of clinically important food hypersensitivity.

Clinical Manifestations

The clinical manifestations of food allergy are listed in Table 15-4. In general, gastrointestinal symptoms are most common, with a frequency between 50 and 80 percent, followed by cutaneous symptoms (in 20 to 40 percent) and respiratory symptoms (in 4 to 25 percent). Symptoms may be mild or severe and most often occur within minutes to 1 to 2 h after the offending food has been eaten.

GASTROINTESTINAL MANIFESTATIONS

ORAL ALLERGY SYNDROME   The syndrome generally occurs in patients with inhalant allergy to birch, mugwort, or ragweed pollen and is associated with the ingestion of various fresh fruits and raw vegetables. Birch pollinosis may be associated with reactions to apples, cherries, peaches, pears, plums, apricots, kiwi, hazelnuts, almonds, pecans, walnuts, raw carrots, and potatoes; ragweed pollinosis with cantaloupe, honeydew, watermelon, and bananas; and mugwort pollinosis with celery, carrots, caraway, dill, parsley, fennel, green peppers, and aniseed. Symptoms include rapid onset of pruritus, burning, and/or angioedema of the lips, tongue,

Table 15-4
Clinical Manifestations of Food Allergy

1. Gastrointestinal manifestations
   A. Oral allergy syndrome
   B. Gastrointestinal anaphylaxis
   C. Food-induced enterocotitis syndrome
   D. Food-induced colitis
   E. Allergic eosinophilic gastroenteritis
   F. Gluten-sensitive enteropathy
   G. Infantile colic
2. Cutaneous manifestations
   A. Urticaria/angioedema
   B. Atopic dermatitis
   C. Dermatitis herpetiformis
3. Respiratory manifestations
   A. Allergic rhinitis
   B. Asthma
   C. Heiner syndrome
4. Generalized manifestations
   A. Systemic anaphylaxis
   B. Food-dependent exercise-induced anaphylaxis
5. Hematologic manifestation
   A. Anemia

palate, and throat. Symptoms usually resolve rapidly, although canker sores sometimes develop and the oral mucosa may feel burnt. Gastrointestinal symptoms such as abdominal cramps, vomiting, and diarrhea may occur. Botanical cross-reactivity (as a result of shared epitopes, profilins, or panallergens) between pollen and such fruits, tree nuts, and vegetables has been suggested as a possible mechanism.

GASTROINTESTINAL ANAPHYLAXIS   Gastrointestinal anaphylaxis is a form of IgE-mediated gastrointestinal hypersensitivity that often accompanies other systemic manifestations of food allergy. This may manifest as nausea, vomiting, abdominal pain, flatulence, abdominal distention, or diarrhea.

FOOD-INDUCED ENTEROCOLITIS SYNDROME   Classic symptoms include protracted vomiting and diarrhea, frequently resulting in dehydration in infants less than 3 months of age. Some infants may have malabsorption, protein-losing enteropathy, and failure to thrive. Cow's milk and soy protein are most often responsible. Stools generally contain occult blood, polymorphonuclear neutrophils, eosinophils, and Charcot-Leyden crystals. Jejunal biopsy usually reveals villous atrophy and increased numbers of lymphocytes, eosinophils, and mast cells. Prick and RAST testings are usually negative.

FOOD-INDUCED COLITIS   Food-induced colitis usually occurs in the first few months of life and is most often due to hypersensitivity to milk protein or soy protein. Infants with food-induced colitis generally appear healthy and have normal weight gain. These infants usually have occult or gross blood in their stools. Colonic biopsy samples reveal mucosal edema, erythema, friability, ulceration, and eosinophilic infiltration.

ALLERGIC EOSINOPHILIC GASTROENTERITIS   Allergic eosinophilic gastroenteritis is characterized by infiltration of the gastrointestinal tract with eosinophils as well as by peripheral eosinophilia and absence of vasculitis. Children with mucosal involvement usually have postprandial nausea, vomiting, abdominal pain, watery diarrhea with or without blood, iron deficiency anemia, occasionally steatorrhea, and failure to thrive. Children with muscular involvement may have symptoms and signs of gastric outlet or intestinal obstruction, depending on the site of bowel involvement. The serosal form is characterized by eosinophilic ascites and abdominal distention and is extremely rare in children. In addition to an IgE-mediated mechanism, cell-mediated immunity may also be responsible. T cells specifically sensitized to antigens may release lymphokines capable of attracting eosinophils.

GLUTEN-SENSITIVE ENTEROPATHY   Gluten-sensitive enteropathy (celiac disease) is a disorder in which mucosal damage to the small bowel is the result of a permanent sensitivity to gliadin. The main clinical manifestations are irritability, anorexia, vomiting, abdominal pain, abdominal distention, digital clubbing, muscle wasting, and failure to thrive. Characteristically, biopsy of the jejunum shows villous atrophy. Both cellular and complement-mediated cytotoxicity and lymphokine-induced damage have been implicated in the pathogenesis of the condition. Antiendomysial or transglutaminase antibodies may be helpful for diagnosis.

CUTANEOUS MANIFESTATIONS

URTICARIA/ANGIOEDEMA   Acute urticaria and, to a lesser extent, angioedema are among the most common manifestations of allergic reactions to food in children. Contact with foods may also cause acute urticaria. However, food allergy is rarely the cause of chronic urticaria unless the offending food is eaten almost every day. Rarely, urticaria is seen as part of the oral allergy syndrome.

ATOPIC DERMATITIS   Food allergy plays an immunopathogenic role in 30 to 50 percent of children with atopic dermatitis. The pathogenesis of atopic dermatitis involves both immediate and late-phase effects of IgE-mediated food hypersensitivity reactions. The immediate or early phase of the reaction results from IgE-mediated cutaneous mast-cell activation. The late phase is characterized by a mixed cellular infiltrate (eosinophils, neutrophils, lymphocytes, and basophils) at 6 to 8 h and thereafter by a mononuclear round-cell infiltrate indistinguishable from that seen in eczematous skin. A single ingestion of a food allergen rarely provokes an eczematous lesion, but chronic ingestion of a food allergen can result in the classic changes of atopic dermatitis.

DERMATITIS   HERPETIFORMIS   Gluten-sensitive enteropathy is found in 75 to 95 percent of patients with dermatitis herpetiformis. The skin lesions may be the result of a local type III reaction. IgA antibodies to smooth muscle endomysium and jejunum have been reported in patients with dermatitis herpetiformis–associated gluten-sensitive enteropathy.

RESPIRATORY MANIFESTATIONS

ALLERGIC RHINITIS   Ingested foods may cause allergic rhinitis. Ingested allergens can activate nasal mast cells in addition to mast cells elsewhere in the body.

ASTHMA   Food allergy may increase airway reactivity, so that other triggers or environmental factors can more readily precipitate an asthmatic attack. Wheezing is often seen with systemic anaphylaxis.

GENERALIZED MANIFESTATIONS

SYSTEMIC ANAPHYLAXIS   Systemic anaphylaxis is almost always IgE-mediated and involves multiple target organs. Early symptoms may include pruritus, urticaria, nausea, vomiting, abdominal pain, angioedema, and wheezing. This may rapidly progress to laryngeal edema, dyspnea, stridor, cyanosis, chest pain, hypotension, cardiac dysrhythmias, diarrhea, and shock. The degree of anaphylactic reactions varies and may manifest in a partial form.

FOOD-DEPENDENT EXERCISE-INDUCED ANAPHYLAXIS
Anaphylaxis has been reported after the ingestion of certain foods (wheat or celery, for example) in association with exercise. Differences in blood flow to the gut, increased food allergen absorption, increased spontaneous leukocyte histamine release, and enhanced mast-cell responsiveness to physical stimuli may have a role in the pathogenesis of this condition.

HEMATOLOGIC MANIFESTATION

ANEMIA   Iron deficiency anemia may develop in children with cow's milk or soy allergy secondary to gastrointestinal blood loss. This may be caused by milk-induced enterocolitis syndrome, milk-induced colitis, allergic eosinophilic gastroenteritis, and Heiner syndrome.

Clinical Evaluation

HISTORY

The history should include a description of symptoms, the type and quantity of food required to evoke a reaction, whether the food is raw, cooked, or otherwise processed, the time elapsed between ingestion and the onset of symptoms, the age at onset, the number of occasions the reaction has been noted, the presence of other factors (exercise or other simultaneously ingested food) required to initiate the symptoms, the length of time since the last reaction, and a description of the most recent reaction. The use of any medication should be determined. Any previous hospitalization or significant illness should be noted. A personal or family history of atopy increases the likelihood that the adverse reaction is due to an allergic reaction rather than some other mechanism.

A dietary diary is a useful adjunct to the medical history. All foods, beverages, and drugs consumed within 12 to 24 h before each occurrence and the character of the adverse reaction should be recorded in chronological order. The diary is then reviewed to determine whether there are any relationships between the foods ingested and the occurrence of symptoms.

PHYSICAL EXAMINATION

A complete physical examination should be done, with particular emphasis on the patient's weight, height, nutritional status, and vital signs. Poor growth may indicate a chronic disease such a gluten-sensitive enteropathy or cystic fibrosis. Eczematous lesion, wheezing, and "allergic shiners" suggest that the adverse reaction is more likely to be due to atopy and food hypersensitivity. Physical examination may also help exclude some disorders in the differential diagnosis. During an acute allergic episode, the following signs may be found: urticaria, angioedema, oropharyngeal edema, increased bowel sounds, wheezing, and hypotension.

Diagnostic Studies

SKIN TESTS

Skin testing with food extracts is often used to screen patients with suspected IgE-mediated food allergies. Details of the skin testing can be found in the previous section under "Seasonal Allergic Rhinitis."

IN VITRO TESTS FOR TOTAL AND SPECIFIC IgE

Many children with IgE-mediated food allergies have elevated serum IgE levels. However, an elevated serum IgE level can also be found in other conditions. Serum IgE antibodies specific for allergens can be measured in vitro by RAST or ELISA techniques, as described earlier in this chapter.

Elimination Diet and Food Challenge Tests

ELIMINATION DIET

The simplest type of elimination diet is elimination of the suspected food(s) from the diet for 2 to 4 weeks or longer. If just a few foods are suspected of causing the reaction, only those foods need to be eliminated (commonly eggs, milk, soy, wheat, peanuts, tree nuts, fish, and shellfish). When no specific allergens can be incriminated but food allergy is suspected, dietary elimination of the common food allergens is helpful (Table 15-5). If symptoms do not subside with the elimination diet, progressively more restrictive diets can be implemented. Great care must be taken to avoid malnutrition due to such severe restriction. Consultation with nutrition services is often necessary if restrictive diets are to be implemented. In severe and unrespon-

sive cases, the use of an elemental diet with the aim of excluding virtually all known food allergens should be considered. Elemental diets with protein hydrolyzed to free amino acids (e.g., Vivonex and Neocate) represent the most restrictive of elimination diets. Confirmation with a food challenge is essential.

FOOD CHALLENGE

An open or single-blind food challenge is acceptable when the resulting symptoms can be objectively observed. The main disadvantage is the increased incidence of false-positive results, primarily because of biased interpretation by the patient, parents, and physician. The double-blind placebo-controlled food challenge has been considered the "gold standard" for the diagnosis of food allergies. Such a food challenge has the advantage of objectivity and must be used if a positive open challenge yields only a subjective response on the part of the patient, if the symptoms are vague or ill defined, or if there is a psychological component to the reaction. Food challenges with foods that have caused immediate or systemic reactions may be dangerous and should be left to trained specialists.

All foods suspected of causing adverse reactions should be eliminated for 10 to 14 days and the symptoms should have resolved before the food challenge takes place. The challenge should be performed on an empty stomach. The offending food is administered in a graded fashion, starting with a small quantity, and the dose is doubled appropriately at intervals of approximately 15 min until symptoms occur or a reasonable serving size (e.g., 8 to 10 g of dry food or 60 to 100 g of wet food) has been ingested. In a blind challenge, the suspected food is hidden in some neutral, tolerated food or in capsules. If the blind challenge is negative, the food must be consumed openly in the usual quantities under observation to rule out the rare false-negative challenge. A positive challenge merely indicates a cause-and-effect relationship but

Table 15-5

Sample Elimination Diet

Foods Allowed	Major Exclusions
Lamb and chicken	Other meat and seafoods
Rice and rice cereals	Bread, cakes, pasta, cereals, and biscuits
Lactose-free and soya-free margarine	Milk, butter, and eggs
Lettuce, carrots, and sweet potato	Other kinds of vegetables
Banana, pear	Citrus fruits
Tap water and mineral water	Tea, coffee, soft drinks, and alcohol
Olive oil	Other cooking oils
Salt and sugar	Confectionery

Instructions:

Stay on basic diet for ———— days.   (Result)

Then on ————, add ————, alone, first thing in morning ————————

Next on ————, add ————, alone, first thing in morning ————————

Next on ————, add ————, alone, first thing in morning ————————

Next on ————, add ————, alone, first thing in morning ————————

Next on ————, add ————, alone, first thing in morning ————————

Continue food additions one at a time. Keep a diet diary as indicated.

---

does not necessarily mean that an immunologic mechanism is responsible. Diagnosis requires the use of clinical skill, skin testing, and appropriate laboratory tests.

Management

DIETARY TREATMENT

The definitive treatment of food allergy is strict elimination of the offending food from the diet. Symptomatic reactivity to food allergens is generally very specific, and patients rarely react to more than one food in a botanical or animal species. The indiscriminate use of elimination diets without a firm diagnosis is a widespread practice pitfall and may lead to psychological dependence on an unsound diet as well as to vitamin deficiencies, malnutrition, and failure to thrive if multiple foods are inadvertently avoided.

As many as 25 percent of infants who are allergic to cow's milk are also allergic to soy. Infants with hypersensitivity to cow's milk or soy should be fed a substitute elemental formula. Formulas whose protein source is free amino acids (e.g., Vivonex and Neocate) are available. These formulas are hypoallergenic and well tolerated by children. Casein hydrolysates (such as Nutramigen, Progestimil, and Alimentum) have also been used successfully. These formulas, however, are expensive and unpalatable. The partially hydrolyzed whey hydrolysate (e.g., Good Start) is less expensive and has a better taste. However, it contains slightly larger peptides and significantly more immunologically identifiable cow's milk protein, thereby rendering it less suitable for the treatment of cow's milk allergy.

MEDICAL THERAPY

Symptomatic treatment of complications resulting from the inadvertent ingestion of food is essentially the same as that for the specific complication resulting from any other cause. Patients with a history of breathing problems, throat tightness, systemic reaction, or anaphylactic reaction after food exposure should be taught how to self-administer epinephrine and should have an epinephrine autoinjector and antihistamine available at all time. Such patients should wear medical bracelets or necklaces containing the statement "Anaphylactic-allergic to . . ."

Prevention

It may be prudent to avoid peanut ingestion during pregnancy and during breast-feeding for all infants, but the efficacy of this strategy is unclear. In high-risk infants, exclusive breast-feeding with delayed introduction of solid foods until 6 months of age may delay or modify the onset of food allergy and related disorders such as atopic dermatitis. It is unclear whether the incidence of allergic disorders after 3 years of age is altered by these interventions. Because small amounts of food antigens ingested by the mother are excreted in breast milk, avoidance of allergenic foods by lactating mothers is often recommended. When breast-feeding is not possible, the use of a partially or completely hydrolyzed hypoallergenic formula is desirable.

Prognosis and Natural History

Approximately 30 to 40 percent of children lose their food hypersensitivity after 1 to 2 years of allergen avoidance and 80 to 85 percent outgrow their food allergies by 10 years of age. The degree of compliance with allergen avoidance and with the responsible allergen may influence the outcome. Hypersensitivity to peanut, tree nut, fish, and shellfish tends to be more persistent, with perhaps only 5 to 10 percent outgrowing peanut allergy.

Acknowledgment

The authors would like to thank Ms. Dianne Leung, Mr. Alexander Leung Jr., and Mr. Sulakhan Chopra of the University of Calgary Medical Library for their assistance in the preparation of this manuscript. The section on food allergy is a modification of the article by Leung AK: Food allergy: a clinical approach. *Adv Pediatr* 45:145–177, 1998, with permission from Mosby-Year Book, Inc.

References

Allergic Rhinitis

Durham SR, Walter SM, Varga EM, et al: Long term clinical efficacy of grass-pollen immunotherapy. *N Engl J Med* 341:468, 1999.

Fireman P: Rhinitis in children, in Nacleno RM, Durham SR, Mygind N (eds): *Rhinitis: Mechanisms and Management*. New York, Marcel Dekker, 1999, p 415.

Leung AK, Robson WL: Sneezing. *J Otolaryngol* 23: 125, 1994.

Noble SL, Forbes RC, Woodridge HB: Allergic rhinitis. *Am Fam Physician* 51:837, 1995.

Meltzer EO: Treatment options for the child with allergic rhinitis. *Clin Pediatr* 37:1, 1998.

Rachelefsky GS. Pharmacologic management of allergic rhinitis. *J Allergy Clin Immunol* 101:S367, 1998.

Food Allergies

Burks AW, Sampson H: Food allergies in children. *Curr Probl Pediatr* 23:230, 1993.

James JM, Burks AW: Food hypersensitivity in children. *Curr Opin Pediatr* 6:661, 1994.

Leung AK: Food allergy: a clinical approach. *Adv Pediatr* 45:145, 1998.

Sampson HA, Metcalfe DD: Food allergies. *JAMA* 268:2840, 1992.

Sampson HA, Bernhisel-Broadbent J, Yang E, et al: Safety of casein hydrolysate formula in children with cow milk allergy. *J Pediatr* 118:520, 1991.

Seidman E: Food allergic disorders of the gastrointestinal tract, in Roy CC, Silverman A, Allagille D (eds): *Pediatric Clinical Gastroenterology.* St. Louis, Mosby, 1995, p 374.

Watson WTA: Food allergy in children: diagnostic strategies. *Clin Rev Allergy Immunol* 13:347, 1995.

John M. Freeman

Seizures

Definitions

Epidemiology

A seizure is a sudden alteration in motor function, behavior, or consciousness due to an electrical discharge within the brain. There are many different types of seizures, depending on where in the brain the electrical discharge begins and on the direction and rapidity of its spread. *Epilepsy is defined as two or more seizures occurring without an identifiable precipitating cause.* Since fever precipitates febrile seizures, febrile seizures, including those that are recurrent, are not considered to be epilepsy.

Seizures are common. Some 10 percent of all individuals will have one seizure during their lives, but only 25 to 40 percent of children who have a first seizure will have a second one. Most (70 percent) children who have a single seizure, febrile or nonfebrile, will not have a recurrence, whether or not they are treated with anticonvulsant medications. Some 2 percent of children and 1 percent of adults will have recurrent unprovoked seizures (epilepsy).

There is no evidence that seizures (or electrical discharges) damage the brain or cause further seizures in humans. Seizures do not of themselves cause mental retardation or cerebral palsy.

The *only* reason to treat seizures is because they interfere with the individual's or family's well-being. The amount of interference will depend on the type of seizure, its frequency, and the time of day when it occurs. Its effects on the child and family will depend on the child's age, developmental level, and activities.

Most epilepsy is not forever. About 60 to 70 percent of those who develop epilepsy will become seizure-free, and most patients will eventually be able to discontinue medications. Therefore treatment of epilepsy should continue for the shortest reasonable time using the lowest dose of the drug that prevents seizure recurrence.

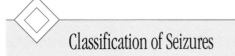

Classification of Seizures

The classification of seizures is shown in Fig. 16-1. The important thing to remember about classification is that recurrent *partial* (focal) seizures strongly suggest that there is a focal abnormality in the brain. Such an abnormality may be due to a tumor, a cyst, a vascular problem, or a developmental abnormality. Most focal seizures in

Figure 16-1

Generalized	
Tonic-clonic	
Absence	
"Minor motor"	
Partial (focal)	
Partial complex	With/without secondary
Partial motor	generalization
Partial sensory	

Classification of seizures.

children are of unknown cause, are not due to one of these lesions, and will *not* require surgery. Only if the seizures persist *and* remain focal is it necessary to consider surgical evaluation. Generalized seizures can also sometimes start focally and spread rapidly throughout the brain, simulating a generalized onset.

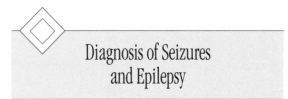

Diagnosis of Seizures and Epilepsy

Since seizures are rarely observed by a physician, the diagnosis of a seizure is usually based solely on someone else's observation of the event and on the physician's interpretation of that observation.

History

The most important part of the evaluation of a child who has had a single suspected "event" is a meticulous history. The history should answer the following questions: Under what circumstances did the event occur? What happened first? What then occurred? Did it start on one side? In one part of that side? How long did it last? What happened during the event? What happened after it was over?

At the end of this history, the physician should be able to say with great certainty that this was clearly a seizure, that this was not a seizure, or that the nature of the event is unclear.

If the event was a seizure, one should provide reassurance (see below) but rarely medication. If it was not a seizure, one should provide reassurance and try to find out what it was and treat that condition if needed.

If, after a careful history, the nature of the event remains unclear, the family should be reassured that it will likely never recur. They should also be told that if it *does* recur, they should carefully observe for the aspects outlined above. In that way, they can make a more precise report and the diagnosis will be facilitated.

Physical Examination

The physical examination after an event is important, although it does not help in establishing whether the event was or was not a seizure. A careful exam may find the source of a fever if the child is febrile. It may find evidence of neurologic dysfunction, which may be either new or old. It may establish evidence of cardiac arrhythmia, a stiff neck suggesting meningitis, or a change in mental status. However, apart from diagnosing an acute process, the main importance of a careful examination at this time is to see if old findings have changed or to establish a baseline should new findings appear.

Laboratory Evaluation

The appropriate laboratory evaluation at the time of the event should be dictated by the findings of the history and the physical exam. *There is no laboratory test or radiologic examination that will diagnose or rule out a seizure. The "full" workup of a seizure does NOT require that every conceivable possible cause of seizure be ruled out!*

Since most initial seizures will not recur, extensive evaluation of a first episode is unnecessary unless there are clinical or historical factors that increase the level of suspicion. Also, since most first seizures will not require treatment, etiology is less important than reassurance.

Magnetic resonance imaging (MRI) or computed tomography (CT) virtually *never* helps in management unless surgery is being contemplated at the time of a first seizure, which never happens.

Metabolic disorders of glucose, calcium, or magnesium are rare causes of seizures and need not be part of the "routine" initial evaluation.

Amino acids and studies for degenerative diseases need not be part of the initial evaluation either unless there is historical or physical evidence of a progressive disorder.

Known causes of new-onset seizures include tumors, vascular malformations, congenital abnormalities, and both metabolic and degenerative diseases. All are, fortunately, rare causes of initial seizures in an otherwise healthy child. Since the treatment of each is difficult, one would prefer, given the choice, to have idiopathic seizures (seizures of unknown cause) to seizures of known cause. Idiopathic seizures are easier to treat, more likely to be controlled, and more likely to be outgrown than seizures of known cause. *When in doubt, choose idiopathic!*

IMAGING

CT and MRI scans are often done at the time of a first event to "rule out a brain tumor." The practice is unwise. Brain tumors are rare in children and rarely present with seizures. Brain tumors that cause seizures are likely to cause recurrent seizures, not just a single seizure. Therefore it is not necessary to do a scan at the time of the first event to diagnose a tumor. Since other lesions such as cysts, malformations, or developmental abnormalities will have been present for a long time, there is rarely any urgency in their diagnosis.

When imaging is needed, CT scans are cheaper and faster than MRIs but less revealing of subtle underlying changes. In a child who has recurrent focal seizures or a progressive or changing neurologic deficit, an MRI scan is preferable.

It therefore should again be emphasized that it is not necessary to image the brain after a first seizure. This may be equally true after recurrent seizures unless the events are clearly focal in origin or progressive in nature.

ELECTROENCEPHALOGRAPHY

An electroencephalogram (EEG) does not diagnose epilepsy nor does it rule out epilepsy. An EEG may be useful, however, in establishing whether the origin of a seizure is focal and what type of seizure it is, so that an appropriate medication can be chosen. However, since one is very unlikely to treat with medication after a first episode, the EEG does not need to be part of the initial evaluation. If the episodes recur, then an EEG may be useful. Although an abnormal EEG at the time of the first seizure does correlate with an increased chance of seizure recurrence, it is unclear that this is sufficient reason to perform one.

PROLONGED EEG MONITORING

It is now fashionable to perform prolonged (sometimes 24-h) EEG monitoring with portable equipment. The patient (or parent) pushes a button when an event is to be monitored. The machine also captures electrical seizures that are not noted by the parents. Such testing is rarely useful unless a child is having multiple events each day and when it is unclear whether those episodes are electrical in origin. Pseudo-seizures and other psychologically caused events (neuropsychophysiologic events in adolescents), cardiac arrhythmias, and fainting spells are among the events that may mimic seizures; their diagnosis can be aided by monitoring.

VIDEO-EEG MONITORING

During video-EEG monitoring, the child's EEG is constantly monitored while the child's activity is simultaneously captured on videotape. This is the only way to be certain that the clinical event is correlated with the electrical abnormality and to ascertain the cause or source of unclear events. The cost of such monitoring is several thousand dollars per day, and unless the child is having very frequent "spells" and has one during the monitoring, the money will be wasted.

Video monitoring at the time of the first event is unimportant because the management of both seizures and nonseizures will be the same. When focal seizures persist and surgery is contemplated, video-EEG monitoring and, at times, the actual placement of electrodes on the surface of the brain may be useful to record the location, determine the limits of the abnormal electrical activity, and locate—by stimulate various areas of brain function—those that may be critical to the accurate removal of the seizure focus and the preservation of normal functions. Such a "grid" (of electrodes) is commonly used at major epilepsy surgery centers.

Management of the Child and the Family After a First "Event"

After a first brief event from which the child has rapidly recovered, it is rarely necessary to admit the child to the hospital or to do extensive testing. A careful history and good physical and neurologic examinations are always indicated. They can (and should) be done by the primary physician and only rarely require a specialist. Instead, whether the event was accompanied by fever and thought to be a febrile seizure or occurred in the absence of fever and was thought to be an afebrile seizure, the management of the child and the family is identical: providing reassurance.

Reassurance of both the family and the child requires time and patience. The family should be helped to understand what a seizure is and what it is not. They should understand the chances of a recurrence and the consequences of such a recurrence. They should be told the risks and side effects of treatment with medication as well as the risks and benefits of nontreatment. It is not the physicians responsibility to tell the family what to do, but rather to help the family to make an intelligent, informed decision.*

For reasons that are not entirely clear, seizures are particularly frightening to parents, family, and observers as well as to health professionals. It is not just the acuteness or unexpectedness of the seizure, since there is not a similar reaction to a heart attack or even to choking. It may be the grotesqueness of the generalized tonic-clonic seizure, the scream at the start of many seizures, the thrashing and movements which accompany the seizure, the helplessness of the observers. There is fear that "the tongue may be swallowed," that the person may stop breathing, or that he or she is in the throes of dying—none of which are true. The ignorance of what to do or not to do may also be a major source of the fear of seizures. *The hardest thing to do during a seizure is nothing, but apart from preventing children from injuring themselves, there is nothing that can or need be done.* Most seizures last less than 5 min, which seems like infinity when one is watching helplessly, and they cease on their own. After the seizure, the patient returns to normal; the seizure will have been only a temporary interruption in the individual's life.

Management of Seizures

Febrile Seizures

Febrile seizures occur in 3 to 4 percent of all children; they are more common when there is family history of febrile seizures and in children over 6 months of age. Such seizures tend to be

outgrown within 2 years of the first event or by 6 years of age. Febrile seizures are the result of the combination of the low seizure threshold of the immature brain, the tendency of the young child to run higher fevers during illness, and the child's genetic seizure threshold. *Febrile seizures are benign! They do not cause death, injury, mental retardation, or cerebral palsy. The ONLY two consequences of a first febrile seizure are another febrile seizure (chance 30 percent) and an anxious parent (chance close to 100 percent).*

Febrile seizures do not cause epilepsy, but 2 percent of children with febrile seizures may go on to develop nonfebrile seizures. There is no evidence that treatment of febrile seizures prevents later epilepsy or that the febrile seizure was the cause of subsequent afebrile seizures.

The risks of recurrence and the factors that influence this risk are shown in Figure 16-2. The risk of recurrence of a febrile seizure is 25 percent within 1 year and 30 percent by 2 years. Children whose first seizure occurred with a

Figure 16-2

Overall Recurrence rate		1 year 25%	2 years 30%
Predictors of recurrence			
Duration of fever before first febrile seizure		*Age*	
< 1 h	44%	< 18 months	35%
1–24 h	23%	> 18 months	19%
> 24 h	13%		
		Height of fever	
Family history of febrile seizures	Yes 35% No 27%	> 38.3 > 40.3	35% 13%
A family history of febrile seizures, complex febrile seizures, or developmental abnormalities did not increase the risk of later epilepsy.			

Chance of recurrent febrile seizures. (Reproduced by permission from Berg AT, et al: *N Engl J Med* 327:1122–1127, 1992.)

---

*We have provided much of this information for parents in book form—Freeman JM, Vining EPG, Pillas DJ: *Seizures and Epilepsy: A Guide for Parents.* 2nd ed, Baltimore, Johns Hopkins University Press, 1997.

higher temperature or a fever of longer duration have a lower chance of recurrence. Younger children and those with a family history of febrile seizures have a higher chance of recurrence. A prolonged first febrile seizure did not increase the risk of recurrence but did increase the chance that any recurrence would be prolonged.

As noted, the chance of the child having later *afebrile* seizures (epilepsy) is also 2 percent. Risk factors associated with later epilepsy are shown in Fig. 16-3.

We do not recommend treating the child with prophylactic anticonvulsant medication after a first febrile seizure and rarely treat such a child even after a second febrile seizure because:

Febrile seizures are benign.
Even if febrile seizures recur, they remain benign.
Later epilepsy is not preventable by treatment of the febrile seizures.
All medications useful in preventing the recurrence of febrile seizures have side effects that are worse than the consequences of the seizures themselves.

If the first febrile seizure is prolonged, there is an increased chance that a second seizure may also may be prolonged. In such a case we

Figure 16-3

Risk factors:	
Seizure > 15 min	More than two seizures on same day
Family history of epilepsy	Neurologically suspect
Chance of recurrence:	
Without any febrile seizure	0.5%
With one febrile seizure	2.0%
With no risk factors	1.0%
With one risk factor	2.5%
With three risk factors	5–10%

Risk factors for later epilepsy after a first febrile seizure.

may give the parent a prescription for rectal diazepam gel (Diastat) to use if a second seizure occurs and lasts more than 10 to 20 min.

Parental anxiety is a clear consequence of a first febrile (or afebrile) seizure. This anxiety is best treated with reassurance of the parent rather than medication of the child. There is no evidence that having a parent keep rectal diazepam on hand, to use "in case the child has another of those awful things," either relieves parental anxiety or is of any benefit to the child.

Afebrile Seizures

Afebrile seizures are seizures that occur in the absence of fever. Since "epileptic" seizures may be precipitated by fever that lowers the child's seizure threshold, it may not be possible to initially distinguish between a febrile seizure and a seizure triggered by fever. Fortunately the distinction is unimportant, because the initial seizure is evaluated and managed identically. If the seizures recur without fever, the diagnosis then becomes obvious.

Febrile seizures are usually tonic or tonic-clonic in form. Afebrile seizures (epileptic seizures) come in far more varieties (see Fig. 16-1). Just as decision making after a first febrile seizure depends on knowing the natural history of febrile seizures, so does decision making after a first afebrile seizure call for a knowledge of their natural history.

NATURAL HISTORY

The natural history of generalized tonic-clonic seizures, of most focal seizures, and of most partial seizures with secondary generalization is shown in Fig. 16-4. After a first afebrile seizure, 60 percent of children will have no more *with or without treatment*. Although treatment after a first febrile seizure decreases the chance of a recurrence, it does not change probability of being seizure-free 1 or 2 years later (see Fig. 16-5). Indeed, more than half of seizures will not recur even without treatment.

Figure 16-4

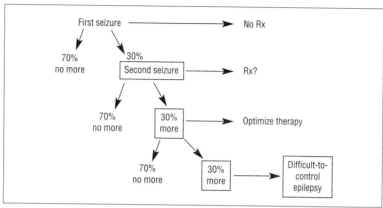

Management of seizures.

Figure 16-5

With immediate Rx: 24% recurrence	**With delayed Rx: 42% recurrence**
87% no seizures at 1 year	83% no seizures at 1 year
67% no seizures at 2 years	60% no seizures at 2 years

There is the same probability of being seizure-free with or without treatment.

More than 50% of first seizures will not recur.

Outcome after a *first* tonic-clonic seizure.

After a second afebrile seizure (now defined as epilepsy), some physicians would recommend starting medications, others would not. The decision should be made with the parents and depend on how long the second seizure occurred after the first, the age of the patient, the type of seizure, and other factors shown in Fig. 16-6.

Approximately 70 percent of generalized tonic-clonic and partial complex seizures will respond to the first anticonvulsant medication, properly used. It is unclear that one medication is more effective than another as the initial and sole treatment for seizures, The difference between many medications lies mainly in their side effects.

Figure 16-6

Risks	Risks will depend on:
Death	• Number of seizures
Injury	• Type of seizure
Anxiety	• Timing of seizures
Intellectual compromise	• Age of patient
Job loss, etc.	• Activities

Risks associated with seizures.

The first medication should be increased gradually until the seizures are controlled or toxicity is evident. When the first medication produces toxicity without controlling the seizures, a second should be added and gradually increased. If the seizures are controlled, the first medication may be gradually tapered.

If two medications have failed to control the child's seizures, there is only a 20 percent chance that any other medication will be effective. Approximately 20 percent of children with epilepsy will be difficult to control and should be referred to an epilepsy specialist. Some would say that all children failing one medication should have such a referral.

The choices for management for these children with difficult-to-control seizures are shown in Fig. 16-7, but a discussion of surgery and the ketogenic diet are beyond the scope of this chapter.*

Other Types of Seizures

Simple absence seizures (called *petit mal* in the past) usually recur many times before they are first recognized. They will continue to recur until treated. This is also true of partial complex seizures, atonic "drop" seizures, and the spasms of infantile spasms. Each of these seizure types requires treatment when they are recognized.

Figure 16-7

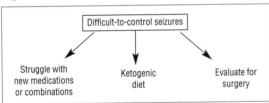

Management of difficult-to-control seizures.

*Further information on the ketogenic diet may be found in Freeman JM, Kelly M, Freeman JB: *The Epilepsy Diet Treatment: An Introduction to the Ketogenic Diet.* New York, Demos-Vermande Press, .

Anticonvulsant Medications

Many physicians rely heavily on drug levels to determine the optimal dosage of anticonvulsant medications. They are deceived. Levels cannot be relied upon to tell when the patient has sufficient medication. Sufficient medication is when the child no longer has seizures. Neither do levels tell when there is too much medication. Too much medication is when the child has behavioral side effects.

Blood levels taken at a trough (before the next dose, as many hours as possible after the last dose) confirm that the child is taking the medicine and is in the range where many children have their seizures controlled or many have side effects. *The proper dose of anticonvulsant medication is enough to control the seizures and not so much that the child has side effects.*

A full discussion of the various anticonvulsant medications is beyond the scope of this article. A brief word about a few of the major anticonvulsants follow:

Phenobarbital is one of the oldest, safest, and by far the cheapest of the medications and is effective for febrile seizures, generalized tonic-clonic seizures, and partial seizures with secondary generalization. Its sedative and behavioral effects make it less desirable than the other, but it is an effective drug.

Phenytoin (Dilantin) is one of the oldest and most effective anticonvulsants. In children, its side effects of gum hypertrophy and hirsutism make it less desirable than some of the newer medications.

Carbamazepine (Tegretol, Carbitrol, Tegretol X-R) is effective in partial complex seizures and generalized tonic-clonic seizures. It has few cosmetic or behavioral side effects and its hematologic side effects, while common, are rarely of clinical importance. The newer forms have slower absorption but are not clearly better than the parent compound.

Valproic Acid (Depakote, Depakene) is effective against cortical and partial seizures. Its wide spectrum and low incidence of side effects make this a useful drug. However, hepatotoxicity occurs in about 1 in 500 patients. The risk is higher in those who are neurologically impaired and on multiple medications.

Other drugs recently approved for marketing include:

Gabapentine (Neurontin) 1994
Lamotrigine (Lamictal) 1995
Tiagabine (Gabitril) 1997
Topiramate (Topamax) 1997
Vigabitrin (Sabril) 1999

The toxicities and the role of these medications in the management of new-onset seizures in children remain to be determined. At the moment, their role as second or third drugs in difficult-to-control seizures is being established. Until more information is available, they should rarely be prescribed by primary physicians.

Counseling the Family

All of life poses a series of risk-benefit analyses. The safest place to raise a child is in a padded cell. However, the consequences of such safety far outweigh the benefits. Children who swim may drown. To make swimming as safe as possible, no one should swim without a lifeguard present, whether or not they have seizures. Bicycle injuries are common, yet we continue to allow children to ride bikes if they wear helmets to minimize head injury.

Children with seizures have a greater risk of injury than those without seizures. The increase in risk is proportional to the frequency of the seizures, their type, the time of day they occur, and the amount of time the child spends in the specific activity (such as swimming). The physician should help the parents and the child to assess the importance of the activity and,

depending on the nature and severity of the epilepsy, should help them to assess the risks involved and the best way to minimize them. Again, the risks and the benefits accrue to the child and the family; therefore the decision about whether or not to participate in the activity belongs to them.

Perhaps the most important information the physician can provide to parents is what they should do if the child has another seizure. (See Fig. 16-8, which can be copied and given to parents.)

Regarding the use of anticonvulsant medication, *parents should be aware that if a child receives medication after the first seizure, there is still a 30 to 40 percent chance that another seizure will take place. If a child is not medicated, there is a 60 to 70 percent chance that*

Figure 16-8

> ### *During the seizure*
> Stay calm
> **Do *not*** put anything in a person's mouth
> **Do *not*** restrain the person.
> **Do *not*** call an ambulance unless the seizure continues for more than 5–10 min
> **Do** *try to place the person on his or her side.*
> **Do** *put something soft (coat, pillow) under the person's head.*
> **Do** *loosen tight clothing around the neck.*
> **Do** *remove sharp objects—chair, table, etc.—from the immediate area.*
>
> ### *After the seizure*
> Stay with the person until he or she is awake and alert.
> Be comforting and reassuring.
> Allow the person to go back to his or her activities upon full recovery.

What to do for a person having a major seizure. (Adapted by permission from Freeman JM, Vining EPG, Pillas DJ: *Seizures and Epilepsy: A Guide for Parents*, 2nd ed. Baltimore, Johns Hopkins University Press, 1997.)

there will never be a second seizure. Since the chance of recurrence is the same, there is no clear reason to start medication after a first event.

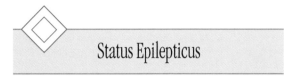

Status Epilepticus

Status epilepticus has been defined as *"a seizure [that] persists for a sufficient length of time or is repeated frequently enough that recovery between attacks does not occur."* Seizures are difficult to watch without intervention, and the observer-parent, bystander, and medical personnel all feel helpless. Once it was thought, based on animal studies, that a generalized seizure lasting longer than 30 min could produce changes in the neurons that might result in neuronal loss. Therefore, status epilepticus was defined as a "seizure lasting more than 30 minutes" and considered as a medical emergency requiring urgent treatment to prevent death or permanent neurologic dysfunction. Although recent studies use different definitions, (e.g., "a seizure lasting > 20 minutes," "a seizure lasting > 10 minutes," "or a seizure in a child older than 5 years lasting > 5 minutes"), there is little scientific basis for any of these new definitions and no evidence of permanent sequelae after such a seizure. Most seizures terminate on their own, in less than 5 min.

Studies have shown that in children, the consequences of prolonged seizures are related to their cause rather than to their duration. Children who have generalized tonic-clonic seizures lasting more than 30 min suffer no residua if the seizures were triggered by fever (febrile seizures) or were due to drug withdrawal. Prolonged seizures due to infections, trauma, anoxia, etc., were more likely to result in neurologic deficits. The deficits were due to the underlying process, not to the seizures per se.

Prolonged seizures (status epilepticus) are often undertreated, overtreated, or maltreated. During a prolonged generalized tonic-clonic seizure, the child should be placed on its side with the head on a soft surface. *Nothing* hard (such as a spoon) should be placed in the mouth, although a soft material such as a sleeve or handkerchief may minimize biting of the tongue. As noted, most tonic-clonic seizures will end on their own in less than 5 min, with a gradual slowing of the clonic movements and then a large expiratory sigh. While mild cyanosis often accompanies such a seizure, there is no evidence that that the degree of hypoxia is associated with any significant cerebral hypoxia. The cyanosis is more related to interference with chest movement due to the seizure rather than to an inability to breathe; therefore it does not require or respond to mouth-to-mouth resuscitation. It is generally believed that before the brain becomes sufficiently hypoxic to result in permanent damage, the seizure, which requires oxygen for continued cell firing, will stop on its own.

If the seizure lasts more than 5 to 10 min (by the clock), I suggest that the family use the appropriate dose of rectal diazepam (if they have it). If the seizure persists 10 min after the rectal diazepam is administered, I usually suggest that they call 911 for the help of emergency services (EMS). If no diazepam is available, *and* the generalized tonic-clonic seizure has lasted more than 10 min, by the clock, then 911 may be called. If, on average, it takes almost 10 min for EMS to arrive and another 10 min for them to prepare the patient and get to the local emergency department, 20–30 min will have passed. At that point emergency treatment should begin by protecting the airway and using intravenous medications.

Calling 911 and EMS represents a mixed blessing, since most seizures will stop on their own either before the ambulance arrives or before the child is transported to an emergency department. Often, calling 911 initiates a cascade of events that may be worse than waiting for the seizure to end on its own. The EMS technicians may or may not administer diazepam intravenously to stop the seizure (if it is still ongoing). The child is then taken to the emergency department and arrives either after the seizure or having been depressed by the medication, in which case oxygen saturation may be lowered. To assure adequate oxygenation, the child is thought to require intubation but may be too alert to permit this. He or she is then paralyzed to enable intubation and then must be admitted to the intensive care unit overnight. The next morning the child is extubated. If, as is usual, the child is then well, he or she is discharged unless—as a consequence of intubation—stridor has developed. This cascade of events is sufficiently common that one wonders whether calling for assistance shortly after the start of a recurrent seizure does not result in more problems that it prevents.

If a tonic-clonic seizure is prolonged, the treatment is intravenous anticonvulsants. After assuring that the blood sugar and electrolytes are adequate, intravenous diazepam (or lorazepam) is administered. Diazepam (Valium) is a rapid-acting anticonvulsant that—unfortunately—(25 to 20 min) rapidly redistributes in body fat and does not retain adequate brain levels. Therefore it must be followed by a longer-acting anticonvulsant such as lorazepam (Ativan), which has a longer half-life. Intravenous phenytoin (or phosphenytoin) and intravenous barbiturates have also been used following diazepam. Some of the newer anticonvulsants have recently become available in intravenous form. Because it has less toxic local effects than intravenous phenytoin, phospheny-toin is especially useful in children divalproex (Depakote) and carlamazepine (Tegretol) are among the newer agents whose place in the management of status epilepticus remains to be established.

Suggested Reading

Freeman JM, Vining EPG: Decision making and the child with afebrile seizures. *Pediatr Rev* 13:305–311, 1992.

Freeman JM, Vining EPG: Decision making and the child with febrile seizures. *Pediatr Rev* 13:298–304, 1992.

Freeman JM, Holmes G: Should Uncomplicated Seizures in Children be Treated?: Point-Counterpoint. *Curr Probl Pediatr* 24:129–156, 1994.

Freeman JM, Vining EPG: Febrile Seizures: A Decision-Making Analysis. *Am Fam Physician* 52:1406, 1995.

Freeman JM: Status epilepticus: It's not what we've thought or taught. *Pediatrics* (Editorial) 83:444–445, 1989.

Freeman JM: Just say no!—Drugs and febrile seizures. *Pediatrics* (Editorial) 86:624, 1990.

Books

Freeman JM, Vining EPG, Pillas DJ: *Seizures and Epilepsy in Childhood: A Guide for Parents.* Baltimore, Johns Hopkins University Press, 1990; 2nd Ed. 1997.

Freeman JM, Kelly MT, Freeman JB: *The Epilepsy Diet Treatment: An Introduction to the Ketogenic Diet.* New York, Demos Press, 1994; 2nd Ed. 1996.

Freeman JM, McDonnell K: *Tough Decisions: A Casebook in Medical Ethics.* New York, Oxford University Press, 1987.

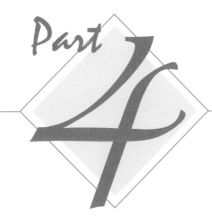

Part 4

Developmental/
Behavioral
Problems

Saul Greenberg

Behavioral Problems

All children display a wide variety of behaviors that concern or upset parents at some time or another. One study showed that 8 percent of preschool children in England were judged to be "behavior problems" by health professionals and parents. Another study in middle-class American families showed that 18 percent of children (up to 5 years of age) were diagnosed as having a behavioral disturbance considered severe enough to warrant intervention. These included problems such as bedtime resistance, food refusal, resistance to toilet training, temper tantrums, aggression, shyness, hyperac-

tivity, and undesirable habits such as thumb sucking.

Individual behavioral symptoms are very common in young children, but whether such behavior is labeled problematic depends on its type, frequency, duration, and severity. One chapter is insufficient to discuss all childhood behavioral problems; many books have been written on the subject. This chapter focuses on several common behavioral and temperamental problems: shyness, aggressiveness, conduct and oppositional defiant disorders, the spoiled child, and food refusal.

Food Refusal

The commonest behavioral complaint that physicians hear from parents is that their child is not eating enough. Some 85 percent of children are rated as being picky eaters. Parents often measure an infant's well-being by his or her weight gain; therefore the amount of weight a child gains becomes, in the parents' minds, an important measure of their success. Although obesity affects between 5 and 25 percent of children and teenagers in the United States, many parents are more concerned that their thin child may be malnourished. This parental anxiety leads some parents to offer the child snacks throughout the day and others to awaken their child with food during the night. Some parents cook special meals for their children, while others will force a child to sit in the high chair or at the table for a long period of time after the meal has ended. This struggle over food often meets considerable resistance from children, and soon mealtime becomes a nightmare.

Causes of Food Refusal

Children gain about 15 lb during the first year of life but only gain 4 or 5 lb per year between the ages of 1 and 5 years. This normal slowdown in growth results in a reduced need for calories and a normal decline in appetite. At the same time the infant becomes more interested in the environment and is often distracted from feeding by the surrounding world. At this point children become more independent and also want to feed themselves. Parents fear that decreased eating might cause poor health or nutritional deficiencies. They may then force the child to eat, which decreases the normal pleasure of eating and actually reduces the child's appetite.

Children's heights often fall off in the first 2 to 3 years as they track lower to their eventual height percentile, corresponding to their parents' height. Once they get to the new growth channel, they continue to grow along it at a normal rate. A similar decline in weight percentiles also accompanies this "catch-down" growth. Some parents feel that the slowing of a child's gain in height and weight is due to inadequate food intake, although the child never appears to be underweight during this gradual shift.

Although this normal appetite slump in toddlers is the most common cause of food refusal, there are some pediatric disorders that can lead to the same result. These include:

Anatomic problems—cleft palate, tracheoesophageal fistula

Gastrointestinal problems—gastroesophageal reflux and esophagitis, celiac disease

Metabolic problems—renal tubular acidosis, inborn errors of metabolism

Neurologic problems—cerebral palsy, familial dysautonomia

Genetic problems—Down syndrome

Systemic problems—cardiac or pulmonary disease

Infection—urinary tract infection, acute viral infections

Treatment of Food Refusal

REASSURE PARENTS ABOUT GROWTH AND NUTRITION

GROWTH CURVES   Parents may be reassured by a demonstration that their child is plotting normally for height and weight on a growth chart. The child who is growing normally is getting enough nutrients.

NUTRITIONAL REQUIREMENTS   Full nutrition does not have to happen at every meal. It occurs over many months, and a child cannot become malnourished between breakfast and bedtime. Parents should not worry if a child eats very little at a meal or even skips that meal.

There is no one food that is essential for good nutrition. Meat is a good source of protein, but the protein in milk, fish, or eggs is just as good. Even cereal and grains can provide adequate protein if they are taken in the right mix.

PROTEIN   Protein is essential for cell growth and repair. However, the average American diet has 20 percent of its calories from protein, although only 7 percent is sufficient to prevent protein malnutrition. A high-protein diet also tends to be high in fat, and the traditional American diet derives 30 percent or more of its calories from fat.

VEGETABLES   Many children dislike vegetables, but vegetables should be encouraged because of their vitamin content and their ability to prevent cancer and heart disease. However, many of the nutritional ingredients and fiber of vegetables can be found in other foods, such as fruits, grains, and cereals. Parents do not have to share this information with young children, but they can worry less about their children who dislike vegetables.

"JUNK FOODS"   Some foods that are usually thought of as junk food can still provide children with basic nutrients. Hot dogs and hamburgers may be high in fat and salt and should not be eaten daily, but they do provide protein. Pizza also provides essential protein and fat in the cheese and carbohydrates in the crust; it certainly provides a way of sneaking in vegetables, in the toppings.

Improving Poor Appetites

1. Let the child decide how much to eat. Children have a great innate ability to know when they need food and when they do not. Parents need to respect a child's internal hunger clock. When a child says "I'm hungry" an hour before dinner, offer food, even if it means giving an appetizer course, like raw vegetables,

that might be part of dinner anyway. Do not insist that the child empty the bottle, finish a jar of baby food, or clean the plate. Children often make up for a small meal or a missed meal at the next mealtime. A parent's responsibility is to provide the variety of foods children need and then allow them to obey their internal clock and eat as much or little as they want.

2. Let children feed themselves.   Parents have a tendency to pick up a fork or spoon loaded with food and try to coerce the child to take it. Teach children to feed themselves from as early an age as possible. Infants at 6 to 8 months of age can start on finger foods; at 12 months of age, they can start to use a spoon. When children are hungry, they will feed themselves.

3. Respect food dislikes.   All children have a few food dislikes. Usually parents are concerned that their child is missing some essential food or ingredient, especially vegetables. There are no essential foods, just essential food groups. If a child has strong food dislikes (e.g., causing gagging), he or she should not be served them. Food is not medicine. For other minor food dislikes, a child can be asked to taste each food.

Even if a child's variety of foods is limited, one can build a child's diet around his or her favorite good foods. A child should be allowed to explore new foods independently; they should be offered in small amounts and with minimal insistence.

4. Do not bribe or force a child to eat. Threats or punishments are not good ideas either. Hard as it may seem to do, parents should try not show that they are upset by a refusal to eat. If a child is seeking attention, he or she may get it from a parent's show of disapproval. Bribes or rewards should not be given for meeting a parent's eating expectations. Occasionally a child can be praised for trying new foods that he or she normally dislikes.

5. Limit snacks to two per day.   If a child eats most of a meal, one can offer a small-sized nutritious snack, such as fruits or vegetables, a few hours later. If the child skips most of the meal, the next snack can be canceled. A snack should be provided only if a child requests it; if the meal is several hours away, a bigger snack can be offered. Some children do well on only two meals a day and no snacks. Do not offer a child treats instead of food out of fear that the child will otherwise starve. The child will just continue to refuse food until he or she obtains the desired treats. A sweet treat can be offered on occasion, since never letting a child have a sweet gives too much significance to those foods; this can cause problems later on.

6. Limit juice and milk intake. Drinking too many fluids can fill kids up and suppress their appetites. Milk contains as many calories as many solid foods, and excessive drinking of juice may lead to obesity later on. Restricting children's intake of fluids, except for water, will increase their appetite.

7. Serve small portions of food. Being served more food than he could possibly eat often turns off a child's appetite. A good rule of thumb is to offer 1 tbsp of each kind of food for each year of age. Children are more likely to finish a small amount of food, and if they are still hungry, more can be offered.

8. Set regular mealtimes. Give children a warning 10 or 15 min before mealtime, allowing them to settle down from activities before eating. If possible, set regular mealtimes. Playing with toys, reading books, or watching television should not be allowed during mealtimes.

9. Make mealtimes pleasant. Try to avoid arguments during mealtime and try to talk about things that you know interest the child. Do not discuss how little children eat in their presence and do not praise them for eating a lot. Children should eat to please themselves. Do not make a child sit at the dinner table after the rest of the family has finished eating. If a parent creates a pleasant, stress-free environment for eating and provides a variety of nutritious foods, which regularly include a child's favorites, some of the food struggles may diminish.

Shyness and Aggressiveness

A child may behave shyly or aggressively in certain situations. The way any child reacts to unfamiliar situations is largely affected by his or her inborn temperament or personality.

After the age of 2 years, when children start to interact with other children, it becomes easier to see a trend toward shyness or aggressiveness. Neither of these should be considered a problem unless it clearly and repeatedly causes the behavior that interferes with the child's life and prevents effective problem solving. It is unlikely that any major problem will result from a child's inherent shyness or aggression before the age of 6 years. With preschoolers, one can intervene by giving a shy child a small push or gently restraining an aggressive child.

After the age of 6 years, a child's shyness or aggressiveness can be more of a problem. At this age, antisocial behavior may be accompanied by some of the features of other, more extreme behavior disorders, such as conduct and oppositional defiant behaviors, and/or attention-deficit disorder with hyperactivity.

Parents cannot expect to change a child's fundamental predisposition to shyness or aggressiveness, but they may be able to change the manner in which the child handles difficult situations.

The Shy Child

Shy children often avoid others and are usually timid, easily frightened, bashful, reserved, and hesitant to commit themselves to things. In social situations they are often silent, speak softly, and do not take the initiative. A shy child under the age of 6 may regularly be bossed by other children or cling to parents, fail to make eye contact, or refuse to come downstairs when company visits. Periods of shyness are normal at

5 or 6 months of age and again at 2 years. However, signs of a child being exceedingly shy include any of the following symptoms lasting more than 2 months.

Repeated refusal to participate with peers
Repeated incidents of being victimized by other children
Preference for being left alone
Excessive clinging to parents
Persistent fearfulness or depression

CAUSES OF SHYNESS

1. Temperament or physical handicaps. Many children appear to be shy almost from birth, and this constitutional shyness may continue for the rest of their lives.

2. Physical handicaps. Any physical difference may cause shyness as children avoid situations in which they are made to feel uncomfortable.

3. Parental Causes. Shy parents often produce shy children (i.e., a tendency to shyness may be inherited). Shyness may also occur in children who are overprotected by their parents or, conversely, overly criticized by them. Children who are threatened frequently with punishment may react with fear and timidity. Children who are frequently teased by parents or siblings may become shy and avoid social contact to avoid ridicule.

4. Lack of self-confidence. Children who feel insecure lack self-confidence. They are preoccupied with feeling safe and not getting hurt and therefore do not develop social skills.

TREATMENT OF SHYNESS

1. Parents can act as a model for outgoing behavior. A child should see his or her parents standing up for their rights when it is necessary, taking social risks, or taking the initiative in difficult situations. When children observe their parents starting conversations, making eye contact, touching, and staying close to people, they will have an example to follow. Parents should give their child examples of how they have overcome their shyness in various situations. For example, parents can discuss how they introduce themselves to a stranger at a party or interact with salespeople or officials.

2. Focus attention on specific behaviors, not overall behavior. Shyness should be considered a set of behaviors that can be tackled individually. One should focus attention on each situation as it happens and not on the child's personality. Parents *should not* call their child shy. They should talk only about a given situation. Blame should never be assigned to shy behavior.

3. Reinforce outgoing behavior. Parents should be encouraged to praise their child's efforts at being more independent and more assertive. They should point out how much they admire acts of self-confidence. For example, when a child says hello to someone, encourage his or her behavior by saying, "You spoke to Mr. Smith very nicely. I liked the way you said, 'It was nice to meet you, Mr. Smith.'" Have the child's teacher help as well, rewarding behavior such as answering questions or raising a hand to volunteer information.

4. Practice social skills and situations. Rehearsing situations that a child finds stressful is helpful. For example a parent should go over every step in meeting a new person, including the introductions and appropriate things to say. Teach the words and techniques to enable a child to enter other children's play. "Can I help you do that?" or "I want to play too. Which team should I join?"

5. Practice ways of handling rejection. If a child is rejected by a friend, practice ways of coping with the rejection. For example, explain to the child when he or she is rejected by a social clique that children who know each other often stick together and do not accept newcomers easily. "It doesn't mean that they don't like you or that you are a bad kid." Remind children of previous successes in social interactions.

6. Ease a child into difficult situations. Children behaving in a shy manner need to be taught how to overcome their lack of self-confidence and fear of rejection. If a child is likely to be shy in a certain situation, one should try subtly to make it less threatening. Arrange an entrance into the situation at a good time and let the child acclimatize before leaving him or her alone. Try to smooth the path but avoid either forcing or coddling. Pushing a child into a situation does not teach the child how to be outgoing, and a child who is ridiculed or ignored will feel rejected.

7. Provide appropriate activities for a child to make friends. Many shy children feel overwhelmed in large groups. Therefore, provide one-on-one or smaller group activities. Pair shy children with younger playmates who are less threatening. Organize special activities in which each child takes a turn, or provide large objects that require cooperation, such as seesaws.

The Aggressive Child

Aggression can be defined as behavior that results in personal injury, psychological or physical, to someone else. For example, an aggressive child under the age of 6 may boss, tease, hit other children and make them cry, or disturb everyone at a social gathering by demanding constant attention. Aggression is commonly triggered by situations in which a child wants something another child has. Some preschool children even attack their parents physically over conflicts about feeding, bedtime, or the denial of something the child wants. Temper tantrums may occur frequently. The aggressive child tends to be impulsive, immature, action-oriented, and inarticulate about feelings. Over-aggressiveness may persist and is present in about about 1 percent of 10 year olds.

CAUSES OF AGGRESSIVENESS

Some believe that aggression is part of a child's inherent temperament, while others feel that young children learn aggressive habits by following examples set by parents, sibs, and peers. Faulty child-rearing practices—such as a combination of lax discipline and hostile attitudes by parents—can produce aggressive and poorly controlled children. Competition, exposure to TV violence, marital strife, and a parent who is absent from home for extended periods are other factors believed to foster aggression.

TREATMENT OF AGGRESSIVENESS

1. Disapprove of specific behaviors, not the child. When correcting a child's aggression, direct remarks at the situation, not the child. Children become angry or resentful if they feel they are being personally criticized.

2. Praise self-control and good behavior and ignore bad behavior. The most direct way to encourage a child to get along with others is to praise him or her for doing so. Use a reward system, such as a star chart or tokens that can be traded in later for concrete rewards. Rewarding good behavior should be combined with ignoring aggressive acts that do not pose a threat to the physical safety of others. By paying attention to fighting or teasing, a parent may inadvertently reinforce this behavior. While ignoring the aggression, give a great deal of attention and show concern and empathy to the *injured* party.

3. Set a good example of fairness and self-control. Children will be influenced by the parents' display of respect for the rights of others. If, for example, parents argue and belittle one another, it is likely children will relate in a similar manner.

4. Teach social skills and rules about the treatment of others. A child should be taught that other people have rights and needs that must be respected. This should be done shortly after a child has ignored or violated someone else's rights. Apart from direct discussion, one way of doing this is through role-playing. Children should be taught how to "talk it out" rather than "fight it out." Give a child a list of things to do besides hitting when he or she feels upset, such as saying "I'm not playing anymore" and leaving the group.

5. Anticipate problem situations. Aggressive children often act before they think. If a child tends to be aggressive in certain situations, a parent should take a few moments to discuss how he or she would like things to go. Teach some aggression-inhibiting sentences the child can use when angry, such as, "Count to ten" or "Talk, don't hit."

6. Intervene when the child abuses another child's rights. Point out what is fair in a given situation, gain everyone's commitment to play fair, and then withdraw. Try not to be punitive, but become involved when a situation seems to be getting totally out of hand.

7. Monitor the child's television viewing. Many studies have shown that television has an influence on the put-downs and aggressive behavior that children use with each other. One study showed that heavy viewers of TV, espe-cially of action adventures and cartoons, were more aggressive and less cooperative with their playmates. After watching even a brief episode of TV violence, children may act out in more aggressive or hurtful ways. Be aware of what a child watches and be prepared to say no.

8. Punishment and discipline. With younger children, a very effective form of punishment for aggression is the use of "time out," whereby a child is isolated from ongoing activity and sent to his or her room or required to sit on a chair for a specified period of time (Table 17-1).

Time out is an effective way of stopping bad behaviour because it removes the child from any likelihood of receiving reinforcement (such as verbal attention or physical contact) or getting any benefits from the inappropriate behavior during the time-out period. If time out is not feasible, a parent might take away privileges or have the child apologize to the injured party. Physical punishment should be avoided, since it

Table 17-1

Time Out

Time out serves to stop misbehavior, convey disapproval, give both parties an opportunity to regain their composure, and decrease the likelihood of repeated misbehavior. Just as attention is the most powerful positive feedback for a child, removal of attention is the most effective negative consequence. For time out to be effective:

1. Introduce time out by 18 to 24 months of age.
2. Only two to three priority behaviors should result in time out, especially those that involve aggression toward people or things.
3. Only one warning should be given; no warnings for aggressive behavior.
4. A brief statement of the offense should be given.
5. Time out should be in a noninteresting but nonfrightening place. Be sure the time-out place does not have built-in rewards, such as a room containing toys or a TV set. One may have the child sit in a chair near the parent.
6. If the child leaves the chair, he or she should be returned to it without talking and restrained if necessary. One may have to return a child to his or her room and hold the doorknob.
7. Limit time out to 1 min for each year of the child's age, to a maximum of 10 min measured with a timer that the child can hear. The timer may be reset until the full time has been served out in silence.
8. Keep time out quiet. This is not a time for teaching, preaching, or discussing the offense.
9. Clear the air afterwards. Do not dwell on the offense, and comfort the child if necessary.

often generates hostility and humiliation in the child and provides an example of the use of aggression at the very time a parent is trying to teach a child to be nonaggressive.

Conduct Disorders

Many young children are disobedient and at times destructive. In preschool children, conduct problems are most commonly manifest by aggressive behavior. In middle childhood, aggressive behavior is still the most common form of antisocial activity, but there may also be episodes of stealing, lying, and fire setting. In adolescence, antisocial activity is manifest by physical aggression, breaking into property and stealing, truancy, drug use, and sexual offenses. In the normal child, these behaviors are isolated, short-lived, mild, and inclined to decrease in frequency with age. In children with conduct disorders, such behavior occurs with greater severity, frequency, and pervasiveness over a variety of settings. The terms *conduct disorder* and *antisocial behavior* are often used synonymously.

The specific behavioural criteria for the diagnosis of conduct disorders are found in Table 17-2.

Conduct Disorders in Older Children

Conduct disorder is one of the most prevalent psychopathologic condition of childhood. In a survey of British children aged 10 and 11, conduct disorders were diagnosed in 6 percent of the boys and 1.6 percent of the girls. In Ontario, Canada, about 5 percent of boys and 2 percent of girls were rated by teachers to show conduct disorders.

Associated Conditions

Children and adolescents with conduct disorders have a higher rate of depression, as well as learning and attentional problems, than other children. They often have specific learning disabilities, particularly reading disorders. However, not all children with learning disabilities have conduct disorders. In spite of normal intelligence, some children with conduct disorders have deficits in language development and problem-solving skills. Poor school performance can lead to low self- esteem and truancy.

Up to 75 percent of these children also have increased activity levels symptomatic of attention deficit–hyperactivity disorder (ADHD). Children with both conduct disorder and ADHD tend to be more aggressive and show a greater variety and severity of antisocial behavior than children with conduct disorders alone. Children with both disorders are at high risk for persistence of antisocial behavior into adulthood.

Causes of Conduct Disorders

The causes are the same as those of aggression in the younger child. There is strong evidence for a genetic influence on the development of conduct disorders. There is a higher-than-expected incidence among children of male and female criminals as well as among identical twins. Family risk factors—such as marital discord and divorce, alcoholism, and psychiatric impairment—are known to be associated with antisocial behavior in children. A child whose friends show antisocial behavior is more likely to become involved in this behavior as well.

Identification of Conduct Disorders

It is possible that early identification of aggression and other warning signs of conduct disorder may allow these children to be treated successfully. The early signs associated with the development of conduct disorder include:

Aggressive behavior
Reports that the child is difficult to control
Hyperactivity

Table 17-2
Criteria for Conduct Disorder

A. A negative and persistent pattern of behavior in which the basic rights of others or age-appropriate societal norms or rules are violated as manifested by the presence of three or more of the following criteria in the past 12 months, with at least one criterion present in the past 6 months:

Aggression to people and animals
1. Often bullies, threatens, or intimidates others
2. Often initiates physical fights
3. Has used a weapon that can cause serious physical harm to others (e.g., a bat, brick, knife, gun)
4. Has been physically cruel to people
5. Has been physically cruel to animals
6. Has stolen while confronting a victim (e.g., mugging, purse snatching)
7. Has forced someone into sexual activity

Destruction of property
1. Has deliberately engaged in fire setting
2. Has deliberately destroyed other's property (other than by fire setting)

Deceitfulness or theft
1. Has broken into someone else's house, building, or car
2. Often lies to obtain goods or favors or to avoid obligations
3. Has stolen items of nontrivial value without confrontation of a victim (including forgery, shoplifting)

Serious violations of others
1. Often stays out at night despite parental prohibitions, beginning before age 13 years
2. Has run away from home overnight at least twice while living in parental or parental surrogate home (or once without returning)
3. Has often been truant from school beginning before age 13 years

B. The disturbance in behavior causes clinically significant impairment in social, academic, or occupational functioning.

SOURCE: American Psychiatric Association: *Diagnostic and Statistical Manual of Mental Disorders*, 4th ed. Washington, DC, APA, 1994.

Oppositional behavior (see below) after age 3
Poor relationships with siblings, including physical aggression, hostility, yelling, and teasing

The more severe the disorder is at 3 years of age, the greater the likelihood that it will persist to 8 years of age. If high-risk children are identified, intervention programs may prevent future behavioral problems. These programs should be aimed at helping the child develop social skills, self-control, and self-esteem. Parent programs should be aimed at improving parenting skills and decreasing marital discord.

Treatment of Conduct Disorders

A family physician or pediatrician may be able to counsel the family, but referral to a psychologist or psychiatrist for treatment is appropriate if the behavior is extreme, unremitting, or violent, the child's daily functioning is significantly impaired, or the family cannot manage the child. The goal of treatment is to help the child comply with age-appropriate rules and decrease the frequency of aggressive behavior.

One of the most effective and best-studied approaches to managing the child with a conduct disorder is training the parents to handle the behavior as outlined above, in the discussion headed "The Aggressive Child." During therapy sessions, these skills may be learned and then practiced at home. An alternative treatment is cognitive therapy, in which the child or adolescent is taught problem-solving skills to be used in instances that previously might have elicited aggressive behavior. Family therapy has also been used to establish clear communication and develop mutual negotiating skills; it may allow the simultaneous treatment of family problems that often accompany the conduct disorder. As well, parents may be advised to improve family relationships, channel the child's energies into positive directions, and improve the child's self-esteem. Marital counseling may also be indicated for the parents.

Medication plays only a small part in the management of these children. Carbamazepine and clonidine have been used in children whose aggressive outbursts take the form of frequent "blind rages," and methylphinidate has been used when ADHD is present. Children with concomitant depression may be candidates for treatment with antidepressant medication.

Prognosis and Outcome

In general, children whose antisocial behavior is limited to minor delinquent acts and whose relationships with other children are positive do reasonably well. However those who have severe antisocial problems and get on poorly with others do not. Long-term studies indicate that 75 percent of these children continue to show antisocial behavior as adolescents and 40 percent to 50 percent have significant problems as adults. These problems include:

Alcoholism and drug abuse
Increased rate of divorce, separation, and remarriage
Criminality
Increased school dropout rate

Increased unemployment
Psychiatric problems, including neuroses and schizophrenia

Other factors that predict problems in adulthood include serious and frequent antisocial behavior, problems in the community as well as at home and school, and any trouble involving the police.

Oppositional Defiant Disorder

Oppositional defiant disorder is a term often used with reference to younger children. The disorder involves negativism and hostility, but, unlike conduct disorders, does not involve the violation of societal norms. It is characterized by stubbornness, tantrums, disobedience, and defiance of authority. This behavior reaches a peak during the "terrible twos" and usually decreases afterwards. Negativism becomes prominent again during the adolescent years. About one-third of the problem behaviors exhibited by children are related to noncompliance. If disobedience becomes a way of life for a child, he or she may be said to have an oppositional or defiant disorder as defined in Table 17-3.

Causes of the Oppositional Defiance in a Child

The degree to which environmental factors contribute produce an oppositional defiant child is unknown. However lax discipline by permissive parents or unduly harsh, restrictive, or inconsistent discipline may lead to persistent noncompliance in children. Parents who are in stress or conflict or who show little regard toward the law will influence a child's proneness to obey. A

Table 17-3

Criteria for Oppositional/Defiant Disorder

A criterion is met only if the behavior is considerably more frequent than that of most people of the same mental age.

A pattern of negativistic, hostile, and defiant behavior lasting at least 6 months during which four or more of the following are present:

1. Often loses temper
2. Often argues with adults
3. Often actively defies or refuses adult requests or rules; e.g., refuses to do chores at home
4. Often deliberately does things that annoy other people; e.g., grabs other children's hats
5. Often blames others for his or her or her mistakes or misbehaviors
6. Often is touchy or easily annoyed by others
7. Often is angry and resentful
8. Often is spiteful or vindictive

SOURCE: American Psychiatric Association: *Diagnostic and Statistical Manual of Mental Disorders*, 4th ed. Washington, DC, APA, 1994.

very creative or strong-willed child will tend to be more stubborn and a child who is tired, ill, or hungry will also be less likely to obey.

Treatment of the Defiant Child

1. Offer choices. To prevent power struggles between parent and child, allow children to maintain power over a situation by offering them choices, with consequences for each choice they make (e.g., "Do you want to brush your teeth before or after you wash your face?"). This allows the child to learn to solve problems, make decisions, and become more independent.

2. Compromise—parent and child. A child must be taught that when two people cannot agree, a compromise will allow both to give up a little and still have at least some of what they want. Parents should also try to alter their position from a demand to a compromise. Use requests and suggestions rather than direct orders. A child who has advance warning, rather than being expected to obey immediately, is more likely to cooperate.

3. Reward compromise. Praise the child when he or she is willing to reach a compromise or comply with your demand. In addition, use a reward system, such as gold stars on a calendar or coupons to be traded in for future privileges or treats.

4. Ignore minor defiance and avoid threats and power struggles. Parental attention, even negative attention such as scolding, can reinforce a child's misbehavior. Threats are often difficult to carry out, and children soon learn to ignore them. Ignore minor defiance and try to avoid head-to-head combat; instead, teach a child ways to cooperate. It is sometimes necessary to back off from confrontations and delay decisions when both parties are angry.

5. Setting and enforcing rules. In making a rule, tell the child exactly what to do and when it should be done. Instead of saying, "Clean up your room," say "Pick up your toys and make your bed." When a parent explains the reason for a rule, children are more willing to comply. Make fewer rules, so that they can be remembered and enforced. State rules in a positive way; that is, tell the child what to do rather than what not to do. Say, "Please use your knife and fork," rather than "Don't eat with your fingers." Rules should be enforced consistently or children will test them at every opportunity. Impose reasonable penalties if rules are not followed and avoid excessively harsh punishments, such as yelling or spanking. For the adolescent, a contract that outlines what he or she will do and what a parent will do in return may strengthen the teen's commitment to behave acceptably.

6. Strengthen your relationship with the child. A child will be more likely to accept a parent's discipline if there is a close relationship with abundant affection between parent and child. Try to show plenty of love and affection and spend lots of time with him or her. Allow a child to exhibit some signs of rebellion and win some disagreements that are not crucial, such as a teen choosing his or her clothes and hairstyle.

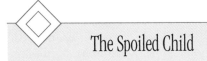

The Spoiled Child

Spoiled children are those who get their way too often, are given too much, have too many things done for them, or want too much attention. Generally, spoiled children are undisciplined, manipulative, and unpleasant to be with. They often do not cooperate with suggestions. They also try to control other people and do not respect other people's rights. Other children do not like them because they are too bossy and selfish. Adults do not like them because they are rude and whiny and make excessive demands.

Most psychologists feel that one cannot spoil a young infant. A new baby needs to have all its needs responded to promptly and gently in order to feel secure and loved. Parents who respond promptly to their baby's crying or hold their baby do not produce a spoiled infant or child. Giving attention to children is also good

for them as long as it is not excessive, given at the wrong time, or always given immediately. Children do not usually cry of fuss deliberately to get something before 5 to 6 months of age. As children get older, however, it will become possible to spoil them.

Causes of Spoiling

Many parents cannot bear to see their children sad or disappointed in any way, so they give them everything they ask or plead for. Children become spoiled when their parents are overly permissive and lenient without setting limits, and when they give in to tantrums and whining.

1. Feelings of guilt. Many working and divorced parents feel guilty that they do not spend enough time with their children. As a result, they tend to avoid setting limits or doing anything that might make the child unhappy.

2. Overindulgence. Overindulgent parents often entertain their children and meet all their needs and wishes even before being asked. This deprives children of the opportunity to think for themselves, make decisions, and develop their own needs and preferences. Overindulged children never have to work for anything or take the initiative to get things for themselves. These children believe that life will provide for them without their own effort and, when grown up, will expect everyone to read their minds and provide for them. For children to grow into successful social beings, they must learn that other people have needs and that those needs count. Children need to learn that there are firm and consistent limits and that they will not be allowed to take advantage of other people.

3. Oversubmissiveness. Oversubmissive parents give into their children's demands, often because they fear the children will not love them. These children learn that whining will give them what they want, and if that does not work, a temper tantrum often will. Always placating children has negative consequences in the long run. It can create unrealistic expectations about getting their own way and it keeps children from being able to acquire the necessary skill of handling disappointment.

Prevention of Spoiling

1. Provide age-appropriate limits or rules. Parents need to set limits for children to keep their child's environment safe. Children need external controls until they develop self-control and self-discipline at around 3 to 4 years of age.

Rules are established for children so that they can learn to live cooperatively with others, to teach them right from wrong, and to protect them from harm. One should expect children to respond to certain rules, such as staying in the car seat, not hitting other children, and going to bed. These rules are not negotiable; however, children should be allowed to have control over decisions such as which cereal to eat, which book to read, and which clothes to wear.

Most children between 2 and 6 years of age have only a limited understanding of cause and effect or another person's feelings. Therefore, one cannot reason about discipline issues with toddlers and it is not necessary to explain the reason for every rule. The physician can suggest ways parents can promote effective discipline (Table 17-4).

2. Say *no* and mean it. If parents are ambivalent about saying no, the children will pick up on it. By not sending a clear message, parents encourage whining, pleading, and tantrums in their kids. Children often test parents to determine if they really mean what they say.

3. Do not give in to manipulation. Children throw temper tantrums to get their parents' attention, to wear them down, and to get their own way. Some children realize that throwing temper tantrums in public places can make their parents change their minds. Parents should make it clear that they will not be manipulated by such actions and not give in to tantrums.

4. Do not be afraid of the child feeling unhappy. Parents can empathize with and acknowledge their child's unhappiness or disappointment, but they should not be moved by the crying and should stick to their decisions. It is more important to help children learn to deal with unhappiness than to give them what they want all the time so that they will not be unhappy.

5. Do not worry about being unpopular with your kids. Some parents want to be their child's friends rather than their parents. Children will often say, "I hate you—you're not my friend" when they can't get their way. Parents should try not to feel guilty, angry, or hurt by these statements.

6. Recognize the difference between needs and wants. Children are not always able to distinguish between what they need and what they want. Needs include dealing with hunger, pain, or fear, and parents should respond promptly. Children often cry because they are refused a want or whim. It can feel uncomfortable to deny children their desires, but children are not necessarily happier when they always get what they want.

7. Teach the child to wait. Delaying immediate gratification is something a child must learn gradually. Children should not be allowed to interrupt parents' phone conversations or conversations with others. Waiting helps children learn to deal with frustration.

8. Teach respect for parents and other people. *For children to grow into successful social beings, they must learn the difference between needs and wants, and that other people, especially parents, also have needs, and that those needs count.* Children's needs for food, love, and safety come first, but their wants (e.g., play) and whims (e.g., an extra bedtime story) should come after a parent's needs are met. It is important for parents to spend quality time with their children, but they should not be expected

Table 17-4

Effective Disciplinary Techniques

1. Begin discipline after 6 months of age.
2. Praise positive behavior frequently.
3. Ignore unimportant behavior; e.g., swinging legs, poor table manners, sulking.
4. Be consistent with rules and ensure that both parents agree on the rules.
5. Set rules that are fair and reasonable; e.g., do not punish thumb sucking or separation fears.
6. State the acceptable or appropriate behavior clearly and briefly (about one word per year of age)—e.g., "Walk, don't run."
7. Prioritize rules—concentrate on only a few rules initially and give priority to safety, preventing harm to others, and then whining or temper tantrums.
8. Commands should not be repeated more than once without subsequent action.
9. Use age-appropriate discipline techniques:
   a. Toddlers and preschoolers—use distraction, ignoring bad behavior, physically moving or escorting, time out and natural and logical consequences for actions
   b. School-age to adolescence—use above plus delay of privileges and negotiation via family conferences
   c. Adolescence—logical consequences and family conferences about house rules; stop using time out.
10. Use consequences effectively:
    a. The consequence should follow the infraction as soon as possible.
    b. Do not enter into arguments with the child while you are correcting him or her—this is a child's way of delaying punishment
    c. Do not give long explanations for the reason for punishment when the child misbehaves; if necessary, they should occur after the punishment is over.
    d. Make the consequences brief (e.g., time out should be 1 min per year of age to a maximum of 10 min).
    e. Administer the consequence before becoming angry—do not yell at, humiliate, or verbally abuse the child.
    f. Consequences should be age-appropriate and not unduly harsh.
    g. Follow the consequences with love and trust; do not insist on an apology afterward.
    h. Criticize the behavior, not the child.

to spend every free moment of the evening or weekend with them. Children should learn to entertain themselves and not expect parents to be their constant playmates.

To avoid raising self-centered children, parents must show them that they were not put on earth to cater only to them. Children must be taught to respect the rights of their parents and thereby learn to be considerate and respect the rights of others.

Bibliography

Canadian Pediatric Society. Effective discipline for children. *Paediatr Child Health* 2(1):29–34, 1997.

Fox AM, Mahoney WJ: *Children with School Problems: A physician's Manual.* Canadian Pediatric Society,

Gottlieb S, Friedman S: Conduct disorders in children and adolescents. *Pediatr Rev* 12:218–223, 1991.

Hoffman J: Spoiled. *Today's Parent* 38–44, Feb. 1999.

Wyckoff J: *How to Discipline Your Six- to Twelve-Year-Old Without Losing Your Mind.* New York, Doubleday, 1990.

Wyckoff J, Unell B: *Discipline Without Shouting or Spanking.* Deephaven, MN, Meadowbrook Press, 1984.

Schmitt BD: *Your Child's Health.* Bantam Books, 1991.

Michael I. Reiff

Chapter 18

Attention-Deficit/
Hyperactivity Disorders

Attention-deficit/hyperactivity disorder (ADHD) is one of the most common and persistent biopsychosocial disorders of childhood and adolescence, affecting approximately 3 to 5 percent of school-aged children in North America. The symptoms associated with ADHD may influence and interfere with many aspects of normal development and functioning throughout childhood, adolescence, and into adult life. Despite a high level of clinical and public interest in ADHD, many areas of knowledge about it remain unclear, and clinical guidelines for its evaluation and treatment remain controversial. The heterogeneity of clinical presentations, the high likelihood of coexisting conditions, and the absence of confirming tests for ADHD all complicate the process of diagnosis. The paucity of carefully controlled long-term outcome studies and the clinical difficulties of obtaining adequate information about individual, home, and school functioning as well as monitoring complex multimodality intervention programs in the community all add to the challenge of facilitating optimal treatment of ADHD and related disorders. This chapter explores present knowledge and controversies regarding this common problem in pediatrics and focuses on clinical issues in evaluation and treatment.

What clinicians and researchers call ADHD is a set of behaviors that represent the final common pathway to a number of heterogeneous biopsychosocial problems. The terms *ADHD* and *attentional disorders* are used interchangeably in this chapter to describe these conditions.

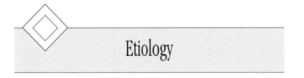

Etiology

Many etiologies have been proposed for ADHD. These known and proposed entities are likely to lead to the same behavioral presentation. Because of the heterogeneity of the disorder and present technologic limitations, suspected

etiologies—including anatomic brain lesions, areas of functional brain impairment, genetic variations, biochemical alterations, and deficits in frontal lobe functioning—have not been consistently demonstrated and no single etiology or validating battery of tests for ADHD has been identified. With increasingly sophisticated techniques, such as functional magnetic resonance imaging, and newer genetic methodologies, it is likely that multiple etiologies will emerge and that at least some will have genetic bases.

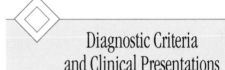

Diagnostic Criteria and Clinical Presentations

ADHD is a diagnosis defined by clusters of behavioral symptoms. The most widely accepted diagnostic formulations for ADHD have been put forth in the *Diagnostic and Statistical Manual* (DSM) of the American Psychiatric Association, which is periodically revised. Since 1980, with the publication of DSM-III, inattention, hyperactivity and impulsivity have remained the core diagnostic dimensions.

CORE DIAGNOSTIC CRITERIA

The DSM-IV (1994) defines inattention and hyperactivity/impulsivity as the core dimensions of ADHD. Nine symptoms are listed for each of the dimensions. The DSM-IV diagnoses require onset before age 7, presence of symptoms for 6 months or longer, pervasiveness of symptoms across two or more settings, frequency and severity of symptoms greater than those of children at a comparable developmental level, *and that the symptoms cause significant impairment in functioning.* Six out of nine symptoms of each dimension are required to be present before a diagnosis is made.

ADHD diagnoses from this model include a predominantly inattentive subtype (six or more inattentive symptoms) a predominantly hyperactive/impulsive subtype (six or more hyperactive/impulsive symptoms) and a combined subtype (six or more symptoms in both dimensions). A category of ADHD/NOS (not otherwise specified) is available for children with significant problems who fall short of meeting full diagnostic criteria. Other ADHD subtypes have been proposed outside the DSM model, including those based on family genetics, cognitive profiles, and subtypes aligned by comorbidity, which may have important implications regarding prognosis and intervention planning.

The DSM-IV diagnostic criteria are presented in Table 18-1. The *Diagnostic and Statistical Manual for Primary Care Practitioners* (DSM-PC) is a recent attempt to recognize the developmental and broad dimensional nature of

Table 18-1

Criteria for Attention-Deficit/Hyperactivity Disorder

Symptoms have persisted for at least 6 months, and were present before the age of 7 years. They are present to a significantly greater degree than is appropriate for age, cognitive ability, and gender of the child. They should be present in two or more settings (e.g., school and home). They present to a degree that is maladaptive and inconsistent with developmental level.

Inattention
- Often fails to give close attention to details, makes careless mistakes in schoolwork or other activities
- Often has difficulty sustaining attention in tasks or play activities
- Often does not seem to listen to when spoken to directly
- Often does not follow through on instructions and fails to finish schoolwork or chores (not due to oppositional behavior or failure to understand instructions)
- Often has difficulty organizing tasks and activities
- Often avoids, dislikes, or is reluctant to engage in tasks that require sustained mental effort (such as schoolwork or homework)
- Often loses things necessary for tasks or activities (e.g., toys, school assignments, pencils, books, tools)
- Is often easily distracted by extraneous stimuli
- Is often forgetful in daily activities

Hyperactivity-Impulsivity

Hyperactivity
- Often fidgets with hands/feet or squirms in seat
- Often leaves seat in classroom or in other situations in which remaining seated is expected
- Often runs about or climbs excessively in situation in which it is inappropriate (in adolescents or adults, may be limited to subjective feelings of restlessness)
- Often has difficulty playing or engaging in leisure activities quietly
- Is often "on the go" or often acts as if "driven by a motor"
- Often talks excessively

Impulsivity
- Often blurts out answers before questions are completed
- Often has difficulty awaiting turn
- Often interrupts or intrudes on others

SOURCE: American Psychiatric Association: *Diagnostic and Statistical Manual of Mental Disorders*, 4th ed. Washington, DC, APA, 1994.

many of the biobehavioral disorders. Symptoms described in the DSM-IV are described in the DSM-PC along as a continuum ranging from developmental variation (variations in behavior that do not cause functional impairment) to problems (problematic behaviors, but falling short of meeting diagnostic criteria for given disorders), to disorders (meeting criteria for the full diagnosis).

INATTENTIVE SUBTYPE

Children and adolescents with predominantly inattentive ADHD subtype are often described as "spacey," "lost in a fog," slow moving, distracted and "daydreamy." They may have a slow cognitive speed and appear to parents and teachers to process information slowly. Learning disorders and auditory and visual processing problems occur frequently in this subtype, as do anxiety and depression. Boys and girls are about equally represented.

IMPULSIVE-HYPERACTIVE SUBTYPE

The predominantly impulsive-hyperactive subtype presents with fidgetiness, difficulty sitting still, and a tendency to be disorganized. Children are frequently observed to act immaturely, to have a poor sense of physical boundaries, and to be belligerent. Rather than depression or anxiety, this subtype more often presents with a tendency toward disruptive behaviors, including oppositionality, defiance, and more serious conduct problems. Academic performance may not be problematic for children with predominantly hyperactive/impulsive ADHD. Although this subtype is described as more prevalent in boys than girls (approximated at 4:1), sex differences in all subtypes may be overstated.

LIMITATIONS OF DSM CRITERIA

The DSM criteria pose problems for researchers as they attempt to recruit subjects "with ADHD" and for clinicians as they attempt to operationalize the criteria for use in assess-ment, considering prognosis and intervention planning.

INTERNAL INCONSISTENCIES IN THE DIAGNOSTIC CRITERIA

The DSM criteria have been criticized as containing surplus meanings, vagueness, and lack of operational definitions. For example, the hyperactivity criteria are a mixture ranging from genetic influences (i.e., general activity level) to normally distributed temperamental style (i.e., leaving one's seat in the class when the work is aversive). Some of the same behaviors could equally result from high arousal, anxiety, or frustration. The inattention criteria are similarly problematic in that they do not match current laboratory models or psychological constructs of attention. So, if parents are asked to rate their children on the individual DSM inattention items, their responses do cluster into a factor of "inattention." However, when these described behaviors are measured in the laboratory, the intercorrelations between measures are low. The relationship between the laboratory measures and the clinical symptoms is also weak. It has been suggested that the reason for so little success in the search for specific etiologic factors or markers for ADHD is that there is too much heterogeneity and vagueness in the ADHD symptom clusters to presume that all children meeting the diagnostic criteria have the same disorder.

LACK OF DEVELOPMENTAL PERSPECTIVE

The DSM criteria have been criticized for lacking a developmental perspective. By adolescence, some of these diagnostic criteria, like the hyperactive behaviors, may be less severe or no longer problematic. It has been suggested that adolescents, because of yearly gains in maturity and self-modulation, should qualify for the ADHD diagnosis by meeting fewer criteria than younger children. The DSM-PC attempts to add this developmental perspective to the DSM diagnoses (Tables 18-2 and 18-3).

Table 18-2
Common Developmental Presentations of Inattention

	Inattention Variation	Inattention Problem	Attention-Deficit/Hyperactivity Disorder: Predominantly Inattentive Type
Early childhood	Difficulty attending, except briefly to a story book or quiet task such as coloring or drawing.	Sometimes unable to complete games or activities without being distracted, is unable to complete a game with a child of comparable age, and only attends to any activity for a very short period of time before shifting attention to another object or activity. Symptoms are present to the degree that they cause some family difficulties.	The child is unable to function and play appropriately and may appear immature, does not engage in any activity long enough, is easily distracted, is unable to complete activities, has a much shorter attention span than other children the same age, often misses important aspects of an object or situation (e.g., rules of games or sequences, and does not persist in various self-care tasks (dressing or washing) to the same extent as other children or comparable age. The child shows problems in many settings over a long period of time and is affected functionally.
Middle childhood	May not persist very long with a task the child does not want to do, such as reading an assigned book, homework, or a task that requires concentration such as cleaning something.	At times the child misses some instructions and explanations in school, begins a number of activities without completing them, has some difficulties completing games with other children or grownups, becomes distracted, tends to give up easily, may not complete or succeed at new activities, has some social deficiency, and does not pick up subtle social cues from others.	The child has significant school and social problems, often shifts activities, does not complete tasks, is messy and careless about schoolwork, starts tasks prematurely and without appropriate review as if he or she were not listening, has difficulty organizing tasks, dislikes activities that require close concentration, is easily distracted, and is often forgetful.
Adolescence	Easily distracted from tasks he or she does not want to perform.		

Source: Wolraich ML (ed): The classification of child and adolescent mental diagnoses in primary care, in *Diagnostic and Statistical Manual for Primary Care* (DSM-PC), child and adolescent version. Elk Grove Village, IL, American Academy of Pediatrics, 1996, by permission.

Table 18-3

Common Developmental Presentations of Hyperactivity/Impulsivity

	DEVELOPMENTAL VARIATION	PROBLEM	ATTENTION-DEFICIT/ HYPERACTIVITY DISORDER: HYPERACTIVE-IMPULSIVE TYPE
Early childhood	The child runs in circles, doesn't stop to rest, may bang into objects or people, and asks questions constantly.	The child frequently runs into people or knocks things down during play, gets injured frequently, and does not want to sit for stories or games.	The child runs through the house, jumps and climbs excessively on furniture, will not sit still to eat or be read to, and is often into things.
Middle childhood	The child plays active games for long periods. The child may occasionally do things impulsively, particularly when excited.	The child may butt into other children's games, interrupts frequently, and has problems completing chores.	The child is often talking and interrupting, cannot sit still at mealtimes, is often fidgeting when watching television, makes noise that is disruptive, and grabs from others.
Adolescence	The adolescent engages in active social activities (e.g., dancing) for long periods, may engage in risky behaviors with peers.	The adolescent engages in "fooling around" that begins to annoy others and fidgets in class or while watching television.	The adolescent is restless and fidgety while doing any and all quiet activities, interrupts and "bugs" other people, and gets into trouble frequently. Hyperactive symptoms decrease or are replaced with a sense of restlessness.

SOURCE: Wolraich ML (ed): The classification of child and adolescent mental diagnoses in primary care, in *Diagnostic and Statistical Manual for Primary Care* (DSM-PC), child and adolescent version. Elk Grove Village, IL, American Academy of Pediatrics, 1996, by permission.

THE DIMENSIONAL VS. CATEGORICAL NATURE OF ADHD

The diagnostic dilemma around ADHD is not so much with children and adolescents who clearly meet criteria for ADHD and have a compatible history and developmental course. The greater diagnostic challenge involves children and adolescents who have more unclear or complex histories or who have significant func-

tional impairments, but who do not meet the full diagnostic criteria. Problems like sustaining attention when classroom material is frustrating, difficulties with homework management, fidgetiness, and, indeed, many of the diagnostic criteria for ADHD can be thought of as *dimensions* of normal behavior at the extremes of a continuum. Because of this, many clinicians and investigators have suggested that ADHD be viewed as a dimensional diagnosis, similar to the diagnosis of mental retardation. In this dimensional model, individuals at the lowest few percentiles in a normal distribution receive a diagnosis, and those who fall short of receiving a diagnosis may still have problems that need to be addressed. The present DSM uses a categorical diagnostic model, most useful for diagnosing disorders like diabetes mellitus, where, with few exceptions, one clearly does or does not have the condition.

DIFFERENCES IN PREVALENCE RATES WITH CHANGES IN DIAGNOSTIC CRITERIA

Because ADHD is defined by behaviors rather than confirmable etiologic or pathophysiologic factors, prevalence rates can change dramatically with changes in the diagnostic criteria. For example, there is greater than 55 percent increase in children endorsed by teachers as meeting the DSM-IV compared to the DSM III-R criteria. In the field trials for the DSM-IV criteria, there was a 15 percent increase in the number of cases identified by the DSM-IV over the DSM-III-R criteria.

USING THE DIAGNOSIS

Diagnosing ADHD by specific behavioral criteria poses some challenges for clinicians. Because of their heterogeneity, children and adolescents meeting criteria for ADHD will present with a diverse set of clinical needs. We generally use diagnoses to predict prognosis and to plan treatment. In the case of ADHD, however, even if criteria for diagnosis are met, this does not necessarily target the specific problems that need to be addressed. In addition, excluding children and adolescents with clear functional disabilities in areas compatible with ADHD from the diagnosis because they fall just short of meeting diagnostic criteria is equally problematic. In a recent survey of pediatricians, we found that only 3 percent of respondents reported using the DSM criteria as their *sole* diagnostic criteria, although the majority re-

ported using these criteria as one component in their own diagnostic algorithms. In addition, they did not consider receiving the ADHD diagnosis essential for choosing candidates for treatment. The majority of clinicians reported using stimulant medication, the primary treatment modality for ADHD, in at least some circumstances where children or adolescents did not meet the DSM criteria for ADHD. Although the DSM criteria remain a useful organizing concept for thinking about ADHD, it may turn out that relying on the assessment of areas of functional disabilities and addressing problems suggested by comorbid conditions may be of equal or greater importance in establishing a prognosis and in planning interventions.

Functional Impairment

The DSM diagnostic thresholds are set up with the assumption that diagnostic criteria are met at the point where individuals experience significant functional impairment. In clinical practice, this is not always the case. Some children meeting criteria for ADHD appear to have minimal functional impairment, and some falling just short of meeting criteria may have significant impairment in one or more areas. The major areas of functional concern for children and adolescents with ADHD include family relationships, peer status, social skills, academic achievement, self-esteem, self-perception, and accidental injury.

Marital discord has been found to be significantly increased in families where a child has been diagnosed with ADHD. Families often describe distress and guilt over ineffective parenting practices, even though it is clear that children with ADHD can present difficult parenting challenges. Parents and siblings of children with ADHD may also have ADHD themselves, in addition to an increased incidence of other behavioral/emotional problems or diagnoses, thus further complicating family relationships and family functioning.

Problems in making and keeping friends and peer rejection can be major and devastating parts of ADHD. Children with ADHD—especially if they are hyperactive, aggressive, or have a poor sense of physical boundaries—are often among the most disliked children in the classroom and tend to be rated negatively by peers at extremely high levels. Because, particularly during adolescence, peer rejection is an important predictor of school dropout, delinquency, and mental health problems, assessment in this area is an important feature of ADHD evaluation and ongoing follow-up. Up to 60 percent of children with ADHD have academic achievement problems, although only 15 to 20 percent have ability-achievement discrepancies large enough to be diagnosed as learning disabilities. These academic difficulties increase throughout adolescence. The failure to complete independent academic work is a hallmark of adolescent ADHD. Adolescents with ADHD may still be fidgety, but functional impairment from hyperactivity is now rare.

Some studies suggest lowered self-esteem and self-perceptions in children with ADHD. Self-esteem issues may arise from difficulty in self-modulation at home, with peers or in the classroom, or around underachievement in school. Self-injury is another area of concern, particularly in children with coexisting aggression.

Ultimately, we treat problems in functioning caused by biopsychosocial disorders rather than the disorders themselves. For purposes of prognosis and treatment, a careful assessment must focus on defining the areas where functioning is most compromised, and these, rather than the defining symptoms of ADHD, become the targets for planning and monitoring the effects of various treatments.

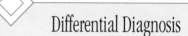

Differential Diagnosis

Since ADHD is defined as a cluster of behaviors, it is first necessary to establish that the behaviors in question are not just variations of normal development or problematic behaviors that fall short of meeting diagnostic criteria. The differential diagnosis must include both conditions presenting with behaviors that would meet criteria for the ADHD diagnosis and conditions that may include significant ADHD behaviors. These are summarized in Table 18-4.

The ADHD behaviors associated with psychosocial factors are presumably maladaptive responses to suboptimal circumstances or conditions at home or school. Medical and neurologic conditions or their treatments can cause behaviors compatible with ADHD. ADHD may present as part of many biobehavioral disorders. For example, over 50 percent of children with Tourette's syndrome also have ADHD. Many behavioral problems, like mood and anxiety disorders, are associated with ADHD but symptomatically discrete and may present like ADHD at some time in their course. ADHD, however, generally presents with an early onset and is generally persistent across childhood and adolescence. Mood and anxiety disorders usually present later and tend to be more episodic.

Other disorders can mimic ADHD in their initial presentation. Juvenile bipolar disorder is a case in point. In young children, it is not unusual for early symptoms to present for an extended period of time as indistinguishable from ADHD. However, the behaviors tend to be refractory to standard treatment modalities and these children ultimately receive a diagnosis of bipolar disorder as other symptoms begin to emerge.

Table 18-4

Differential Diagnosis of ADHD

DIMENSIONAL FACTORS	NEUROLOGIC
Behaviors are within the spectrum of normal developmental variation Behaviors are problematic but fall short of meeting full criteria for diagnosis	Auditory and visual processing disorders Seizure disorder Neurodegenerative disease Posttraumatic head injury Postencephalitic disorder
PSYCHOSOCIAL	**DIAGNOSES WITH ASSOCIATED ADHD BEHAVIORS**
Response to physical or sexual abuse Response to inappropriate parenting practices Response to parental psychopathology Response to acculturation Response to inappropriate classroom setting	Fragile-X syndrome Fetal alcohol syndrome Pervasive developmental disorders Obsessive compulsive disorder Tourette's syndrome Attachment disorder Psychosis or schizophrenia Adjustment disorder with mixed emotions and conduct
MEDICAL	**COMORBID CONDITIONS WITH POSSIBLE ADHD PRESENTATIONS**
Thyroid disorders (including general resistance to thyroid hormone) Heavy metal poisoning (including lead) Iron deficiency Glucose-6-phosphate dehydrogenase deficiency Side effects of medications Effects of abused substances Sensory deficits (hearing and vision)	Oppositional defiant disorder Conduct disorder Depressive disorders Anxiety disorders Learning disorders Language disorders

Comorbidity and Family Genetics

COMORBIDITY

ADHD rarely exists in isolation. Because of this, an evaluation "for ADHD" must include an assessment of ADHD *and* possible coexisting conditions. Many conditions in the differential diagnosis for ADHD can mimic ADHD symptoms as well as exist as independent comorbid problems. These associated conditions may assume equal or greater importance than the ADHD, even if ADHD symptoms are the presenting concern. Up to two-thirds of children and adolescents diagnosed with ADHD have at least one other biobehavioral diagnosis, about one-third have two, and over 10 percent have three or more additional biobehavioral diagnoses. The conditions most commonly occurring with ADHD and their estimated frequencies include oppositional defiant disorder and conduct disorder (50 to 67 percent); mood and anxiety disorders (30 percent); underachievement, learning disabilities, and language disorders (20 to 60 percent); and impaired fine motor functioning (50 percent). In some samples, encopresis and enuresis appear to be about twice as common in children diagnosed with ADHD.

Comorbid conditions can strongly influence outcomes. For example, the risk for antisocial behaviors, delinquency, and substance abuse in children with ADHD is predicted by comorbidity with conduct disorder and not by ADHD itself. Comorbid conditions, including behavioral mood and anxiety disorders, have been found to increase markedly over time in children diagnosed with ADHD. Because comorbid conditions can arise after initial diagnosis, periodic screening for symptoms of these disorders must be an essential part of any ongoing care plan.

GENETICS

Children of adults with ADHD have been found to be at up to 10 times greater risk for ADHD than children of controls. First-degree relatives of individuals with ADHD, including siblings of children with ADHD, have been found to be at about five times the risk for ADHD. First-degree relatives of probands with ADHD are also at significantly greater risk for other emotional and behavioral disorders, including major depressive disorder, oppositional defiant and conduct disorder, overanxious disorder, generalized anxiety disorder, and alcohol and drug dependence.

Evaluation

The discussion above should help lay the groundwork for evaluating children and adolescents for attentional disorders. Since ADHD and other comorbid diagnoses are difficult to establish, it can be helpful to use measures that are normed and validated to compare individuals to their peers along any behavioral or developmental dimensions. Family history and dynamics should be explored in detail, especially because of the high association of similar diagnoses in other family members. The DSM criteria for ADHD provide a useful heuristic framework for help-ing to arrive at a diagnosis, but the degree of functional impairment must be considered in selecting children and families for particular interventions. These functional disabilities should be viewed in a developmental perspective, as they can change considerably through the life span. Because of the lack of established etiologic factors and externally validating laboratory measures for diagnosing ADHD, any tests and procedures should be carefully selected.

A working checklist of dimensions to be assessed during an initial evaluation for ADHD is presented in Table 18-5. Because these dimensions span a broad spectrum of biopsychosocial areas, evaluations are often done with the pediatric clinician included as a member of a multidisciplinary team. Primary care pediatricians, on the other hand, should also be prepared to at least screen in all of these areas and, subsequently, refer as indicated. Available diagnostic tools include structured questionnaires and interviews; behavioral rating scales; parent-child observations; parent and child interviews; physical, neurologic, and neurodevelopmental examinations; laboratory findings; neuropsychological findings; and psychoeducational findings. With careful planning, primary care

Table 18-5

Primary Care Evaluation and Treatment Format

DIMENSION	CONFIRMATORY MEASURES[a]	DEVELOPMENTAL VARIATION	PROBLEM BEHAVIOR	DIAGNOSIS	TREATMENT IMPLICATIONS*
ADHD Behaviors/Disorders					
Inattention	History/Interview				Patient and parent education/mentoring
Impulsivity/Hyperactivity	Behavior rating scales				Cognitive-behavioral strategies
	Continuous Performance Task (CPT)[b]				Medication management
	Neurodevelopmental findings				Individual Educational Plan (IEP) (Other Health Impaired/Section 504)
Disruptive Behaviors/Disorders					
Oppositional and Defiant Behaviors/Disorder	History/Interview				Parent training (contingency management)
Conduct Disturbances/Disorder	Behavior rating scales				Classroom contingency management
					Problem-solving training
					Impulse-control training
					Anger-control training
					Medication management
Learning Status					
Underachievement	Cognitive testing (IQ)				Educational management
Learning problems/disabilities	Achievement testing				Classroom environmental management
					Individual Educational Plan (IEP)
					Learning-style interventions
Language Status					
Language Disorder	Standardized language measures				Referral to language clinician
Cognitive Status					
Mental Retardation	Cognitive testing (IQ)				Parent education and resources
	Achievement testing				Medical evaluation and follow-up plan
					Individual Educational Plan (IEP)
Atypical Development					
Atypical Behavior	History/Interview				Parent education and resources
Pervasive Developmental Disorder (PDD)	Behavior rating scales				Medical follow-up planning
	Observation				Individual Educational Plan (IEP)
					Medication management as indicated
Internalizing Behaviors/Disorders					
Depressive Symptoms/Disorders	History/Interview				Psychotherapy referral
Anxiety Symptoms/Disorders	Rating scales				Medication management as indicated
Family Functioning					
General Functioning	History/Interview				Family therapy
Behavior Management	Rating scales/Family Stress Index				Marital therapy
					Family skills training
Social Functioning/Self Modulation					
With Adults	History/Interview				Problem-solving training
With Peers	Rating scales				Social skills training
School Considerations					
Quality	History/Interview				Counseling around locating appropriate school and classroom settings
Fit					

[a]Assessment and interventions should be individualized. Not all items are indicated for all individuals.

[b]Routine use remains controversial,

SOURCE: Adapted from Reiff MI: Adolescent school failure: failure to thrive in adolescence. *Pediatr* Rev 19:199–207, 1998.

evaluations for ADHD can be carried out within the practical constraints of available time, resources, and reimbursement. An optimal evaluation includes obtaining a comprehensive history; making careful observations; assessing physical, neurologic, neurodevelopmental, and mental status; looking at family risk factors; and reviewing academic and learning-style considerations. If, by the end of an evaluation, the practitioner has either evaluated or screened for the dimensions listed in Table 18-5, a thoughtful prognosis and intervention plan can be developed.

History

DATA COLLECTION AND PREVIEW

ADHD, unlike many medical conditions, cannot be diagnosed solely by office-based observations or tests. It is a diagnosis based on behaviors present over time and pervasive across settings. Since so much of the diagnostic process is based on history and interpretations of behaviors, gathering reliable, organized and comprehensive information from parents and teachers is essential to the evaluation process. This can be done through questionnaires, which can be filled out by parents and teachers prior to an initial visit. Relying on information from one source only can be misleading and inadequate. Table 18-6 reviews important elements that individual clinicians can incorporate into structured histories for parents and teachers that can be previewed before an initial evaluation visit.

RATING SCALES

Behavioral rating scales have come into wide use as tools for the assessment of attentional disorders. These scales can be extremely helpful in gathering information more systematically than is usually possible during the time restraints of an office visit. They also have the dis-

Table 18-6

Elements of Structured History Questionnaires

- Current concerns
- Current functioning
- Demographic data
- Medical history
- Neurologic history (including tics)
- Developmental landmarks
- Developmental history (including behaviors compatible with atypical development)
- Behavioral history (infancy, toddler, preschool years)
- School history (including academics, work habits, behavior, peer interactions, interactions with teachers)
- Family functioning
- Family stressors
- Parenting history (including examples of present behavioral management)
- Rating scales for internalizing, externalizing, and atypical behaviors

tinct advantages of being normed and validated, which allows for quantitative comparisons of children and adolescents to same-age peers. Rating scales can also be used during triage to help determine the level of diagnostic services that might be appropriate for a given child and her or his family. A growing number of these rating scales are available and appropriate for clinical use in primary care settings. Several of these scales, their descriptions, and sources from which they can be obtained are reviewed in Table 18-7. These rating scales, like any other evaluation tools, should not be used exclusively for establishing diagnoses, even though some are based on DSM diagnostic criteria.

Having previewed questionnaires from parents and teachers and reviewed rating scales from home and school, the clinician can then use the evaluation visit to clarify this information; obtain more spontaneous histories from the child or adolescent, parents, or significant others; make behavioral observations; and observe parent-child dynamics, styles, areas of conflict, and affective responses. Using this approach, a thorough primary care assessment visit can usually be conducted within 1 hour of direct clinical time. This may take place over 2-3 visits depending on demand on the clinician.

Table 18-7

Behavioral Rating Scales/Screening Tools

SCREENING TOOL	DESCRIPTION	WHERE AVAILABLE
GENERAL MULTIDIMENSIONAL BEHAVIOR RATING SCALES		
Behavior Assessment Scales for Children (BASC)	A multimethod system including a self-report scale, a teacher rating scale, parent rating scales, a structured developmental history, and classroom observation forms.	American Guidance Service Circle Pines, MN 55014-1796
Child Behavior Checklist (CBCL)	Parent and teacher scales measuring social competence, internalizing and externalizing behaviors.	Thomas M. Achenbach, PhD Department of Psychiatry University of Vermont Burlington, VT 05401
Children's Global Assessment Scale (C-GAS)	A clinician rating system for overall child functioning. Ten categories from superior functioning to needing constant supervision.	*Archives of General Psychiatry*, Vol. 44, September 1987
RATING SCALES FOR EXTERNALIZING BEHAVIORS (ADHD, OPPOSITIONAL-DEFIANT AND CONDUCT-DISORDERED BEHAVIORS)		
Conners Parent and Teacher Rating Scales	Several sets of widely used parent and teacher rating scales. Scales are non-diagnostic.	Multi-Health Systems, Inc. 908 Niagara Falls Blvd. N. Tanawanda, NY 14120
ADHD Rating Scale IV	Normed and validated rating scale for ADHD based on DSM diagnostic criteria.	George DuPaul, Ph.D. Iacocca Hall, Room A-219 111 Research Drive Bethlehem, PA 18015
ACTeRS	Teacher rating scales measuring attention, hyperactivity, social skills, and oppositionality.	Meritech Inc. 111 N. Market St. Champaign, IL 61820
ADDES	Parent and teacher rating scales standardized on a broad normative sample	Hawthorne Educational Services P.O. Box 7570 Columbia, MO 62505

(continued)

Table 18-7 (cont.)

Behavioral Rating Scales/Screening Tools

SCREENING TOOL	DESCRIPTION	WHERE AVAILABLE
RATING SCALES FOR INTERNALIZING BEHAVIORS (DEPRESSION, ANXIETY)		
Children's Depression Inventory (CDI)	A self-endorsed 27-item scale composed of statements regarding affective, cognitive behavioral, and somatic symptoms of depression.	Multi-Health Systems, Inc. 908 Niagara Falls Blvd. N. Tonawanda, NY 14120
Revised Children's Manifest Anxiety Scale (RCMAS)	A self-endorsed 37-item scale yielding a total anxiety score and subscales for physiologic, worry, oversensitivity, social concerns, and concentration.	Western Psychological Services 12031 Wilshire Blvd. Los Angeles, CA 90025
SCHOOL FUNCTIONING		
Academic Performance Rating Scale	A 19-item teacher rating scale for academic productivity and accuracy, learning ability, impulse control, academic performance, and social withdrawal.	George DuPaul, Ph.D. Iacocca Hall, Room A-219 111 Research Drive Bethlehem, PA 18015
SOCIAL SKILLS		
Social Skills Rating System (SSRS)	Parent, teacher and self-report scales.	American Guidance Service Publishers' Building Circle Pines, MN 55014-1796
FAMILY FUNCTIONING		
Abiden Family Stress Index	A 101-item questionnaire exploring general parenting stress, child characteristics, parent characteristics, and life stress.	Pediatric Psychology Press 320 Terrell Road West Charlottesville, VA 22901
The Home Situations Questionnaire–Revised	Assessment of social interactions, oppositional-unfocused, oppositional-focused, and self-engaged situations.	Russell A. Barkley, Ph.D. Department of Psychiatry University of Massachusetts Medical Center 55 Lake Avenue North Worcester, MA 01655

(continued)

Table 18-7 (cont.)

Behavioral Rating Scales/Screening Tools

SCREENING TOOL	DESCRIPTION	WHERE AVAILABLE
The Family Adaptability and Cohesion Scales (FACES) II	A 30-question self-endorsed questionnaire measuring family cohesion, adaptability, and communication.	D. Olsen, Ph.D. Family Social Science University of Minnesota St Paul, MN 55108
The Family Assessment Measure (FAM)	A series of 50 statements about family functioning rated by children and parents from "strongly agree" to "strongly disagree."	Multi-Health Systems, Inc. 908 Niagara Falls Blvd. N. Tonawanda, NY 14120
The Parent-Adolescent Communication Scale	A 20-item scale from "strongly agree" to "strongly disagree in which an adolescent endorses items for each parent.	D. Olsen, Ph.D. Family Social Science University of Minnesota St Paul, MN 55108
STRUCTURED NEURO-DEVELOPMENTAL EXAMINATIONS		
PEER, PEEX 2, PEERAMID 2 (Levine)	A series of structured neuro-developmental examinations for ages 4–6, 6–9, 9–15. Training available.	Educators Publishing Service 75 Moulton St. Cambridge, MA 02138

SOURCE: Adapted from Reiff MI: Adolescent school failure: failure to thrive in adolescence. *Pediatr Rev* 19:199–207, 1998.

Physical, Neurologic, and Neurodevelopmental Evaluation

Careful behavioral observations are generally important parts of a medical evaluation. In the case of ADHD, however, any conclusions from these observations should be interpreted cautiously. Only about 20 percent of children show signs of ADHD in an unfamiliar office setting. In addition, whether or not signs of ADHD are observed has little predictive value regarding subsequent severity or outcome. Observations of stereotypic movements, poor eye contact, and tactile defensiveness have more clinical efficacy and are compatible with the pervasive developmental disorders (autism and related diagnoses).

Routine physical examinations are usually noncontributory unless indicated by suggestive findings from a careful history. Physical findings can be helpful, however, for establishing such diagnoses as fetal alcohol syndrome and fragile-X syndrome. Nonspecific dysmorphic features and minor physical anomalies such as hair whorls, hyper- or hypotelorism, low-set ears, or high arched palate are both nonspecific and nondiagnostic, although they may suggest more prenatal or genetic etiologies.

Standard neurologic examinations are likely to yield few significant findings unless static or progressive neurologic conditions, seizure disorders, or loss of previously obtained developmental landmarks or cognitive skills is suspected. The presence of neurologic soft signs is nonspecific and not helpful in diagnostic formulation. The presence of motor and/or vocal tics should be noted, as they relate to the diagnosis of Tourette's disorder and need to be considered carefully in the planning of psychopharmacological interventions.

An examination profiling neurodevelopmental strengths and weaknesses can be quite helpful and may provide an excellent format for observing children and adolescents. A typical neurodevelopmental examination should include the evaluation of fine motor, graphomotor, and gross motor skills; visual-perceptual-motor (hand-eye) functioning; receptive and expressive language abilities; temporal-sequential organization and short-term memory abilities; and observations of cognitive (work production) speed. Findings of difficulties with short-term and active working memory across auditory and visual modalities can help support the diagnosis of attentional disorders. Neurodevelopmental findings can be used to screen for developmental problems associated with ADHD, such as motor and language delays and auditory or visual processing problems. Clinicians may elect to devise their own battery of neurodevelopmental findings or use more field-tested formats such as the Pediatric Examination of Educational Readiness (PEER), Pediatric Early Elementary Examination-2 (PEEX-2) and the Pediatric Examination of Educational Readiness at Middle Childhood-2 (PEERAMID-2) (Table 18-7). These examinations provide a structured format for neurodevelopmental findings, give estimates of age appropriate responses, and enumerate the neurodevelopmental processes involved in each subtest.

Laboratory Measures

Screening of hearing and vision should be done routinely, as sensory losses in these modalities can both mimic and exacerbate attentional disorders. Laboratory screening for the medical conditions reviewed in Table 18-4—including

thyroid profiles; lead, iron, and hemoglobin levels, G-6-PD assays, chromosome analyses, etc.—are not warranted unless suggested by history or physical findings. Routine neuroimaging studies and electroencephalograms (EEGs) are likewise not indicated unless seizure disorders, neurodegenerative disorders, or other neurologic conditions are suspected. Because of the absence of proven etiologic factors, there is no justification at present for including magnetic resonance imaging or other functional brain imaging techniques, EEGs or EEG brain mapping, neurochemical assays, or a battery of neuropsychological tests of executive function as routine parts of an evaluation for ADHD.

The routine use of computerized measures of attention remains controversial, since consistently strong relationships have not been demonstrated between the DSM behavioral symptoms of ADHD and the psychological construct of attention. These tests, such as the Conners' Continuous Performance Tests (CPT), the Gordon Diagnostic System, and the Test of Variables of Attention (TOVA) have false-negative rates typically of 15 to 35 percent, while false positive rates are lower. These tests should never be used in isolation to diagnose ADHD and are not a substitute for other diagnostic measures. Results in the clinically significant range may reflect anxiety, mood disorders, processing problems, or generally low cognitive abilities as well as ADHD. The administration of CPTs can have clinically useful advantages. The format of CPT administration provides an excellent opportunity to observe a child during the clinically significant condition of attempting to sustain attention and inhibit responses during a boring task where no reinforcement is being received. CPT results can also be helpful in reviewing evaluation results with parents and adolescents who would feel more comfortable about proceeding with an intervention plan after considering more objective evidence. In addition, CPT findings can be useful for demonstrating moment-to-moment fluctuations in attention, helping to explain inconsistency in performance, often interpreted by teachers as a lack of motivation and framed as "he can do it when he really wants to." Although CPT results are sensitive to stimulant medication effects, it is not clear that they predict behavioral changes in home and school settings, and it is not recommended that they be used for assessing medication response.

Academic Achievement, Learning Style, and Learning Disorders

About 20 percent of children with ADHD have significant learning disabilities. Another 40 percent of children and adolescents with ADHD experience learning challenges, including suboptimal learning and/or work production prob-

lems. Examples of some of the academic difficulties posed by elements of attentional disorders are summarized in Table 18-8.

Learning disabilities are diagnosed when significant discrepancies (>1.5 standard deviations or 22 points) exist between measured standard scores of cognitive abilities (IQ) and individual achievement scores in reading, mathematics, and written expression. Other ways of defining learning disabilities include significant discrepancies between achievement in different areas for the same individual or significant discrepancies between a given child's achievement compared that of same-grade peers. Because ADHD and learning disabilities can exacerbate each other, any children or adolescents with significant academic difficulties should have psychoeducational testing. Communication disorders

Table 18-8
Academic Difficulties Posed by ADHD Dimensions

AREAS OF DIFFICULTY	ACADEMIC IMPLICATIONS
Attention	Inattention and distractibility limit learning Difficulty with task persistence Easily bored in routine or unstimulating learning environments, large class size, and considerable "downtime"
Impulse control	Rushing through work, impulsive responses, difficulty self-correcting mistakes
Activity level	Limits ability to take advantage of instructional techniques
Sense of time	Difficulty with time-limited tasks, test taking, and long homework assignments
Organizing, planning, and sequencing	Problems with homework flow and work completion Difficulty with previewing planning and executing long assignments Difficulty with note taking, underlining Difficulty using planners
Short-term memory and consolidation of information	Difficulty memorizing lists, math facts, etc.
Motor planning	Sloppy and slow printing and cursive writing Limited ability to take notes Difficulty with expressive writing if simultaneously struggling with writing mechanics

may also be present and may be related to learning disabilities. The DSM-IV includes categories for expressive language and mixed receptive and expressive language disorders.

Where achievement is clearly below grade expectation, schools are generally mandated to administer a battery of psychoeducational tests, including standardized individually administered IQ and achievement tests. In a team model, an educational or clinical child psychologist would review academic functioning, and, if indicated, administer and interpret psychoeducational testing unless this had already been done through the school system.

Primary care clinicians should be familiar with the major cognitive tests, including the Wechsler Intelligence Scales for Children III (WISC-III) and the Kaufman Assessment Battery for Children (K-ABC) as well as the major achievement tests including the Woodcock Johnson Battery—Revised (WJR-R), the Wechsler Individual Achievement Test (WIAT), and the Kaufman Test of Educational Achievement (KTEA). Some excellent references for primary care clinicians on these and other psychoeducational evaluation tools are available (see Aylward reference at the end of this chapter).

The psychoeducational evaluation should provide the information to establish the diagnoses of borderline intellectual functioning (IQ 71 to 84), mild mental retardation (IQ 50 to 70), moderate mental retardation (IQ 35 to 50) or severe mental retardation (IQ 20 to 35). If borderline intellectual functioning or mental retardation are diagnosed as comorbid conditions to ADHD, and dysmorphic features are also present, diagnoses like fragile X and fetal alcohol syndromes should be considered. IQ scores should be contrasted to the results of achievement tests to establish the diagnosis of learning disorders.

An assessment for academic difficulties should include a review of teachers' observations and any prior testing, including estimates of abilities (IQ testing) and measures of academic achievement including grades, any stan-

dardized group testing (like Iowa Basics, Stanford Achievement tests, etc.), any individually administered achievement tests, and any formal tests of language abilities. The Academic Performance Rating Scale, a systematic questionnaire around multiple issues regarding school functioning is referenced in Table 18-7. An interview around school functioning should include an assessment of the match between the learner and the teacher, classroom setting, school format, and school culture. If intake questionnaires, interview, or neurodevelopmental screening suggest language disorders, formal language evaluation should be requested from a speech and language specialist.

Mental Health Screening

In a team diagnostic model, a clinical child psychologist would conduct this part of the evaluation by assessing the current status of a child's emotional and behavioral functioning. A psychological evaluation includes behavioral observations, assessment of the child or adolescent's perceptions of his or her functioning in different settings, a structured history regarding symptoms of specific emotional or behavioral disorders from parents and older children and adolescents where appropriate, and an appropriate diagnostic formulation.

Primary care physicians and nurse practitioners can and should be able to carry out screening in this domain. The review of multidimensional rating scales (Table 18-7) can help identify major areas of concern, including externalizing behavior disorders (oppositional defiant disorder and conduct disorder) and internalizing behaviors (dysthymia, major depressive disorder, and other mood and anxiety disorders). These scales also screen for aspects of social competency and adaptive behaviors. Both parents and teachers may be good sources of information about different aspects of a child's disruptive or externalizing behavior problems and disorders. Parents and children may be the best sources for information about internalizing behavior problems, which may be more masked in settings outside the home. Because depression and anxiety problems or disorders are particularly common comorbid conditions, it can be helpful to use self-report rating scales, such as the Children's Depression Inventory and the Revised Children's Manifest Anxiety Scale (Table 18-7). These can be easily administered and scored at the time of the visit.

Having reviewed these rating scales, part of the initial visit can then be used for interviews and observations of both parents and children or adolescents around these issues. Table 18-9 summarizes important elements of a primary care interviews around mental health issues comorbid with ADHD. The interview with the child can provide the opportunity to observe interactional skills, speech, use of language, and general mood as well as to explore perceived explanations for difficulties, subjective distress associated with them, and coping strategies.

At times it is difficult to determine whether behaviors arise as part of the attentional disorder or from comorbid conditions, and this can be an important consideration for prognosis and treatment. Demoralization and low self-esteem, for example, may be secondary to chronically poor functioning associated with ADHD or to comorbid dysthymia (chronic low-grade depression). Oppositional behaviors and defiance can easily arise from ADHD-driven impulsivity rather than originating from a separate comorbid diagnosis of oppositional and defiant disorder. Serious conduct problems can evolve from ADHD as an extension of oppositional and defiant behavior or as part of a major depressive disorder comorbid with ADHD. The risk of antisocial and substance abuse disorders is predicted by the comorbidity with conduct disorder at baseline and not by ADHD itself. These and other such associations stress the importance of exploring these emotional and mental health concerns in some detail. Where individuals appear at high risk and comorbid mental health disorders are suspected, referrals can be made to a mental health professional as indicated.

Family Functioning and Psychosocial Risk

Optimal family functioning is integrally related to good outcome for a child with ADHD.

Table 18-9

Mental Health Screening

PARENT INTERVIEW	CHILD/ADOLESCENT INTERVIEW
• Oppositional behaviors and their management • Serious conduct problems • Agression and its management • Fears and worries • General mood • Ritualistic behaviors • Compulsive behaviors • Unusual thoughts • Tics • Substance use/abuse	• Self-esteem and coping style • Sense of self-efficacy and locus of control • Developmentally appropriate and/or atypical interests • Perceptions of school, peer, and family functioning • Self-perception of ADHD symptoms • Anger, temper, and methods of anger control • Significant worries, fears, panic • Significant periods of sad mood or irritability • Rituals (including counting, washing, etc.) • Concerns about being talked about behind one's back • Hearing or seeing things that are not there • Substance use/abuse

Because of this, and, since family members of a child with ADHD are at significantly high risk for ADHD and other comorbid conditions, an exploration of family functioning and psychosocial risk is an essential part of an evaluation for ADHD. In a team diagnostic model, a clinical social worker or psychologist would generally conduct this part of the evaluation by taking a family history, exploring family strengths and functional problems, reviewing family beliefs and attributions to their child, and reviewing behavior management practices and coping styles.

Tools are available to aid primary care practitioners in assessing this area. Some of the rating scales that can be used for this purpose are included in Table 18-7. A family evaluation should include a history for biopsychosocial disorders in family members, including: ADHD, major depressive disorder, oppositional and defiant disorder, conduct disorder, antisocial personality disorder, anxiety disorders, alcohol and drug dependence, and learning problems and disabilities.

Family functioning can be assessed by asking questions about family activities, family member interactions, mutual support, and areas of concern to individual family members. Parenting styles and attributions should be explored in some detail. It is important to understand whether parents perceive their child's behavior as intentional. Of equal importance is whether parents place inappropriate blame for their child's behaviors on themselves or their parenting techniques. Negative attributions of parents may lead to negative interactions and ongoing frustration. Positive beliefs and attributions can encourage problem-solving approaches.

Assessment Formulation and Intervention Plan

If some level of evaluation has been done regarding each of the areas reviewed above, an initial diagnostic formulation can be made. The formulation should include an enumeration of significant problems, diagnoses, and areas of significant functional impairment (Tables 18-5 and 18-10). It should also include an estimation of the cumulative stressors on the family system, since this can have considerable impact on prognosis and prioritization of interventions as well as an estimation of overall (global) functioning of the child or adolescent. Once this is done, individual interventions can be formulated for each area of concern. An overview of possible interventions is presented in Table 18-5. These are developed more fully in the following discussion of treatment.

Table 18-10
Assessment of Functional Impairment

Areas of Functioning	Levels of Impairment
• Family relationships • Peer status • Social skills • Academic achievement • Self-esteem • Self-perception • Accidental injury	*Mild:* Symptoms are present but unlikely to cause serious developmental difficulties. Symptoms are manageable at home, at school, in social situations. *Moderate:* Symptoms cause some developmental difficulties and poor adjustment in at least 1 major area of functioning. *Severe:* Symptoms are causing serious developmental difficulty and dysfunction. They are largely unmanageable.

Treatment

Many treatments have been tried and are used for ADHD. Medication management, behavioral treatments, and education remain the mainstays of empirically based intervention plans. Other modalities have been proposed for treating ADHD, including allergy treatments, restrictive and supplemental diets, optometric vision training, sensory integrative training, chiropractics, biofeedback, treatment for inner ear problems, and pet therapy, as well as traditional psychotherapy. Where these modalities have been studied, they have been shown to have minimal or no evidence of efficacy.

COMBINED TREATMENT APPROACHES

Surprisingly little is known about combined treatment approaches for attentional disorders or about which subgroups of children with ADHD might benefit from such combined approaches. The largest study to date is the recently completed Multimodal Treatment Study of children with ADHD (the MTA study). In this 14-month study, almost 600 children were randomly assigned to either medication management alone, behavioral treatment alone, a combination of both, or routine community care. The results indicated that carefully monitored medication management with frequent visits and input from teachers is more effective than intensive behavioral treatment for ADHD. For some outcomes, such as academic performance or positive family relationships, the combination of behavioral therapy and medication was necessary to produce improvements. The study also found significant differences between the medication management following the study protocol and that provided in the community. These differences mostly related to the quality and intensity of the medication management

treatment. These findings strongly argue for a consistent and intensive approach to treatment, much in the same way that "asthma pathways" and treatment guidelines for other medical conditions have recently been established.

COMPREHENSIVE TREATMENT

It is generally recognized that the treatment of ADHD and comorbid conditions requires an effective partnership among children, families, significant school personnel, medical and mental health care clinicians, and other community resources. Wherever possible, offering assessments and ongoing management through a consistent interdisciplinary team is optimal for children, families, and professionals. This format provides opportunities for ongoing joint staffing and communication among families and team members and a chance for the team to develop an evolving but consistent approach and interdisciplinary language. The use of compatible medical records and databases can also afford the opportunity for systematic case review and clinical research. If this approach is not possible or practical, it can be helpful for practitioners to develop a pool of consistent professionals with whom to achieve some of these same goals. Community professionals can team with parent support groups to extend networking opportunities. General treatment goals and modalities are reviewed in Table 18-11. It is important for families to view attentional disorders as chronic conditions where equal attention must be paid to fostering normal development and coping with ongoing symptoms as well as normalizing problem behaviors.

Treatment appropriately begins during the evaluation process. Much of this has to do with the language in which the evaluation is framed and the ways in which the conceptual issues around attentional disorders are conveyed to children, adolescents, and their parents. The evaluation should remain as child-centered as

Table 18-11
Treatment Objectives and Modalities

TREATMENT OBJECTIVES	TREATMENT MODALITIES

• Foster normal development
• Foster positive self-esteem
• Promote self-efficacy
• Involve children and adolescents in decision making as is developmentally appropriate
• Remove problematic behaviors
• Treat associated problems
• Develop coping strategies for ongoing problems
	• Educational counseling
	• Support groups
	• Educational resources: literature, videos, Internet sites
	• Psychological and behavioral therapies
	   Cognitive behavioral techniques
	   Behavioral therapies
	   Treatments for family dysfunction
	   Assessment and treatment of
	      parental biobehavioral issues
	• Academic Interventions
	• Medication management

possible. Areas of concern should be addressed within the context of coexisting strengths. It should be made clear that the evaluation is a way to delineate areas of suboptimal functioning and to begin a problem-solving process. Parents must understand that this is a different approach to diagnosis than that customary with more discrete and self-contained conditions that can be more readily verified by specific historical and physical findings or laboratory measures. The family should understand that the evaluation process is organized to look at overall functioning within the context of ADHD symptoms *and* associated problems. Children's only prior contact with medical evaluations may have been within the context of medical illness, where their full participation and cooperation may not have been critical for successful diagnosis and outcome. Here, their level of comfort with the process, their participation and optimal performance, and their understanding of their own issues and others' concerns will be key factors in successful evaluation and outcome.

At the completion of the evaluation, a separate visit can be scheduled to review the results and begin to develop a multimodality intervention plan. Children, as developmentally appropriate, and certainly preadolescents and adolescents, should be part of these meetings. To the extent possible, treatments should be empirically based. *The litmus test for any intervention should be whether it promotes self-efficacy and good self-esteem. A well-conceived treatment plan must be achievable.* It must be formulated within families' economic and functional capacities to successfully carry it out. Interventions must be prioritized and tailored to meet a child's clinical and developmental needs. Some factors influencing these priorities include: how readily the interventions can be communicated, taught, and monitored; how easily they can be combined with other proposed treatments; and how available the treatments are in a given community. Other considerations should include how long the treatment effects are expected to last after the intervention is terminated, how well the positive outcomes generalize outside the treatment setting, whether the child will be stigmatized by family or peers because of participation in a given treatment, and how a given treatment plan coincides with other family goals and values.

FACTORS PREDICTING SUCCESSFUL TREATMENT

Factors predicting positive outcomes for children and adolescents include early evaluation and interventions, self-understanding of problems and issues, having a supportive family, gaining an understanding of the school system, having an appropriate IEP if indicated, and willingness to participate in counseling, mentoring, and coaching. Factors predictive of negative outcomes include delayed diagnosis; an ongoing cycle of treatment failures; parents and teachers making characterologic attributions around ADHD behaviors; ongoing substance abuse; medication refusal; unwillingness to participate in counseling, mentoring or coaching; and remaining undereducated around problems and possible interventions. Some parents may not want to pursue a treatment program even after a through evaluation process. In this case they should be informed about the possible consequences of nontreatment, including low self-esteem, social and academic failure, and a possible increase in the risk of later antisocial behavior.

Educational Counseling, Demystification, and Reframing

The material reviewed earlier in this chapter can provide the background for the ongoing education of children, adolescents, and families around ADHD-related issues. *Education is the mainstay of successful treatment at every stage.* During childhood, parents and children can be seen together, but it is important to address a portion of the counseling at each visit toward the child at his or her developmental level. Older children should be educated to understand and be progressively responsible for elements of their treatment plan. It is essential to establish a knowledge-base before adolescence, so that adolescents can begin to "own" their sta-tus and take progressive responsibility for the identification of their problems, successes, and treatment plans. It is advisable to see adolescents separately from parents for at least part of the visit and gear education to promote self-efficacy and self-esteem. Adolescents should be involved in decision making as much as is developmentally appropriate.

The language used during visits and the reframing of negative ideas can be powerful components of educational interventions. Non-facilitating statements such as "I'm different from 'normal' students, and this limits what I should expect of myself" can be reframed into facilitating statements like "I'm not (qualitatively) different, but I do have learning style issues that need to be addressed because they interfere with my optimal functioning." It can be helpful to engage in the process of "motivational interviewing" as part of the treatment process. The principles of motivational interviewing include developing discrepancies, avoiding argumentation and "rolling" with any resistance, eliciting self-motivational statements, and summarizing and supporting those statements that favor change. This approach can be particularly rewarding with adolescents, but it can and should also be used with preadolescents and younger children when developmentally appropriate.

Support groups

Support groups such as CHADD (Children and Adults with Attention Deficit Disorder) [National Office.499 NW 70th Ave, Plantation, FL 33317 (http://www.chadd.org/)] can be important resources for parents. Local chapters can connect parents to appropriate experts, advocates, and resources within the community and school systems and provide a forum for speakers and discussions. The national organization holds annual educational meetings and makes responsible information and materials available to parents.

Educational Resources: Literature, Videos, Internet Sites

A plethora of ADHD-related educational resources and materials are now available for parents and children. The quality of these materials varies so significantly that they can almost be considered an embarrassment of riches. Health professionals can help parents locate empirically and clinically sound and responsible materials compatible with or complementary to their own views and practice.

Psychological and Behavioral Therapies

PSYCHOTHERAPY

Traditional psychotherapy has not been found to be useful in the treatment of attentional disorders, although it may certainly be indicated for comorbid conditions, including depressive and anxiety disorders.

COGNITIVE-BEHAVIORAL TECHNIQUES

Cognitive-behavioral therapies, where children are taught to "stop and think" before acting, have a great deal of intuitive appeal as treatments for impulsive children with attentional disorders. Cognitive-behavioral programs are designed to facilitate self-control and reflective problem solving. These therapies—including verbal self-instructions, problem-solving strategies, cognitive modeling, self-monitoring, self-evaluation, social skills training, and self-reinforcement—have all been used and studied. Despite their appeal, they have generally been found to be ineffective with children who have ADHD. Gains from these therapies and programs have generally been short-lived, and children have had difficulty generalizing these skills outside of the specific therapeutic setting and using the skills independently. When behavioral goals are highly specific, however, such as increasing a child's on-task behavior during periods of independent work, self-monitoring approaches coupled with self-reinforcement have demonstrated positive results in school contexts. Training for greater self-awareness of one's own anger cues and the use of these cues as signals to enact various coping strategies has also been found successful.

BEHAVIORAL THERAPIES

Behavioral parent training and behavioral classroom interventions for children with ADHD have been used successfully. A typical parent training program aims to increase parents' understanding of their child's behavior and the unique self-regulation difficulties posed by attentional disorders and to offer techniques for giving commands and for reinforcing and extinguishing behaviors. These programs often last 8 to 12 weeks, are done individually or with groups of parents, and cover techniques including contingency management, how to give clear commands, use of time outs, point systems, and cost-response. Treatment modalities include direct instruction, modeling, role playing, discussion readings, and "homework" designed to give parents experience in using these techniques to help shape their child's ability to regulate his or her own behavior. Classroom management programs are similar, where teachers and paraprofessionals are taught similar techniques and also learn to administer daily report cards, which provide feedback to children and their parents and allow parents to provide consequences at home. Children with ADHD often need more reinforcement of these procedures and more intensive programs than noncompliant children without attentional disorders.

The general rules of behavior modification include (1) giving positive attention (praise, attention, hugs, smiles, privileges, points, chips . . .) to behaviors parents wish to encourage, (2) actively ignoring behaviors that are not intolerable but which parents wish to extinguish, and (3) giving negative attention (punishments) for behaviors which are intolerable and need to be stopped. The most effective praise or punishment procedures are short and immediately connected to the positive or negative behaviors. Parents may need specific suggestions about giving commands. Components of an effective command, after establishing good eye contact, include (1) a well-modulated terminating statement ("You have to stop doing that"), (2) a warning ("If you don't stop doing that within 3 minutes . . ."), and (3) a statement of the consequences of both the negative response (". . . you'll be in time out) and a positive response (". . . then you and your sister can continue playing). Standard behavioral techniques such as time-out procedures and loss of privileges can also be taught. If these are to be used, they should be discussed first at a family meeting and understood by the child before implementation. A typical time-out procedure is activated when a child chooses the negative response to a command after being told that time out will be the consequence. The child is then removed from the opportunity to get adult attention and sent to a quiet, nonentertaining location. The door to that space is shut. A timer is set for from 2 to 5 min, depending on age. The time, when set, is not negotiated, and the parent does not respond to any attention-seeking behavior. If the child is quiet and self-modulated when the timer goes off, he or she is allowed out of time out and the first positive behavior is acknowledged. If the child is not quiet when the timer goes off, it is set for an additional minute and the same procedure is followed until the child is quiet and time out is over. Response cost, or loss of privileges, can also be instituted for noncompliance. The most effective consequences are logically related to the inappropriate behavior. For example, loss of TV or video-game privileges may be instituted for failure to complete homework. Loss of car privileges may be enforced for returning home late.

Although the most powerful effects of behavior management programs come from the more intensive systematic approaches, pediatric clinicians can and should teach, reinforce, and use the language of these techniques as part of any treatment program. If this more informal approach remains suboptimal, referrals can be made to community mental health therapists for behavioral parent training or even more intensive summer school programs where available.

TREATMENT FOR FAMILY DYSFUNCTION AND ASSESSMENT OF FAMILY PSYCHOPATHOLOGY

Where significant parental or marital discord is present, parents may not be able to successfully carry out parent-training strategies because of more fundamental issues. These families should be referred for family and/or marital therapy. Because of the high frequency of ADHD and other biobehavioral problems and disorders in parents of children with attentional disorders, these conditions should be considered in situations where there is significant family conflict and appropriate referrals for individual evaluation and treatment made.

Academic Interventions

The greatest functional disabilities for many children and adolescents with ADHD arise in the school setting. Students with attentional disorders may experience many of the problems reviewed in Table 18-9.

Many sets of sound recommendations are available to clinicians, teachers, and parents. These interventions tend to be practical but somewhat less evidence-based than the behavioral recommendations discussed above. Systematic neurodevelopmental examinations, such as those developed by Levine (Table 18-7), can help the practitioner assess strengths and areas of concern from a task-analysis perspective. Resources (such as the book *Educational Care*, by Levine, referenced at end of chapter) are available for translating these findings into strategies that can be used in school and at home to help remediate or bypass targeted areas of concern.

Federal laws are in place relating to the education of students with attentional disorders. Public Law 94-142 of the Individuals with Disabilities Education Act (IDEA) and Section 504 of the Rehabilitation Act of 1973 require that special education and related services be available for children who have disabilities that impair their educational performance. Children with attentional disorders are eligible under part B of the IDEA and section 504, as they fall into the law's "Other Health Impaired" category. The law requires that the special education and related services be specifically designed to meet the needs of the specific child. To do this it calls for the development of an individual education plan (IEP), which identifies each disability and the interventions that will be activated in the least-restrictive setting. The law also mandates that children suspected of having disabilities receive prompt identification and evaluation through a multidisciplinary team. Titles II and III of the Americans with Disabilities Act (ADA) also require public and nonsectarian private schools to meet the needs of children with attentional disorders. Primary care clinicians can play a key role in getting parents to request these services by writing a dated letter to the school principal.

Medication Management

GENERAL CONSIDERATIONS

Medication management has been the most prevalent and effective single treatment modality for children with attentional disorders. In general, medication management alone has been found consistently superior to psychosocial treatments alone across all comparison studies. The results of the Multimodal Treatment Study of Children with ADHD (MTA) study strongly confirm this. In this study, outcomes from medication management using the study protocol were significantly better than outcomes from

medication management in community practices. Several factors that appeared responsible for these differences should be considered for incorporation into routine clinical management. In the first weeks of treatment, special care was taken to find an optimal dose of medication for each child. After this period, the prescribing physician met with the child and family monthly for half-hour visits to assess concerns and, at the same time, review monthly teacher input. This information was used to make necessary changes in the child's treatment. If the child was experiencing any difficulties, the physician was encouraged to adjust the medication. In contrast, community physicians generally saw the child face to face only one or two times a year for short periods of time, interactions with teachers were not generally sought, and lower doses of stimulant medication were generally prescribed. When used, psychopharmacologic agents should be one part of a well-conceived intervention plan as described above. They are somewhat more effective when used in conjunction with behavioral, social and educational interventions, especially when comorbid conditions are present. Over the last several years clinicians have become much more comfortable and familiar with using both a range of psychostimulant agents other than methylphenidate and non-stimulant psychopharmacologic medications. Characteristics of the most common medications used for treating ADHD are summarized in Table 18-12. Clinicians and researchers have also gained increasing experience with using medication to also treat ADHD in combination with comorbid conditions. These issues will be discussed below.

STIMULANT MEDICATIONS

An array of medications has been used to treat ADHD. Stimulant medications, methylphenidate (Ritalin) in particular, have been the most prescribed, and their use has captured a great deal of public interest and debate. Between the years 1990 and 1995, for example,

Table 18-12

Psychopharmacologic Agents for ADHD

MEDICATION	DOSE	ONSET	DURATION	MAJOR SIDE EFFECTS/COMMENTS
		STIMULANTS		
Methylphenidate (Ritalin) 5, 10, 20 mg tablets	0.3–1.0 mg/kg/dose BID to TID	20–30 min	3–5 h	Common: Loss of appetite, insomnia, stomachaches, headaches, irritability, dizziness, weight loss. Behavioral "rebound" as medication wears off. Rare: tics. Staring, daydreaming, and irritability decrease with increasing dose. No relationship between dose and rebound, tics, emotional and cognitive constriction, growth delays. Blunted affect and social withdrawal if dose is too high. If growth velocity deceleration occurs at all, it is with higher doses. Most side effects dissipate with time. Tolerance is rare. SR form can be unreliable
Ritalin SR (sustained-release) 20 mg tablets	0.6–2.0 mg/kg/dose QD (may supplement with metylphenidate for additional 4-h coverage)	30 min–1.5 h	3–8 h	
Dextroamphetamine (Dexedrine/ Dextrostat) 5 mg (Dextrostat also 10 mg) tablets	0.15–0.5 mg/kg/dose BID to TID		4–6 h	Same potential side effects as methylphenidate. Spansule form is often more reliable and effective than Ritalin SR.
Dexedrine Spansules 5, 10, 15	0.3–1.0 mg/kg/dose QD (may supplement with dextroamphetamine for additional 5-h coverage)	30–60 min	6–10 h	

(continued)

Table 18-12 (cont.)

Psychopharmacologic Agents for ADHD

MEDICATION	DOSE	ONSET	DURATION	MAJOR SIDE EFFECTS/COMMENTS
Adderall 5, 10, 20, 30 mg tablets	0.4–1.5 mg/kg/dose QD to BID	20–40 min	6–8	Same potential side effects as methylphenidate.
Methamphetamine (Desoxyn) 5 mg tablets	0.15–0.5 mg/kg/dose BID to TID	20–40 min	4–6 h	Same potential side effects as methylphenidate. Use limited by high cost
Pemoline (Cylert) 18.75, 37.5 mg chewable tablets	2 mg/kg/day QD to BID	1–2 h	7–10 h	Same potential side effects as methylphenidate. Obtain and monitor liver function tests with use. Use limited by potential hepatotoxity.
HETEROCYCLIC ANTIDEPRESSANTS				
Imipramine (Tofranil) 10, 25, 50 mg tablets	2–5 mg/kg/day BID–TID	Initial dose 0.5– 1.0 mg/kg QD and advance by 10–25 mg Q5–7d		Constipation, decreased appetite, dry mouth, blurry vision, tachycardia, fatigue, dizziness, effects on cardiac conduction. Weight gain with the exception of Desipramine. Drowsiness on Nortriptyline. Baseline EKG and EKG and blood levels at dosage changes exceeding 3 mg/kg/d Increased levels if used with methylphenidate. Gradually taper to avoid "flu-like" symptoms
Desipramine (Norpramin) 10, 25, 50, 75 mg tablets	2–5 mg/kg/day BID to TID	Initial dose 0.5–1.0 mg/kg QD and advance by 10–25 mg Q5–7d		
Nortriptyline (Pamelor) 10, 25, 50, 75 mg tablets 10 mg/5cc liquid	1–3 mg/kg/day	Initial dose 0.5 mg/kg QD and advance by 10–25 mg Q5–7d		

(continued)

Table 18-12 (cont.)

Psychopharmacologic Agents for ADHD

Medication	Dose	Onset	Duration	Major Side Effects/Comments
Amino-ketone Antidepressants				
Bupropion (Wellbutrin) 75, 100 mg tablets	50–100 mg/dose TID	Takes 4–6 weeks to see initial effects		Dry mouth, constipation, drowsiness. Potential for lowering seizure threshold.
Wellbutrin SR 100, 150 mg tablets	100–150 mg/dose BID			
Alpha₂ Adrenergic Agonists				
Clonidine (Catapress) 0.1, 0.2, 0.3 mg tablets	0.05–0.15 mg/dose TID	May take 4–6 weeks to see initial effects		Sedation, especially when inactive or bored, weight gain, temporary worsening of tics. Effects seen with dose increase: headache, dizziness, abdominal pain, nausea or vomiting. Patch may cause contact dermatitis. Taper gradually to avoid rebound hypertension
Catapress TTS Transdermal patch 1, 2, 3	1 patch Q 5–7 days			
Guanfacine (Tenex) 1,2 mg tablets	0.5–1.5 mg/dose BID to TID			

methylphenidate production in this country increased five-fold. This has sparked considerable discussion about whether ADHD is over-diagnosed and medication over-prescribed, and whether this increase in production represents a diversion to recreational use by teenagers. In this debate Ritalin has taken on the properties of a social metaphor for how our society thinks about the pressures of the 90's and issues of child-rearing, parenting, schooling, and the diversity of learning styles. Although the debate continues, the majority of responsible studies have shown that the percentage of youth being treated with psychostimulants is well within the estimates of the prevalence of ADHD, and that more legitimate "cases" are being diagnosed and treated. This does not mean, however, that in some circumstances ADHD is *not* over-diagnosed, and stimulants over-prescribed. Annual surveys of drug use and emergency room visit monitoring, however, have not shown substantial increases in MPH abuse.

Stimulant medications have been the most used agents in treating the core symptoms of ADHD and are generally the most effective. It is important for parents and children to gain a perspective on what these medications will and will not do. Overactivity; attention span; impulsivity; self-control; compliance; physical and verbal aggression; social interactions with parents, teachers, and peers; academic productivity and accuracy; handwriting; on-task behavior; and reduction in aggression have all been shown to improve with stimulant treatment. About 75 percent of parents and teachers have immediate and dramatic positive perceptions of children's behavior when they are started on stimulants. Comorbid oppositional and conduct symptoms may also improve. Children may also show improved participation in leisure-time activities, like playing baseball. Of course, all of these do not improve in all individuals. On the other hand, reading skills, social skills, learning, long-term academic achievement, antisocial behavior, and arrest rates have not been found to consistently improve, although many of these issues are still under investigation.

Stimulant medications are thought to work through effects on central norepinepherine and dopamine pathways. Clinically, they appear to enhance the functioning of executive control processes by helping to overcome deficits in inhibitory control and working memory. These medications are rapidly absorbed and metabolized. Effects are brief and do not continue after the medication has been stopped. Because the short-acting forms last less than the length of a schoolday, many children and adolescents choose to take the longer-acting preparations.

The choice of stimulants must be tailored to the individual. A suboptimal or nonresponse to one stimulant should not discourage the clinician from recommending another. About 70 percent of children will show a positive response to the first stimulant tried. About 85 to 90 percent will respond to at least one of the stimulants. In addition, the side-effects profile may be more favorable on one medication than another for any given individual. There is no evidence of superior effectiveness of one psychostimulant over another and no way to predict which individuals will experience side effects or be a nonresponders to any specific preparation. This argues strongly for trying several of these medications in a systematic way until an optimal treatment and side-effect profile is achieved.

CONTROLLED TRIALS

Stimulant medication can be initiated using a double-blind, placebo-controlled trial, or by starting at a low dose and gradually adjusting it upward until optimal effects are observed. A typical double-blind placebo-controlled trial can be set up over a 3-week period. Estimated low and medium doses and placebo can be given daily for 1-week periods on consecutive randomized weeks. At the end of each week, parents, teachers, and older children and adolescents can rate the week on a scale such as the ADHD Rating Scale IV (Table 18-7), which is normed and validated. After the trial is completed, the order of weeks is reviewed along with the rating scale results, and, if significant improvement over placebo is seen, medication can be continued at an appropriate dose. This kind of trial can incorporate parents, older children, and adolescents into the decision-making process before the actual decision to start medication is made. It can particularly facilitate adolescent "buy-in" by providing a somewhat objective assessment of medication efficacy. Some parents, however, are reluctant to even try stimulants because of concerns about possible side effects and perceived dangers of medication. In these cases it may be prudent to start medication at very low doses to avoid side effects and rebound. All factors being equal, a double-blind placebo-controlled trial is recommended. Computerized continuous performance tests (CPT's) measuring the abilities to pay and sustain attention do not accurately predict stimulant-induced gains in behavior or achievement, and CPTs should not be used to identify medication responders or to titrate medication dosage.

DOSAGE

There is no "right dose" of psychostimulants for weight or age. The optimal dose for on-task behavior, classroom productivity, and teacher ratings varies from individual to individual and does not appear to correlate with body weight. Some few individuals require very large doses without any indication of being overmedicated. A small subgroup of children may experience "cognitive toxicity" at doses that seem optimal for behavioral control.

Stimulants can enhance functioning at home and at play as well as in school. Just like wearing glasses to enhance focus in all activities, optimal stimulant coverage includes use throughout the day and on weekends. Use after school can cut down on behavioral conflicts as well as enhance homework production and focus during sports, music lessons, etc. It can also help children convert their activities from more passive TV watching and video-game playing to those requiring more active processing of information such as reading and becoming involved in projects. Daily use may also help to minimize the ups and downs of side effects and behavioral rebound in some cases. Competent medication follow-up takes careful planning.

General parent feedback and even teacher behavioral rating scales are often insufficient indicators of the success or failure of medication management. For example, up to 45 percent of children are endorsed as having significantly improved or completely normalized their behavior on placebo on typically used teacher behavioral rating scales for ADHD, and over 90 percent of children are endorsed by teachers as having improved or normalized behavior on some dose of stimulant medication. On the other hand, efficiency of work production has closer to a 5 percent placebo effect, and, when classroom productivity is actually measured, only about half of children improve or normalize on some dose of medication. Observed on-task behavior in the classroom is again different. About 10 percent of children improve on placebo, and around 75 percent of children improve or normalize on some dose of medication compared to peers. *Because of this, medication management should be directed toward specific target behaviors.* The targets should be those where medication efficacy has been demonstrated in evidence-based studies. The clinician should then establish ways to measure changes in those target behaviors by enlisting teachers, school psychologists, and school social workers to assess progress as objectively as possible. Parents also should be provided with structured and countable observation formats or rating scales directed at specific target behaviors at home. This kind of feedback from home and school should be reviewed as part of any follow-up visits for medication management.

On medication, the correspondence between accurate self-evaluation and performance increases. On medication, children also pick their effort or ability more often as an explanation for their success than medication. This issue of what children and adolescents attribute to medication and what they attribute to themselves is an important subject for discussion during visits for medication follow-up. It can be productive to discuss medication as a tool that can be used effectively or ineffectively for producing a product or achieving a goal. This can be explored in academic, social, and behavioral domains. Children should become knowledgeable about effects and side effects of medication and should progressively take more and more responsibility for their own medication regimens by preadolescence. New issues around medication management are likely to arise during adolescence. At that time medication can take on street value. Medication dosage can become less predictable during adolescence. Later-afternoon and evening doses of medication often become more essential for the production of school-work. Adolescents who are unclear about medication efficacy should be offered a systematic medication-placebo trial that includes self- and teacher-endorsed rating scales and comments. Adolescents need to be involved in all decision making around medication management issues.

SIDE EFFECTS

Several controversies have arisen regarding the side effects of stimulant medication. A number of studies have examined the issue of whether stimulant medications reduce growth. The vast majority of studies show that stimulant medications do not cause significant or persistent reductions in height. This suggests that "drug holidays" on weekends or summers are not necessary on this account. Since stimulant medications can exacerbate tics, their use in children with Tourette's syndrome and other tic disorders has been controversial. Recent studies have shown that not only are stimulant medications effective in reducing ADHD behaviors of children with Tourette's syndrome, independent of tic severity, but also, at moderate doses, tic frequency or severity are unlikely to be affected. Even with chronic use, usual doses of stimulant medications do not appear to exacerbate tics, but they should be carefully monitored when used.

Nonstimulant Medications

The use of nonstimulant medications for the treatment of attentional disorders has been increasingly studied. They have been used particularly when stimulants are contraindicated or ineffective because of excessive side effects, short duration of action, suboptimal response, or exacerbation of tics or Tourette's disorder.

Some of these medications have the advantage of also treating mood, anxiety, and tics.

Tricyclic antidepressants have been the most studied nonstimulant medications for the treatment of ADHD. Positive effects on inattention, impulsivity, hyperactivity, anxiety, and depression have been found. The effects on learning are unclear. Possible advantages over stimulants include a longer half-life and a more sustained action, no behavioral rebound effects, and no associated risk for substance abuse. Positive and sustained effects on ADHD symptoms have been found in up to 70 percent of children for doses in the range of 4 to 5 mg/kg of desipramine and imipramine and 2 mg/kg of nortriptyline. Lower doses are often not as effective or as sustained. The use of these higher doses in some children is limited by side effects such as headaches, insomnia, somnolence, or gastrointestinal distress. The most important side effects are cardiovascular, including the possibility of inducing arrhythmias. Several reports of sudden and unexplained deaths in children treated with desipramine have raised questions about the safety of these agents, although it is likely that this number of deaths falls in the range of baseline risk for age. Because of this, and the potential for lethal overdose, heterocyclics should be considered second-line medications for attentional disorders, and their use should be carefully monitored with levels and electrocardiograms.

Bupropion is an amino-ketone antidepressant that has effects on both dopamine and norepinepherine. Bupropion has been subject to few studies, but in these investigations—which includes one large, controlled multisite study—it has been shown to be effective in reducing ADHD symptoms at doses comparable to its use for depression. Side effects are minimal, although at higher doses it can lower the seizure threshold of some individuals.

Alpha$_2$ adrenergic agents, including clonidine and guanfacine, can also be effective for treating aspects of attentional disorders, particularly children who are very hyperactive, display outbursts of impulsivity, and are oppositional and defiant. Direct effects on attention and distractibility remain unclear, and it does not appear to be particularly useful for children with primarily the inattentive type of ADHD. Since it can also be effective in the treatment of tics associated with Tourette's disorder, it is often used where Tourette's is a comorbid condition. The use of these medications has been limited by sedating effects, particularly with clonidine. Other side effects, including hypotension are rare. Discontinuation of medication should be done gradually to avoid rebound hypertension. These medications have also been used at bedtime to counteract insomnia and rebound effects of stimulants. The combination of clonidine and methylphenidate has been implicated as a factor in five cases of sudden death in children, although this remains unproven.

ADHD with Comorbid Conditions

ADHD WITH AGGRESSION OR CONDUCT DISORDER

Stimulants have been shown to be effective in improving ADHD symptoms in aggressive children and adolescents with ADHD, in addition to suppressing physical and verbal aggression, negative peer interactions, stealing, and property destruction. They do not appear to help social information processing. Some studies of children with comorbid conduct disorder indicate improvement of ADHD and aggressive symptoms with antidepressants. Clonidine and stimulants have also been used to treat this combination of symptoms.

ADHD WITH DEPRESSION AND ANXIETY

Children with comorbid anxiety or depression have been found to demonstrate a reduced response to stimulants. Tricyclic antidepressants have been found to reduce both symptoms of

ADHD and anxiety and depression symptoms. Clinical experience suggests the efficacy of bupropion, bupropion in combination with stimulant medication, or stimulant medication used in conjunction with SSRIs for ADHD with depression or anxiety.

ADHD WITH TICS OR TOURETTE'S DISORDER

Stimulants have been found to be effective in treating ADHD behaviors, aggression, and social skill deficits in children with Tourette's disorder or chronic tics without exacerbation of tics. Some studies, however, have shown worsening of tics. Tricyclic antidepressants have been found to be effective in improving ADHD symptoms in children with tics or Tourette's disorder with a generally neutral effect on tics. Clonidine and guanfacine have been found useful in decreasing ADHD symptoms and tics in some situations.

ADHD WITH MENTAL RETARDATION OR PERVASIVE DEVELOPMENTAL DISORDERS

Stimulant medication can be effective for the treatment of ADHD accompanied by these disorders, although the response may be more variable. Stimulants have been described as occasionally precipitating psychotic-like behaviors in children and adolescents with PDD. Risperidone at doses of 2 mg/day has been used successfully in ameliorating overactivity, aggression, social relatedness, and anxiety in children and adolescents with PDD.

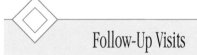

Follow-Up Visits

Follow-up visits should include an interim history, a review of any ongoing interventions, and periodic screening for new comorbid problems;

Table 18-13
Agenda for ADHD Follow-Up Visits

- Review of newly collected teacher and parent narratives and rating scales
- Interim history
- Review of ongoing interventions
- Periodic screening for new comorbid problems
- Medication management: height, weight, blood pressure, heart rate, review of side effects, discussion of attribution to medication, appropriate laboratory tests as indicated
- Review home functioning: behavioral functioning, relational issues
- Review school functioning: academic, behavioral, and social-relational functioning
- Review self-esteem and behavioral, social, and academic self-efficacy issues
- Review understanding of attentional disorders, comorbid problems, and all interventions with children and adolescents at a developmentally appropriate level
- Problem-focused discussions around timely issues: organizational skills, study skills, homework management, self-modulation skills, anger management, etc.
- Updated reading materials and handouts for children, adolescents, and parents
- Review and revision of intervention plan

they should always include components of support and educational counseling, as discussed above. Visits can be preceded by the collection of new narratives and rating scales from teachers and parents and generally be conducted within a half-hour of clinical time. A review of agenda items for follow-up visits is found in Table 18-13.

Summary and Conclusions

The etiology of ADHD remains unknown, although new functional neuroimaging and genetic studies continue to hold promise in this area. The difficulties that the heterogeneous presentations, the dimensional nature of the symptoms, and the lack of confirming diagnostic tests pose in establishing diagnostic criteria for ADHD and making the diagnosis of this condition have been discussed in detail. These issues make an assessment of functional impairment at

the child's given developmental level an essential step toward a careful diagnostic formulation and development of a treatment plan. The high occurrence of comorbid conditions makes "an evaluation for ADHD" really an evaluation for ADHD *and* these comorbid problems. Because the diagnosis cannot be made solely from office-based history, observations, and procedures alone, the use of rating scales and other structured input from parents and teachers can be of indispensable value. A multidisciplinary team or other collaborative approach can be an optimal way of conducting such a broad-based evaluation for ADHD in some circumstances. This chapter has emphasized a primary care approach with referrals to specialists in other disciplines as indicated. It has stressed the ongoing importance of careful psychopharmacologic management, and the growing array of agents available to practitioners has been reviewed. A treatment approach consisting of education, support, behavioral treatments, and medication management and focusing on self-esteem and self-efficacy is sound and empirically based. More and longer-term studies, such the

MTA study, are essential to help shape future practice.

Suggested Readings

Cantwell DP: Attention deficit disorder: a review of the past 10 years. *J Am Acad Child Adolesc Psychiatry* 35:978–987, 1996.

Conners CK: Is ADHD a disease? *J Attent Disorders* 2: 3–17, 1997.

Culbert TP, Banez GA, Reiff MI: Children who have attentional disorders: interventions. *Pediatr Rev* 15: 5–15, 1994.

Miller KJ, Castellanos FX: Attention deficit/hyperactivity disorders. *Pediatr Rev* 19:373–384, 1998.

Reiff MI, Banez GA, Culbert TP: Children who have attentional disorders: diagnosis and evaluation. *Pediatr Rev* 14:455–464, 1993.

Reiff MI: Adolescent school failure: failure to thrive in adolescence. *Pediatr Rev* 19:199–200, 1998.

References

American Psychiatric Association: *Diagnostic and Statistical Manual of Mental Disorders*, 4th ed. Washington, DC, APA, 1994.

Aylward GP: *Practitioner's Guide to Developmental and Psychological Testing*. New York, Plenum Press, 1994.

Book and Video Catalogue. ADD WareHouse, 300 Northwest 70th Avenue, Suite 102, Plantation, FL 33317. (http://www.addwarehouse.com)

Kutcher SP: *Child and Adolescent Psychopharmacology*. Philadelphia, Saunders, 1997

Levine MD: *Educational Care*. Cambridge, MA, Educators Publishing Service, 1994.

Mercugliano M, Power TJ, Blum NJ: *The Clinician's Practical Guide to Attention-Deficit/Hyperactivity Disorder*. Baltimore, Paul H Brookes, 1999.

The MTA Cooperative Group: A 14-month randomized clinical trial of treatment strategies for attention-deficit/hyperactivity disorder: multimodal Treatment Study of Children with ADHD. *Arch Gen Psychiatry*, 56:1073–1086, 1999.

The MTA Cooperative Group: Moderators and mediators of treatment response for children with attention-deficit/hyperactivity disorder: The Multimodal Treatment Study of children with attention-deficit/hyperactivity disorder. *Arch Gen Psychiatry* 56:1088–1096, 1999.

National Institutes of Health: *NIH Consensus Development Conference on Diagnosis and Treatment of Attention Deficit Hyperactivity Disorder*. Washington, DC, National Institutes of Health Continuing Medical Education, 1998.

Wolraich ML (ed): The classification of child and adolescent mental diagnoses in primary care, in *Diagnostic and Statistical Manual for Primary Care (DSM-PC)*, child and adolescent version. Elk Grove Village, IL, American Academy of Pediatrics, 1996.

Frances Page Glascoe

Developmental Delay

Approximately 6 million children, about 12 percent of those between birth and 21 years of age, receive services under the Individuals with Disabilities Education Act (IDEA).[1] An additional 3 to 6 percent have disabilities that are undiagnosed. Even larger numbers of children, between 7 and 10 percent, have serious difficulty with academic tasks and cannot read or comprehend at grade level. Overall, between 22 and 28 percent of America's children fail to graduate from high school.[2–4] Clearly, developmental problems including seriously substandard school performance, are among the most common and pressing problems of pediatric patients.

Who are these children and how should clinicians best care for them? This question is addressed via a discussion of the nature and causes of disabilities and developmental delays. Included is a description of the challenges and rewards these conditions present to health care providers. Finally, effective methods are presented by which pediatricians can readily fulfill the tasks of detecting and addressing developmental problems.

Definitions, Etiology and Ontology

The term, *disability*, conjures up images of overt dysmorphology and incapacitation. Yet among children with handicapping conditions, most are considered "mild": approximately 51 percent have learning disabilities, 21 percent have speech-language impairments, 12 percent have mental retardation, and 9 percent have emotional disturbance. The more physically overt conditions—such as physical and health impairments, traumatic brain injury, and sensory impairments—represent only 7 percent of disabling conditions.[4] It is important to note, however, that the term *mild disabilities* does not mean that such problems are insignificant. All include, as part of the eligibility criteria for special education services, serious difficulties benefiting from regular classroom curricula. For children to receive needed services under IDEA, they must first meet the criteria for diagnosis. Although criteria and categories vary from state to state, differences are slight. Table 19-1 contains a list of typical categories and eligibility criteria.

The fact that mild disabilities are prevalent means that most developmental problems are not overtly visible. Most children with disabilities talk, although they may not talk well. Most have at least some level of literacy, although they may not read well. Those with emotional or behavioral disabilities may at times be attentive, cheerful or cooperative. Few children with disabilities or delays have any dysmorphic features, neurologic dysfunction, or other physical signs and symptoms. Only rarely does birth or developmental or family history of disabilities serve as an adequate harbinger of problems.

There are, however, associations between children's developmental status and the degree to which their families can provide enriching environments. In one seminal study, children with four or more psychosocial risk factors were shown to have significantly elevated odds of disability or academic failure. Risk factors included parental mental health problems (including depression and anxiety), parents with less than a high school diploma, a single-parent household, three or more siblings in the home, poverty, frequent household moves or other life events, and an authoritarian parenting style (a high number of commands with minimal responsiveness to child-initiated interactions).[5] A recent study showed that while intermittent hearing loss in children with otitis media is a strong predictor of language delays and academic problems, psychosocial risk factors were even stronger predictors, such that children with both intermittent hearing loss and a lack of developmental stimulation had substantially greater developmental deficits.[6]

Just as language, motor, social, behavioral, self-help, and academic skills develop over time, developmental problems also develop. This phenomenon is usually referred to as development's "age-related manifestations." For example, it is not possible to identify disordered syntax or many other features of language impairments until children are old enough not only to talk but also to combine several words. This means that a an 18-month-old who appears normal because of an appropriately sized single-word vocabulary may be considered impaired by 24 to 30 months if word combinations fail to emerge or fail to emerge in an orderly manner. A student entering kindergarten who can identify most letters of the alphabet may appear to be developing normally but may be diagnosed with learning disabilities if she has not mastered the sounds of letters by 6 to 7 years of age. During the first 1½ to 2 years of life, children with psychosocial risk factors tend to develop normally. By the third year, however, delays in linguistic and cognitive skills often become apparent.

Table 19-1

Criteria for Special Education Classification

CATEGORY	CRITERIA
Speech-language impaired	Performance 2 or more standard deviations below the mean on diagnostic measures of expressive and receptive language.
Mental retardation	IQ or DQ less than 74, and performance 2 or more standard deviations below the mean on adaptive behavior measures.
Specific learning disabilities	Performance 1 or more standard deviations below the mean and 1 or more standard deviations below IQ on measures of reading, math, or written language.
Emotionally disturbed	Meets criteria from *Diagnostic and Statistical Manual of Mental Disorders*, 4th ed. (DSM-IV) (e.g., anxiety disorder, depression, thought disorder) with evidence that emotional difficulties adversely affect academic achievement.
Physical impairment	Presence of a physical disability (e.g., motor coordination disorder or cerebral palsy) and academic performance 1 or more standard deviations below the mean.
Health impairment	Presence of a significant health problem (e.g., chronic illness, seizure disorder, attention-deficit/hyperactivity disorder) and academic performance 1 or more standard deviations below the mean.
Visual impairment	Acuity less than 20/200 after correction or need for visually adapted teaching methods or materials.
Autism and other developmental disorders	Meets DSM-IV criteria including disturbed developmental rates, sequences, sensory response, language, and socialization.
Hearing impairment/ deafness	Loss of hearing, with or without amplification, that adversely affects language or academic achievement.
Traumatic brain injury	Temporary or permanent insult to the brain that results in physical, speech, vision, hearing, cognitive, psychosocial, behavioral, or emotional deficits and deficits in academic achievement.
Multiple disabilities	Two or more severe impairments, inability to profit from programs designed for only one impairment.
Developmental delay (used in 0–3 programs, although states may opt to serve children under this category until age 9)	2 or more 25% delays relative to chronological age or 1 or more 40% delay in physical development, cognitive development, communication development, social or emotional development, or adaptive development.

Diagnosis

Early Detection

Because developmental problems are subtle and emerge slowly over time, the American Academy of Pediatrics (AAP)[9] suggests that development and behavior should be assessed at each well visit, beginning with the newborn and continuing through young adulthood. Although these policies are wise because they are designed to ensure that children receive the benefits of early intervention, many clinicians have difficulty complying. Barriers include increasingly large patient panels, minimal reimbursement for in-office screening, limited behavioral compliance in young children (which makes it challenging to administer screening tests), the time required to administer screening tools, and the poor attendance at well-child visits of many at-risk patients. These challenges all contribute to the tendency of pediatricians to rely heavily on clinical judgment and informal checklists rather than on validated screening tools.

What is so wrong with informal approaches? There is substantial evidence that informal methods lead to vast amounts of underdetection. Palfrey et al.[10] showed that fewer than 30 percent of children with disabilities were detected prior to school entrance. Put another way, more than 70 percent of children with developmental and behavioral problems are not detected by their primary care providers. A closer look at checklists, such as those imbedded in age-specific encounter forms, provides insight into the problems of informal approaches. Most checklists include four to five tasks per age level (e.g., climbs stairs, drinks from a cup, combines words, scribbles, follows commands). If a child misses one, should he be referred for evaluation? If two are missed? Three? Four? Conversely, if all listed skills are observed or reported, can we be truly confident that a child

is developing normally? Indeed, many checklists rely on items from the Denver Developmental Screening Test—Revised (DDST-R), which itself missed 70 percent of children with speech-language impairments and 50 percent of children with mental retardation, suggesting that children who demonstrate all skills on DDST–R–based checklists may still have substantial problems. Ultimately, though, there are no known answers to questions about the appropriate cutoff to use in scoring checklists. Such an unproven approach would be completely unacceptable for detecting lead levels, phenylketonuria (PKU), or any other medical condition. Why, therefore, do we accept such guesswork for something as vital and treatable as developmental and behavioral problems?

Lest the 25 percent of pediatricians who actually use routinely standardized developmental/behavioral screens assume they are effectively screening for disabilities, there is often compelling evidence to the contrary. For example, many providers use inaccurate measures (e.g., the Denver-II will either miss 60 percent of children with problems or identify 60 percent of normal children as deficient, depending on how the questionable score is interpreted).[11] Still other clinicians administer screens only after noticing a problem. This is a practice at complete odds with the rationale for screening in the first place, because symptomatic patients do not need screening; only asymptomatic ones do. Still other clinicians use screens in a nonstandardized manner (e.g, administer only key items on the Denver-II). All this again leaves professionals without clear information on children's developmental and behavioral status.

Selecting Effective Methods for Detecting Developmental Delays

Fortunately, there are many viable alternatives to unvalidated, informal methods that produce ambiguous results and to validated but overly lengthy measures that are difficult to use correctly in busy primary care settings. In fact, there are hundreds of measures on the market, some good, some not. Because the test publication industry is not regulated professionally or federally, clinicians must acquire skills in selecting wisely among the vast and competing array of screening tools. Well-accepted standards for quality instruments are shown in Table 19-2.[12–14]

The two final points on screening test accuracy in Table 19-2 are the most critical and also the most difficult to attain. This fact narrows the list of viable instruments to fewer than about 20, and the better of these are described below. It may not be necessary to point out that standards for screening test accuracy, sensitivity and specificity are lower than for most medical screens. This is due to limitations inherent in the one-time measurement of child development (which is somewhat akin to hitting a moving target), to development's age-related manifestations, and to children's changing psychosocial risk status. Screens are designed to be administered longitu-

dinally; therefore it is anticipated, although not yet proven, that repeated administrations (e.g., at each well-child visit) will lead to higher detection rates. Nevertheless, sensitivity of 70 to 80 percent represents a dramatic improvement over the below-30 percent detection rates found in epidemiologic studies.[10]

Effective Screens for Primary Care

Some of the most efficient tools for primary care rely on information from parents. Parent-based measures circumvent the challenges of trying to directly elicit skills from children who may be uncooperative, fearful, asleep, or even sick. Such instruments can be mailed home along with appointment reminder letters; or they can be completed in waiting rooms and sent home in preparation for a follow-up visit in response to the unexpected "oh by the way" query that disrupts patient flow. They can be administered by interview when translators are needed or when literacy is a problem, or completed over

Table 19-2

Criteria for Accurate Screening Tools

- Have a clear set of directions so that different examiners can administer the test in an identical manner.
- Are standardized by administering the measure to hundreds if not thousands of children around the country. The collective performance of this group forms the test's "norms," establishing what is average or typical for each age level.
- Have been administered alongside diagnostic measures of development including measures of intelligence, language, and motor skills. The relationship between these criterion or "gold standard" measures is shown via correlations that ideally approach .70 or greater. This process is also used to eliminate redundant items and/or to help calibrate test scoring.
- Are tested for reliability across examiners and over short time intervals. Ideally agreement should be 80% or better.
- Show adequate sensitivity to psychosocial problems (meaning that at least 70 to 80 percent of children with disabilities are detected).
- Have adequate specificity to normal development (meaning that at least 70 to 80 percent of children without disabilities are correctly identified by passing scores).

the telephone with families who fail to seek well-child care routinely. The flexibility with which parent-based measures can be administered has tremendous advantages for busy practices, substantially reducing the time required for professionals to administer tests.

Nevertheless, some providers worry about the accuracy of tools relying exclusively on responses from parents. How well can parents with limited education, minimal experience at parenting, or high levels of anxiety or depression provide quality information about their child? A substantial amount of research shows that parents—despite differences in well-being, experience, and education—are well able to give accurate information provided that the questions asked of them are well constructed. In addition, almost all parents compare their child to others and often do this in pediatric waiting rooms. Because comparisons are a simple task cognitively and involve only matching and discriminating (in contrast with having to recall milestones, invoke Piagetian developmental theory, etc.), this phenomenon seems to explain why parents, regardless of differences in education levels and experience, are able to provide quality information about their children.

Even so, dependence on parent-based instruments can be a problem when literacy is limited and parents are asked to complete measures in writing. Many such parents will omit items in questionnaires, respond randomly (e.g., by circling yes or no capriciously), or fail to return their questionnaires in an attempt to conceal their own reading difficulties. To circumvent this, some test authors advise asking parents, prior to giving them a questionnaire, a question such as, "Would you like to complete this form on your own or have someone go through it with you?" Another way to limit the effect of poor reading skills is to select measures written at the fifth-grade level or below. This will ensure that more than 90 percent of parents will be able read and comprehend them.[15]

Developmental and Behavioral Screening Tools for Primary Care

MEASURES RELYING ON INFORMATION FROM PARENTS

Below is a brief description of several tools that meet standards for screening test accuracy, rely on information from parents, and take 10 or fewer minutes to complete. All are broad-band tools, meaning that they measure almost all developmental domains: language, motor, cognition, socialization, and adaptive behavior. Few of the developmental tools also measure behavioral and emotional problems; therefore two separate measures of this domain are presented below.

Ages and Stages Questionnaire, 2nd ed., 1996. Paul H. Brookes, Publishers, P.O. Box 10624, Baltimore, MD 21285 (phone: 1-800-638-3775, fax: 1-410-337-8539) ($190). (http://www.pbrookes.com/catalog/books/asq2.htm)

For children 0 to 5 years of age, the ASQ provides clear drawings and directions for eliciting thoughtful responses. Separate forms in English, Spanish and French include 36 to 37 items for each age within in the American Academy of Pediatrics well-child visit schedule. The ASQ provides separate cutoffs in each of five domains: communication, gross motor skills, fine motor skills, problem solving, and personal social skills. Scoring modifications are available for screening children whose ages fall between the specified intervals. Well standardized and validated, the measure produces high levels of sensitivity and specificity. A separate behavior measure was also developed by the same authors for children in the 0- to 5-year age range. Training videos are also available.

Child Development Inventories (CDIs), 1992. Behavior Science Systems, Box 580274, Minneapolis, MN 55458 (phone: 1-612-929-6220) ($41).

Developed by the Department of Family Practice Medicine at the University of Minnesota, the CDIs include three separate measures with 60 items each (the Infant Development Inventory, 0 to 21 months; Early Child Development Inventory, 15 to 36 months; and the Preschool Development Inventory, 36 to 72 months). All are completed by parental report in about 5 to 10 min. The CDIs can be self-administered in waiting or exam rooms or mailed to families. The CDIs screen for language, motor, cognitive, preacademic, social, and self-help skills.

The forms for older children have a behavior and health checklist. Although these items do not provide cutoff scores, the individual items are helpful in making referral and intervention decisions on patients with problematic performance on the developmental portion of the measures.

The infant version provides a cutoff score in each domain while forms for the older two age groups produce a single cutoff score tied to 1.5 standard deviations below the mean. Clinicians must then analyze errors to determine the domains in which children are having the most difficulty in order to make appropriate referrals (e.g., fine motor deficits might dictate an occupational therapy referral, while global deficits dictate the need for comprehensive assessment).

Parents' Evaluation of Developmental Status (PEDS)(1997). Ellsworth and Vandermeer Press, Ltd., PO Box 68164, Nashville, TN 37206 (phone: 1-615-226-4460, fax: 1-615-227-0411) (http://www.pedstest.com)

This 10-item measure for children 0 to 8 years of age makes use of parents' concerns or judgments about their child's developmental and behavioral status. This is an important approach because parents often need encouragement to answer sensitive questions and may not respond the first time they are asked. Across several studies, about 40 percent of parents report having concerns but not sharing them with their child's health care provider. PEDS addresses this by providing multiple opportunities for parents to share concerns. To these concerns are assigned probabilities of delays or disabilities linked to optimal responses from health care providers. PEDS takes about 2 min to elicit and score, less if parents complete it on their own. Items are written at the fifth-grade level in both Spanish and English and more than 90 percent of parents can complete it independently. PEDS is both a developmental/behavioral screen and a surveillance tool that helps clinicians make a broad range of evidenced-based decisions about the kinds of in-office services to provide: when to refer and where, when to give parents advice about child-rearing and developmental stimulation, when reassurance is needed, when children should be monitored more vigilantly than usual, and when additional screening is needed.

One of the two PEDS forms is used to follow children longitudinally and enables professionals to keep track of decision making and activities related to detecting and addressing difficulties. A detailed manual provides direction for counseling parents, offers sources of patient education materials, gives guidance on explaining screening and diagnostic test results, and includes information about the tool's validity, standardization, sensitivity (74 to 79 percent) across age groups, and specificity (70 to 80 percent).[16]

MEASURES THAT DIRECTLY ELICIT SKILLS FROM CHILDREN

Some providers are less than comfortable relying on information from parents, despite the accuracy, validity, brevity, and flexibility of the approach, especially for busy clinics. Others have the time and personnel to deploy lengthier measures that require children to demonstrate their skills overtly. Pediatric training programs often require residents and medical students to administer directly elicited measures as a way to teach development and behavior. Many physicians also serve on advisory boards for agencies that serve developmentally delayed children, and may need to recommend a range of tools. To address the needs and interest of these professionals, the following is a description of tests that meet standards for screening measures and rely either completely or in large part on eliciting skills from children.

Battelle Developmental Inventory Screening Test (BDIST) (1984). Riverside Publishing Company, 8420 Bryn Mawr Avenue, Chicago, IL 60631 (phone: 1-800-767-8378) ($99.00 + $270 if materials kit is purchased but test stimuli can be obtained for about $50 by shopping at discount department stores).

For ages 12 to 96 months, these items use a combination of direct assessment, observation, and parental interview. The receptive language subtest may serve as a brief prescreen. The BDIST is difficult to administer and users will need training and/or should work through practice exercises. The measure takes 15 min for younger children and 35 min for older ones. Well standardized and validated, the BDIST has appropriate levels of sensitivity at all age groups (70 to 80 percent) when using the cutoffs tied to performance at 1.5 standard deviations below the mean. The BDIST also produces age-equivalent scores, although these appear deflated especially in the motor domains.

Brigance Screens (1997). Curriculum Associates, Inc. (1985) 153 Rangeway Road, P.O. Box 2001, North Billerica, MA 01862-090 (1-800-225-0248) ($248.55). (http://www.curriculumassociates.com/)

Designed for children between 21 and 90 months of age (a 0- to 24-month version will be available in the year 2001), the Brigance Screens have separate forms, one for each 12-month age range. Items tap speech-language, motor, readiness, and general knowledge at younger ages and also reading and math at older ages. The measure has been translated into multiple languages including Vietnamese, Laotian, Tagalog, Spanish, etc. The Brigance Screens produce cut-off and age-equivalent scores for motor, language, and readiness and an overall cutoff. Well validated and standardized, the measure also meets standards for screening-test accuracy at all age levels. In conjunction with teacher ratings, the Brigance Screens can also identify children who are academically talented and intellectually gifted. Often used in Head Start and other early stimulation programs, the Brigance Screens include a method for monitoring progress and for deciding when at-risk and delayed children who are already in early stimulation programs need further assessment. The tests take 10 to 15 min to administer. Training videos are also available.

Bayley Infant Neurodevelomental Screen (BINS) (1995). The Psychological Corporation, 555 Academic Court, San Antonio, TX 78204 (1-800-228-0752) ($195). (http://www.psychcorp.com)

The BINS is designed for children 3 to 24 months of age and involves 10 to 13 directly elicited items per 3- to 6-month age range. The BINS assess neurologic processes (reflexes and tone), neurodevelopmental skills (movement and symmetry), and developmental accomplishments (object permanence, imitation, and language). For each area, the BINS produces cut scores of low, moderate, or high risk. The test has high levels of specificity and sensitivity. Excellent training videotapes are available that can greatly assist naive examiners in learning to give the test accurately. Assuming reasonable cooperation on the child's part, the measure takes 10 to 15 min. A parent report version is under development.

Developmental Detection Tools for Use with Older Students

It is difficult to justify the administration to older patients of developmental screening tests. The reason is that most students of first-grade age or older are administered, annually or biannually, group achievement tests through the schools.

These are comprehensive and detailed and often involve 3 to 9 hours of testing across broad academic areas. This is far more information than a busy physician could hope to derive during even an extended office visit. However, it is worthwhile for physicians to obtain and interpret the results of group achievement tests (scores can be readily obtained by calling the school). Schools rarely use the scores to screen individual children. Instead, the results are used to evaluate the performance of entire schools, counties, and states. Teachers, because they generally work with children for only 1 year at a time, do not often have the background information—family and developmental history—to interpret the results meaningfully for each of their students.

The process of scrutinizing group achievement test scores for possible evidence of learning disabilities, slow learning, giftedness, language problems, mental health difficulties, attention-deficit hyperactivity disorder, poor study skills, and the host of other deterrents to good school performance have been described in detail elsewhere.[17,18] Even so, not all states offer annual or biannual group achievement testing. In these cases or when gathering information from parents or teachers is less than helpful, pediatricians may want to consider having, as part of their screening test arsenal, a measure of academic skills such as the one described below.

Comprehensive Inventory of Basic Skills-Revised (CIBS-R) (1996). Screener Curriculum Associates, Inc., 153 Rangeway Road, P.O. Box 2001, North Billerica, MA 01862-090 (1-800-225-0248) ($214) (http://www.curriculumassociates.com/)

The CIBS-R screener is designed for students in first through sixth grades (ages 6 to 13). The screener requires the examiner to obtain teacher ratings (below average, average, above average) and to administer three subtests (reading comprehension, sentence writing, and calculation), two of which can be administered in a group setting. In addition to standard scores, per-

centiles, and age and grade equivalents for these subtests, it is also possible to derive a score for information processing—the rate at which students read, compute, or write. The measure takes 10 to 15 min to give and has high levels of accuracy in detecting a range of developmental disabilities.

Screening Tests of Behavior/ Emotional Development

There is substantial overlap between behavioral and developmental problems. Children referred to psychiatric services have a 50 percent risk of communication problems and children referred to speech-language centers have a 44 to 50 percent chance of having psychiatric problems. Conditions such as learning disabilities also carry a high psychological comorbidity, often manifest as loss of self-esteem or depression. Thus, children observed to have emotional and behavioral difficulties should be carefully screened for developmental problems, while those with developmental problems need careful assessment of their psychological well-being and behavior. The following two measures are useful for evaluating behavioral and emotional status. Both are broad-band and screen for a range of difficulties.

Eyberg Child Behavior Inventory (2000). Psychological Assessment Resources, Inc. P.O. Box 998, Odessa, Florida 33556 ($68.00) (http://www.parinc.com) (1-800-331-8378)

Designed for children 2 to 11 years of age but best used only in the 2 to 6-year age range, the ECBI consists of 36 short statements of common behavior problems responded to by parental report. Items sample internalizing (depression, anxiety, or adjustment) and externalizing (attention, conduct, aggression, etc.), although the measure has been validated only against externalizing disorders. More than 16 problems suggests the need to refer to either mental health or behavioral interventions. Fewer than 16 enables the measure to function as a problems list that can be addressed with in-office counseling and handouts.

Jellinek MS, Murphy JM, Robinson J, et al: Pediatric Symptom Checklist [PSC]: screening school age children for psychosocial dysfunction. *J Pediatr* 112: 201–209, 1988 (the test is included in the article) or freely downloadable at http://dbpeds.org/screening.html

The PSC is designed for children 4 to 16 years of age and consists of 35 short statements of problem behaviors (including those which are internalizing versus externalizing). For children above age 6, the PSC also serves as a developmental screen and identifies children with school failure. Parents rate items as never/sometimes/often. A value of 0, 1, or 2 is assigned and a score of 28 or more dictates the need to refer.

Screening Home Environments

The clear relationship between the child-rearing skills of parents and children's emotional and developmental health suggests that it is advisable to stay abreast of environmental contributors to children's developmental and behavioral status. For example, knowing whether parents are divorcing, bereaved, struggling with depression, or have limited child-rearing skills can help providers make decisions about families' needs for counseling or other supportive services. Some pediatric clinics use screens such as those described below as routine intake questionnaires. One advantage to this approach is that parents may be more likely to disclose problems such as depression or history of physical/sexual abuse as a child in paper-pencil questionnaires than in verbal interviews.[19]

Kemper, KJ, Kelleher KJ: Family psychosocial screening: instruments and techniques. *Ambul Child Health* 4:325–339, 1996 (the measure is included in the article. (http://www.achjournal.org) or can be freely downloaded at http://www.pedstest.com

The Family Psychosocial Screen includes a series of validated items drawn from several studies conducted by Dr. Kathi Kemper and colleagues. The validated questions include: (1) a four item measure of parental history of physical abuse as a child,[20] (2) a six item measure of parental substance abuse,[21] and (3) a three item measure of maternal depression.[22]

Coons CE, Gay EC, Fandal AW, et al: *Home Screening Questionnaire* (HSQ). (1981). Denver Developmental Materials, Inc. P.O. Box 6919, Denver, CO 80206 (1-303-355-4729) ($18).

Designed for children 0 to 6 years of age, the HSQ uses parental report to identify children at risk for delays due to negative environmental influences. Items were selected to be predictive of the HOME Inventory (which requires a home visit). The HSQ was standardized on 1501 children from low-income families. Subsequent studies found it to correlated highly with developmental status and social competence after the age of 15 months. The test has good sensitivity but only fair specificity to developmental/behavioral status and may be best used to assess home environment in order to refine intervention plans.

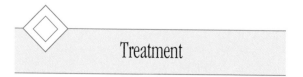

Treatment

Early Intervention and Early Stimulation

Early intervention is the optimal treatment for children with disabilities and for those at risk for disabilities due to psychosocial disadvantage. Although intervention services can take many forms, most are multidisciplinary in nature and the better programs have a strong family training component.

Research shows a strong dose-response relationship for treatment. Those who attend longer and more frequently have substantially better outcomes. For children who are at risk, early intervention or early stimulation, as most such programs are designated (e.g., Head Start, Even Start, Success by Six, or even good-quality day care), usually elevates IQ and school achievement, although these gains may "wash out" if not supported by ongoing family training and subsequent individualized educational programming. However, even when short-term IQ and academic gains are not maintained, early intervention continues to have substantial long-term benefits. Participants are much more likely to graduate from high school, hold jobs, and avoid teen childbearing and criminality.[7] Indeed, for every 2 years of early stimulation services prior to kindergarten, society saves approximately $100,000.[8]

Much like children at risk, those with disabilities also benefit from early and ongoing intervention. For this group, the savings to society for early intervention carry a value of about $30,000, which reflects lessened need for intensive and expensive special education programs later in life, increased likelihood of living independently, and of being employed. This price tag does not reflect the many improvements in family functioning and well-being that usually accompany involvement in early intervention programs. Overall, the value of early intervention is sufficiently clear that Congress, through IDEA and the Americans with Disabilities Act (ADA), has invested heavily in programs ensuring that every young child with a disability has access to a free and appropriate public education. In recent years, early stimulation programs have also enjoyed an improvement in congressional largesse that has enabled a modest expansion of Head Start services, federally subsidized day care centers, and special education services through the public schools.

Diagnostic Services

Schools have a range of diagnostic services (i.e., speech-language pathologists, psychologists, occupational and physical therapists), which can be facilitated by a letter from a physician to the school's psychologist, principal, and/or district special education director. Ideally such correspondence should document hearing and vision status, since schools must have information on this before testing for other disabilities. If there is a medical diagnosis (e.g., spastic diplegia), it is important to mention the possible category of eligibility (e.g., physical impairment) to ensure communication. Schools also have, under IDEA, 40 days in which to complete testing and arrange for placement. Mentioning this in a referral letter should promote expeditious service delivery. Schools may opt first, however, to attempt modifications in the classroom before offering testing.

Interventions

Services through the public schools cascade from least restrictive, meaning that children are completely mainstreamed or included in the activities of nondisabled peers, to most restrictive, which refers to a virtual absence of contact between children with and without disabilities. There are essentially ten options for special education placements. These are listed in Table 19-3, along with a brief description of each. In addition, there are numerous "related services" that can be added to each child's program, as shown in Table 19-4.

Placement and service decisions are made by a Multidisciplinary (M-)Team, an ad hoc group consisting of teachers, parents, sometimes the child, and often other relevant professionals (e.g., the school psychologist, special education director, pediatricians, speech-therapists, etc.). The M-Team devises an Individual Family Service Plan (IFSP) for children between ages 0 and 3 or an Individual Educational Plan (IEP) for children between 3 and 22 years of age. These plans list placement(s) and related services. Each child's IFSP/IEP also includes goals and objectives, to which a responsible person is

Table 19-3

Program Options for Students Receiving Special Education Services

PLACEMENT	EXAMPLE/DESCRIPTION
Special teacher consults with regular classroom teacher	Designs a behavior management program for a student with ADHD.
Special materials in the regular classroom	Tape-recorded or large-print books, access to a computer with checking of spelling and grammar, reduced writing assignments, oral tests, weekly progress reports, etc.
Special teacher works with student in the regular classroom	Instructional aide, nursing services, inclusion model services
Speech-language therapy	Student leaves regular classroom for typically 1–2 h per week for individual or small group instruction.
Resource services	Student leaves regular classroom for typically 1–4 h per week for individualized and remedial instruction, ideally at studentís current level of achievement (which may be substantially below grade placement, requiring instructional materials usually not available to regular educators).
Self-contained special classroom	Student attends a regular public school and may have mainstreaming often during nonacademic activities such as art, music, library, physical education. Self-contained classrooms may have kitchens, showers, laundry facilities and other equipment necessary for teaching critical life skills to students with comprehensive disabilities.
Consultation from outside agency	Can include on-site and direct intervention from mental health or other professionals or advice to educators from specialists in rarer conditions such as autism. In some (often rural settings) students may leave the school building for services.
Special school	More common in urban areas, special schools may be devoted exclusively to students—for example, with physical disabilities and mental retardation or severe emotional disturbance—and enable school systems to amalgamate needed resources (e.g., the P.E. coach may be a physical therapist, a nurse may be on the staff prepared to assist with gastrostomy-tube feedings, catheterization, tracheostomy-tube cleaning, etc.
Residential school	Provides continuous (24 h per day) intervention for students with severe disabilities. Often such placements are temporary and devoted to highly-intensive instruction that enables students to return to less restrictive placements (e.g., toilet training, reduction of self-injurious, violent, or combative behavior)
Home-bound instruction	Involves a visiting educator who comes to each student's home, usually for 3–9 h per week at most. Because home-bound instruction is less than intense and requires the family to be present, it is best reserved for students who are immunocompromised, in traction, or otherwise temporarily but nonacutely ill.

Table 19-4

Related Services Offered through the Individuals with Disabilities Education Act

- Physical therapy
- Occupational therapy   } must be ordered by a physician
- Medications or medical interventions at school
- Speech-language therapy
- Parent training
- Parent counseling
- Social work services
- Psychotherapy
- Special transportation
- Extended school year (usually requires evidence of regression or failure to maintain skills)
- Rehabilitation counseling (career/employment preparation, orientation and mobility training, etc.)
- Recreational therapy
- Audiologic evaluations
- Assistive technology (communication devices, wheelchairs, word processing, training of families and school personnel in the use of augmentative systems, etc). Note that hearing aids are not included.

assigned (e.g., the child's teacher). IFSPs/IEPs are reviewed annually by the M-Team to assess progress, determine new goals, and decide whether changes in services and placements are needed.

Challenges and Issues

Despite IDEA's many strengths, there are some noteworthy weaknesses. The first is that certain developmental problems are addressed only partially or not at all. For example, a child with cerebral palsy or other motor coordination disorder whose written language problems are surmounted with an adaptive word processor may also have substantial difficulties with activities of daily living (e.g., buttoning, feeding, dressing) due to fine motor deficits. However, the school's occupational therapist is not obligated to address these nonacademic difficulties, especially in higher-functioning students. An even more disturbing omission is visible for students who are considered slow learners—i.e., IQs

between 74 and 85 (4th to 16th percentiles). These children, in a classroom of 30 or fewer, are likely to be the lowest performers and to be working several grade levels below grade placement—which means that most are given work that is too difficult for their levels of skills—a phenomenon that usually leads to very little if any new learning. Serious secondary problems with self-esteem are a common result and can lead to aggressive and/or depressive behavior and often to high school dropout. Yet, such children are rarely eligible for special education services, since they do not meet eligibility criteria for learning disabilities, mental retardation, language impairment, etc.

A second challenge arising from IDEA is that one of its central goals, as with any other civil rights legislation, is to integrate disabled children, a segregated minority, into the larger society. This means that special education personnel must strive for mainstreamed placements. The fact that mainstream placements are almost always less expensive often prompts schools to recommend them to excess. This may result in a child receiving services that are insufficient to promote learning.

A final and related challenge in special education laws is that parental advocacy is needed to ensure that children receive optimal services. Parents who are intimidated, depressed, lacking in self-efficacy, or too trusting may not be able to argue adequately for sufficient interventions.

To address the limitations of public school services, primary care physicians may need to consider a range of responses. Table 19-5 contains suggestions for helping address unmet student needs.

Table 19-5

Suggestions for Tailoring Educational Interventions to Meet Patients' Needs

1. Look for low- or no-cost programs for children who need help but are not eligible for special education services and for those at risk. These may include after-school literacy programs (e.g., through community centers), Head Start, summer school, Title 1 Reading and Math (remedial programs available in low-income elementary schools), etc. In addition, children who are at chronic risk of school failure need opportunities for success in other areas and may benefit from opportunities to volunteer or participate in sports, fine arts or music, to learn vocational and prevocational skills, etc.
2. Marshal private resources when needed. For example, insurance may cover private physical therapy, which can focus on daily living skills, sensory intergration, and other needs not addressed in school-based physical therapy. For parents with fiscal resources, after-school tutoring and summer school can help speed progress.
3. Refer parents for advocacy training or provide patient education materials for parents of special education students. A website that has information for parents on Individuals with Disabilities Education Act is available (http://www.nectas.unc.edu/); it includes information on where to locate service providers.
4. Refer families to parenting organizations for help with advocacy and for practical support/information. A website (http://www.hood.edu/seri/assoc.htm) is available for information on parenting groups, such as the Orton Dyslexia Society, Children and Adults with Attention Deficit Disorders (CHADD), the Autism Society, and the American Speech-Language-Hearing Association (ASHA). In addition, another website (http://www.nectas.unc.edu/) offers information about state-wide Parent Training and Information Centers (PTI's) and Community Parent Resource Centers (CPRCs) in the United States.
5. Communicate directly with school personnel via letters and phone calls in order to share recommendations regarding placement, obtain information on patient functioning, and build collegial relationships with educators.
6. For students not qualifying for special education, request Screening-(S-)Team services under the Americans with Disabilities Act (ADA). This law allows for modifications in the regular classroom that should help students benefit more completely from instruction (e.g., access to a calculator or word processor checking of spelling and grammar, tape-recorded books, reduced writing assignments, and altered curricula—for example provision of second-grade material for students with delays who have been passed on to higher grades, a behavior management programs in the regular classroom, peer tutoring, extra time to complete assignments, help with organizational skills such as daily or weekly progress reports sent from school to home, etc. Such modifications can help to avoid in-grade retention, a common recommendation for students with academic delays and one that may incur benefits when offered in kindergarten or first grade but is otherwise associated with increased rates of high school dropout.

Prevention

Anticipatory Guidance and Developmental Promotion

Parents view physicians as a primary source for information about child development and behavior, even more so when children have developmental delays.[2] Recognizing this, the American Academy of Pediatrics[8] and the *Bright Futures* guidelines[23] encourage providers to offer anticipatory guidance and to otherwise promote optimal development during each well-child visit. The goals of these efforts are to teach parenting skills, facilitate family functioning and well-being, and promote children's learning, development, and behavioral self-control. In so doing, it may be that many emerging developmental and behavioral problems will be averted and prevented.

Although these are lofty goals, there are brief and effective methods for accomplishing these tasks. Much of this has to do with giving parents information when and how they need it via clear verbal advice, written information, modeling and role playing, videotapes, and group well visits.[24] Table 19-6 provides information about such methods and the materials needed. When these methods are not effective (e.g., when

Table 19-6

Providing Developmental Promotion, Anticipatory Guidance, and Surveillance in Primary Care Settings

1. Ask parents to complete parent-report instruments while in waiting or exam rooms and arrange for office staff to routinely distribute these to every family.
2. Mail parent-based tests in advance of well visits so that the visit itself can be devoted to interpreting results, devising treatment plans, identifying resources, etc. Allowing parents to complete measures at home often improves the quality of parent report because families have additional time to respond. Advance mailings can also be helpful with families whose English is limited because they can usually find someone in the community to help translate items.
3. Tape-record directions and items on parent-report instruments and use of simplified answer sheets to circumvent illiteracy. Tape-recorded translations may be a helpful approach in practices where many parents speak little English.
4. Train office staff to administer and even score screening tests.
5. Set up return visits devoted to screening when developmental concerns are raised unexpectedly toward the end of an encounter. A similar alternative is to have office staff call families after an encounter and administer a screen over the telephone.
6. Maintain a current list of telephone numbers for local service providers (e.g., speech-language centers, school psychologists, mental health centers, private psychologists and psychiatrists, parent training classes, etc.).
7. For children in the 0- to 3-year age range, refer to your local early intervention system under Part B of the Individuals with Disabilities Education Act (see http://www.nectas.unc.edu). This program provides diagnostic testing and arranges for early intervention, social services, mental health programs, etc. For children 3 years of age and older, contact the department of special education at your school board to obtain screening, diagnostic, and intervention services. These are provided without cost to families.

(continued)

Table 19-6 concluded

8. Acquire brochures from local service providers. Making these available to families when needed may promote parental follow-through on referral suggestions.

9. See Glascoe et al.(1998) in the electronic pages of *Pediatrics* for a list of hypertext links to on-line patient education materials, many of which can be downloaded and used as information handouts. (http://www.pediatrics.org/cgi/content/full/101/6/e10)

10. Several texts that include patient education handouts are listed below: Schmitt B: *Instructions for Patient Education*, 2nd ed., contains several hundred 1- and 2-page handouts. (W.B.Saunders Co., Independence Square West, Philadelphia 19106); (phone: 1-800-545-2522)($42.95) (http://www.patienteducation.com). Dr. Schmitt contributes a new handout to almost every issue of *Contemporary Pediatrics*. [To subscribe, call 1-800-432-4570, or write to Circulation Department, Medical Economics, Five Paragon Drive, Montvale, NJ 07645 ($89.00 per year)].

Wycoff J, Unell B: *Discipline Without Shouting or Spanking*. This simple and inexpensive text ($6.00) is written at the fourth- to fifth-grade level and includes short 2- to 5-page chapters on behavioral problems that make very effective handouts. These give not only guidance but also very helpful examples. (Simon & Schuster, 1230 Avenue of the Americas, NY, NY 10020; phone: 1-800-223-2336. (www.amazon.com)

11. Keep parent information sheets handy. Some clinics keep them in plastic binders (so that originals are not lost). When an issue arises, the originals can be easily retrieved, copied (reread on the way back to the exam room in order to provide a refresher on the contents), and then highlighted and delivered to parents.

12. Collaborate with local service providers (e.g., day care centers, Head Start, public health clinics, department of human services workers, etc.) to establish communitywide child-find programs that use valid, accurate screening instruments.

13. Consider having a website for your office on which parents can complete and send forms prior to a visit.

SOURCE: Glascoe FP: *Collaborating with Parents: Using Parents' Evaluation of Development Status to Detect and Address Developmental and Behavioral Problems.* Nashville, TN, Ellsworth & Vandermeer Press, Ltd, 1998, by permission.

parents need more intensive assistance), health care professionals also need to have a list of local resources such as parenting groups, mental health centers, early stimulation programs, and developmental/behavioral assessment centers. Although many health care professionals lack confidence that such services are available in their communities, it is important to remember that most are mandated under federal law (e.g., Head Start, community mental health centers, services under ADA and IDEA). Brief investigation with the director of special education at the local school board or even through the yellow pages will yield a surprising number and range of referral options. Arranging for professionals from unfamiliar services to present briefly at a pediatric society meeting can help bridge gaps among providers. Ultimately such efforts will create a more seamless mesh of developmental/behavioral services that flow readily to and from health care professionals and that ultimately ensure quality intervention for children with developmental and behavioral problems.

References

1. U.S. Department of Education. *Eighteenth Annual Report to Congress on the Implementation of the Individuals with Disabilities Education Act.* Washington, DC, US Government

Printing Office, 1996. (http://www.ed.gov/pubs/OSEP96AnlRpt)

2. Boyle CA, Decouflé P, Yeargin-Allsop, M: Prevalence and health impact of developmental disabilities in us children. *Pediatrics* 93:399–403, 1994.

3. Newacheck PW, Strickland B, Shonkoff JP, et al: An epidemiologic profile of children with special health care needs. *Pediatrics* 102:117–123, 1998.

4. US Bureau of the Census. *School Enrollment* Washington, DC, US Government Printing Office, 1998.

5. Sameroff AJ, Seifer R, Barocas R, et al: Intelligence quotient scores of 4-year-old children: social-environmental risk factors. *Pediatrics* 79:343–350, 1987.

6. Roberts JE, Burchinal MR, Zeisel SA, et al: Otitis media, the caregiving environment, and language and cognitive outcomes at 2 years. *Pediatrics* 102:346–354, 1998.

7. Ramey CT, Bryant DM, Wasik BH, et al: Infant health and development program for low birth weight, premature infants: program elements, family participation, and child intelligence. *Pediatrics* 89:454–465, 1992.

8. Glascoe, FP, Foster M, Wolraich ML: An economic analysis of developmental detection methods. *Pediatrics* 99:830–837, 1997.

9. American Academy of Pediatrics. Committee on Practice and Ambulatory Medicine: Recommendations for preventative pediatric health care. *Pediatrics* 81:466–470, 1988.

10. Palfrey JS, Singer JD, Walker DK, Butler JA: Early identification of children's special needs: a study in five metropolitan communities. *J Pediatr* 111:651–655, 1994.

11. Borowitz KC, Glascoe FP: The insensitivity of the Denver Developmental Screening Test in speech and language screening. *Pediatrics* 78:1075–1078, 1986.

12. American Psychological Association: *Standards for Educational and Psychological Tests*. Washington, DC, American Psychological Association, 1985.

13. Barnes KE: *Preschool screening: The Measurement and Prediction of Children at Risk*. Springfield, IL: Charles C Thomas, 1982.

14. Squires J, Nickel RE, Eisert D: Early detection of developmental problems: strategies for monitoring young children in the practice setting. *Journal of Developmental and Behavioral Pediatrics*, 17:420–427, 1996.

15. Davis TC, Mayeaux EJ, Fredrickson D, et al: Reading ability of parents compared with reading level of pediatric patient education materials. *Pediatrics* 93:460–468, 1994.

16. Glascoe F P: *Collaborating with Parents: Using Parents' Evaluations of Developmental Status to Detect and Address Developmental and Behavioral Problems*. Nashville, TN: Ellsworth & Vandermeer Press, Ltd., 1998.

17. Glascoe FP. Detecting developmental and school problems, in Wolraich ML (ed). *Disorders of Development and Learning: A Practical Guide to Assessment and Management*, 2nd ed. Chicago, Mosby–Year Book, 1996.

18. Glascoe FP: Developmental, behavioral and educational surveillance, in Green M, Haggerty B, Weitzman M (eds). *Ambulatory Pediatrics*, 5th ed. Philadelphia, Saunders, 1999.

19. Kemper KJ: Self-administered questionnaire for structured psychosocial screening in pediatrics. *Pediatrics* 89:433–436, 1992.

20. Kemper KJ, Carlin AS, Babonis T, Buntain-Ricklefs J: Screening for maternal experiences of physical abuse during childhood. *Clin Pediatr* 33:333–339, 1994.

21. Kemper KJ, Greteman A, Bennett E, Babonis TR: Screening mothers of young children for substance abuse. *J Dev Behav Disord* 14:308–312, 1993.

22. Kemper KJ, Babonis TR: Screening for maternal depression in pediatric clinics. *Am J Dis Child* 146:876–878, 1992.

23. Green M (ed): *Bright Futures: Guidelines for Health Supervision of Infants, Children, and Adolescents*. Alexandria VA; National Center for Education Materials and Child Health, 1994.

24. Glascoe FP, Oberklaid F, Dworkin PH, Trimm F: Brief approaches to educating parents and patients in primary care. *Pediatrics* 101:10, 1991. (http://www.pediatrics.org/cgi/content/full/101/6/e10)

Ronald L. Lindsay

Chapter 20

School Failure/ Disorders of Learning

How Common are School Failure and Learning Disorders?

Disorders of learning and school failure are the most common disorders of higher cortical function in childhood. In the United States in 1998, special education programs served 5.1 million school age children, ages 6–17, or 11 percent of the estimated population. In the past decade (1987–1997) the number of children involved in programs for students with disabilities increased by 30 percent. In 1998, some 2.6 million children or 5.6 percent of the estimated enrollment had specific learning disabilities. This prevalence is probably an underestimate because it does not account for children who have not been identified, children with learning disabilities who do not meet state criteria to qualify for special education services, those who receive services under a different category, and those who drop out of school. Roughly twice as many boys are diagnosed formally, a ratio that is possibly biased. In a typical pediatric practice, if a clinician sees 20 to 25 patients a day, at least 2 or 3 patients will be enrolled in special education services in school. Their learning problems can be subtle and can be undetected into adulthood, becoming symptomatic in college or graduate school. In fact, with their neurologic basis, learning disorders are now considered to be lifelong conditions rather than exclusively pediatric problems. *Indeed, instead of* outgrowing *learning disabilities, it would be more true to say that children* grow into *them.*

The Roles of Clinicians

Developing success in school is critical for children and adolescents. Needless anxiety occurs when a child performs inadequately in school.

Children who experience learning problems and school failure are especially prone to behavioral and emotional problems that outweigh the learning difficulties that generated them. Among these problems are a loss of self-confidence, discouragement, and decreased effort, all contributing to a downward spiral that can lead to lifelong tragic consequences. Despite this relevance to and impact on general well-being, many parents simply do not view the clinician's office as an appropriate setting in which to raise concerns about their child's learning. Unfortunately, many clinicians share this view.

HISTORY

It has been a quarter-century since the recognition of the "new morbidity," i.e., the need by clinicians to give greater attention to the prevention, early detection, and management of developmental and behavioral problems encountered in primary care. Yet many clinicians remain uncomfortable dealing with these issues. Clinicians vary widely in the nature and extent of their experience with school failure and learning disabilities. It was not until 1987 that pediatric residency programs were required to include training in developmental and behavioral problems. It took 12 more years, to 1999, for the fields of developmental disabilities and developmental/behavioral pediatrics to be officially recognized as subspecialties.

The concept of learning disabilities grew out of the medical constructs of dyslexia, dyscalculia, and developmental aphasia. Late in the nineteenth century, select cases of a rare medical disorder referred to as *congenital word blindness* began to be reported. The conceptualization of specific neurologically based deficits in reading (dyslexia) would need to wait a decade for the development of a psychology of reading. The concept of a congenital arithmetic disability in children was first proposed in 1937. The term *dyscalculia* was coined in 1960 to refer to difficulties with numbers.

THE ROLE OF CLINICIANS IN DIAGNOSIS

With the increased number of children suspected of or diagnosed as having learning problems, clinicians have an increasingly important role in their early identification, diagnosis, and management. Clinicians are the professionals whom parents most commonly encounter in the care of infants and toddlers. The clinician is in a position to identify the developmental precursors to learning problems prior to school entry (see Chap. 19, "Developmental Delay").

Primary care clinicians are often asked to make or confirm the diagnosis of a learning disability. Parents of children encountering difficulty in school will turn to clinicians to help them deal with an educational "system" that is intimidating. Often referrals are made for the evaluation of a child with an attentional problem or to rule out other medical disorders that may mimic or be associated with learning problems. Attentional symptoms observed by parents and teachers might be a primary problem or secondary to an undiagnosed learning problem. Because there is a significant degree of comorbidity between attention-deficit/hyperactivity disorder and learning disabilities (15 to 25 percent), a medical evaluation of a child for school failure should explore for the presence of both diagnoses.

A primary care clinician can be an asset in the evaluation process as a member of or a contributor to an interdisciplinary evaluation team. After the diagnosis of a learning or attentional problem is established, the clinician may be called on to participate in the management and monitoring of the child's learning problems.

With appropriate intervention, most children can be expected to adjust to and compensate for learning problems. If the diagnosis of learning problems is made later in a child's school career and appropriate intervention is delayed, the prognosis will be more guarded. The effectiveness of schools in screening for and diagnosing learning disabilities is subject to local variation in funding and expertise and to differences in the way state boards of education define learning disabilities. In the face of this variability, it is imperative for the clinician to assume a monitoring and advocacy role in children's academic progress.

Principal Diagnoses

There is no universally accepted definition of a learning disability, which complicates the diagnosis and management of learning disorders. The lack of a common nosology is due to the multiple disciplines that contribute to the field of learning disorders: developmental pediatrics, education, psychology, occupational therapy, speech and language pathology, child neurology, and child psychiatry.

A definition of learning disabilities developed by the National Joint Committee on Learning Disabilities (NJCLD) in 1990 stated the following:

> *Learning disabilities* is a generic term that refers to a heterogeneous group of disorders manifested by significant difficulties in the acquisition and use of listening, speaking, reading, writing, reasoning, or mathematical abilities. These disorders are intrinsic to the individual, presumed to be due to central nervous system dysfunction, and may occur across the life span. Problems in self-regulatory behaviors, social perception, and social interaction may exist with learning disabilities, but do not by themselves constitute a learning disability. Although learning disabilities may occur concomitantly with other handicapping conditions (for example, sensory impairment, mental retardation, serious emotional disturbance), or with extrinsic influences (such as cultural differences, inappropriate or insufficient instruction), they are not the result of those influences or conditions.

Although considerable debate exists, educators generally accept that a fundamental characteristic of a learning disability is a discrepancy between ability and academic achievement. This is usually quantified as a difference between performance on an IQ test and tests of academic content areas (reading, mathematics, etc.), although there are varying interpretations on the size of the discrepancy sufficient to make the diagnosis. While the discrepancy approach is increasingly found to be invalid in recent research, it is the approach in common use and clinician need to be familiar with the criteria used by their state to qualify a child for services for learning problems. *Each state board of education uses its own definition; some states use a 15- or 20-point discrepancy between IQ and performance scores while others use a formula that derives the criteria based on a regression of IQ and achievement. Thus it is possible for a child to move from one state to another and either "develop" or "be cured" of a learning problem.*

In general, *learning disorders* refers to difficulties with the three R's ("reading, 'riting, and 'rithmetic"). This chapter focuses on disorders of reading (dyslexia) and arithmetic/mathematics (dyscalculia). Considerable research has been focused on dyslexia, with less attention to dyscalculia.

Various approaches to classifying these learning problems have been proposed. The neuropsychological approach involves the subtyping of learning disorders and the relationship of these subtypes with other forms of learning disorders. Research into the cognitive components of learning problems focuses on experimental studies of academic function rather than the performance of students on achievement tests. A phenomenologic approach examines the neurodevelopmental underpinnings of learning, including memory, sequential processes, language competency, higher-order cognition (problem-solving skills and strategy use), visuospatial skills, and attention.[1] A combination of these approaches can provide a reasonable framework for the clinician.

Prevalence of Learning Disorders

About 1 in 20 children are thought to have a learning disorder. The prevalence of dyscalculia is estimated to be at least 6 percent.[2–4] In one study, 6.4 percent of students demonstrated dyscalculia, while 4.9 percent had dyslexia.[3] There was some overlap in delayed skills: 2.7 percent of students were poor in both reading and mathematics, 2.2 percent were low in reading alone, while 3.6 percent were low in mathematics alone. In a nonreferred sample of students in Connecticut, 7.5 to 7.8 percent of second and third-graders respectively, were diagnosed as dyslexic.[5]

Dyslexia

Dyslexia, a language-based disorder of learning characterized by difficulties in single-word decoding, is highly associated with disorders of phonological processing abilities. A phoneme is the smallest unit of functional sound. Phonological processing has three component skills: phonological awareness (assessed by rhyming tasks), phonological recoding (assessed by rapid naming tasks), and phonemic recoding in working memory (assessed by digit- and word-span tasks). Of these three phonological processing skills, phonological awareness appears to be the most deficient language skill in children with dyslexia.

Phonological awareness is the ability to translate printed symbols or graphemes (letters or letter patterns in English) into sound. To be successful in reading, children must perceive individual language sounds with precision and speed. Children with difficulties with phonological awareness do not appreciate that speech is composed of sounds that join together to form syllables and words. If a child cannot perceive the "at" sound in *rat* and *cat* and understand that the difference is in the first sound or phoneme, then the child will not be able to decode the written word accurately and fluently.

Slow, labored, and inaccurate decoding of words will lead to poor reading comprehension.

Dyscalculia

There are at least three different profiles of neuropsychological assets and deficits leading to impaired mathematics performance in children. Children with dyscalculia fall into three categories: (1) children with difficulties with visuospatial skills, (2) children with difficulties in arithmetic fact retrieval, and (3) children with difficulties in the use of arithmetical procedures.

One group of mathematics-impaired children have relatively intact reading and spelling skills. Their poor performance on measures of visuospatial skills is suggestive of right hemispheric dysfunction and a nonverbal learning disability. The second group of mathematics-impaired children have functional deficits in procedural skills such as counting strategies, carrying, and borrowing. These procedural deficits are mediated by poor attentional and active working memory skills. The computational errors committed by these children are due to their tendency not to monitor their work when solving problems.

The third group of mathematics-impaired children have memory retrieval deficits in which they could not call up mathematics facts in an efficient, timely, and automatic manner. These children have problems such as the memorization of multiplication tables and appear to have a generalized deficit in representation or retrieval from long-term memory. Children in the last two groups (procedural and memory deficits) do well on nonverbal problem-solving tasks, have deficiencies in verbal/auditory-perceptual tasks, and have both poor arithmetic and poor reading performance.

Other Learning Problems

Two learning disorders that can frequently accompany the above patterns are dysgraphia and pragmatic language disorders. When these occur in isolation, however, they can easily be missed. Thus, children with dysgraphia or a pragmatic language disorder can receive a fairly comprehensive psychoeducational assessment through the school and not receive a diagnosis or qualify for classification as learning-disabled. It is therefore especially important for the clinician to make note of signs and symptoms of each of these disorders and encourage the parent to make sure that they are specifically addressed when appropriate.

DYSGRAPHIA

A child with dysgraphia may have a history of difficulties with drawing during preschool. Poorly structured drawings, distorted shapes, or missing details in drawings can be clues to problems with visuomotor ability or fine motor control, which can contribute to dysgraphia and impede school performance. The parent should be asked if the child has labored or sloppy handwriting. Sometimes teachers deduct points from assignment grades because of sloppiness. Asking the child to draw or, if older, having the child copy a few sentences will allow the clinician to evaluate several aspects of performance, including pencil grasp; ease of finger, hand, and wrist movement, accuracy of copying, attention to detail; and task persistence.

PRAGMATIC LANGUAGE DISORDER

Pragmatic language refers to the use of language in social contexts. It includes the nonverbal aspects of tone, rate of speech, and turn taking. Good verbal pragmatic ability on the part of a listener allows him or her to understand the true desires or intentions of the speaker or the audience.

Children with poor verbal pragmatic ability are often unable to discriminate the tone of a speaker and are thus unable to change their tone of voice, change the topic, or use appropriate language. They do not wait for or observe the nonverbal cue that it is their turn. Instead, they impulsively jump in whether or not the other person has yielded his or her turn. And frequently their rate of speech is so fast and "cluttered" that is it difficult to understand what they are attempting to say or to get a word in. This is also a form of nonverbal learning disability and frequently accompanies dyscalculia. By engaging the child in conversation during an evaluation, a clinician can gain a sense of a child's pragmatic language skills.

Comorbidity of Learning Problems with Attentional Problems

Even in the absence of cognitive processing deficits, significant educational delays can be attributed to the inability to sustain attention. There are significant relationships between dyslexia, dyscalculia, and attention. Several population studies have shown that attention deficits may be more strongly associated with dyscalculia than with dyslexia. In a nonreferred cohort of Israeli fourth graders, 26 percent of those with dyscalculia had symptoms of attention-deficit/hyperactivity disorder (ADHD)[4]; while in a nonreferred sample of students in Connecticut, only 15 percent of third-grade children diagnosed with dyslexia exhibited inattention.[5]

Although attentional problems can exacerbate the severity and consequences of dyslexia, these two disorders appear to have different etiologies. Dyslexia is now considered to be highly associated with disorders of phonological awareness. Attentional factors have only a limited association with such phonological deficits. Arithmetic computation is the area in which students with attentional problems are most likely to show diminished classroom performance, even when holding IQ, reading ability, and problem structure constant.

Nonetheless given the strong relationship between attentional and learning problems, it is prudent for students suspected of having attentional problems also to be screened for learning disorders, especially dyscalculia. Moreover, students who are encountering significant difficulty with arithmetic should have inattention ruled out as a contributing factor.

Typical Presentation

When parents call for an appointment for an evaluation of their child's difficulties at school, a number of chief complaints may be voiced. They include:

Not keeping up with classmates
Forgetting to bring home assignments or failing to turn in completed homework
Problems in following directions or failing to pay attention in class
Not being able to read or spell
Problems in solving arithmetic problems
Not having friends at school
Acting up in school
Complaints of somatic symptoms (stomachache, headache, leg pains) on school days
Distress caused by anxiety, depression, substance abuse, or sleep disorders

Here is an example of a child presenting to the office of a primary care clinician:

Jack is an 8-year-old boy who is having difficulty with reading. His parents have tried to work with him and wonder if he needs more testing. They attempted to help him by the use of flash cards. He is starting to associate single sounds with letter combinations but cannot combine the letters and sounds in order to read words. Jack's teachers report that he is very fidgety during reading lessons and does not listen at story time. The teachers want Jack started on medication immediately. Further questioning of Jack's teachers by the clinician reveals that Jack attends well in math class and enjoys participating in science projects in class. Jack is popular with his peers but refuses to accept a reading partner. When asked, Jack admits that he is worried that the reading partner will make fun of him. Jack's father also had difficulties with reading in the elementary grades.

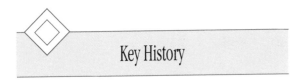

Key History

The Routine Well-Child Visit

When a parent calls the office to schedule a routine visit for a school-age child, one approach is to request that the parent bring to the appointment the child's current report card *and* the most recent full-year school report, including scores from the most recent standardized achievement battery. The receptionist can be provided with a script to inquire about possible learning concerns. If these are hinted at, the parent should be asked to bring in a letter from the child's class or home-room teacher detailing current learning and behavior. If the school has formally evaluated the child for a learning problem, it is important to obtain a copy of that assessment. Some practices request this material a week or more before the scheduled visit. Requesting this information sends a message to the family that the clinician is seriously interested in this aspect of development and can be considered an ally and a resource should problems occur.

The key item for which one should scan school records is discrepancy (1) between grades in different subject areas (the child with dyslexia will consistently perform more poorly in reading-dependent subjects while doing much better in reading-free subjects such as elementary mathematics and art); (2) between the teacher's grading of a child's performance and the effort grade for the same subject; (3) between the class grades for a subject and the standardized achievement scores (such will occur when the child has difficulty demonstrating learning achievement according to one method of grading or testing but can show that

learning has been successfully accomplished when other methods are used); and (4) in the child's performance from year to year (especially when the tendency is toward a decline in achievement over several years). Certain discrepancies, such as fluctuations in day-to-day classroom performance across all subjects, may be more suggestive of attention deficits than of learning disabilities.

During the well-child visit, the clinician should ask the parent and child about homework and extracurricular activities. It is an important sign of learning disabilities for children to be spending an unusually long time devoted to homework, especially when it interferes with life outside of school. When a large part of this homework is incomplete classwork, there is almost certainly a problem.

Prior to the Office Evaluation of Learning Difficulties

Teachers, parents, and preteen or teenage students are all valuable sources of detailed information on learning difficulties. This gathering of information from multiple sources can be a time-consuming process, but it will earn dividends at the end of the evaluation. Clinicians have limited time for history taking, so the use of questionnaires and rating scales can facilitate the gathering of this information (Table 20-1). Questionnaires and rating scales can allow some parents to air their concerns in a format that is less threatening than a formal interview. However, questionnaires should not be relied on as the sole source of information. With information from multiple sources, the clinician can develop a more complete picture of the child's current functioning in multiple environments. This information can help validate examination findings with observations from home and school. The clinician may find that there may be some disagreements between observers. Observations at home and school or by parents can be markedly different. Usually it is not that the reporters are

Table 20-1

Questionnaires and Rating Scales

Tool	Description
ACTeRS	Teacher rating scales measuring attention, hyperactivity, social skills, and oppositionality
ANSER System (Levine)	Detailed parent, school, and child (over age 9) questionnaires assessing education, health, development and behavior
Conners' Parent Symptom Questionnaire and Teacher Questionnaires	Several sets of widely used parent and teacher rating scales
Child Behavior Checklist	Parent and teacher scales measuring social competence and internal and externalizing behaviors
Levine Neurodevelopmental Examinations (PEER, PEEX 2 PEERAMID 2)	Series of structured neurodevelopmental examinations for ages 4 to 6, 6 to 9, 9 to 15
Yale Children's Inventory	Parental rating scales for school-related problems of children (11 narrow-band and two broad-band scales, behavioral and cognitive)

unreliable but that the conditions in which the observations are being made differ. One child may perform better at school because of the structured setting. Another child may perform better at home with more one-on-one help from a parent and fewer distractions (*if* the television is turned off). A father may have different perceptions of his child if most of his observations are made on the weekends or the late evenings, when there is no homework.

During the Office Visit

If the clinician can obtain and review historical data prior to the office visit, the time spent with the parent in the office can be utilized to clarify certain points. This review can also allow the clinician to structure the evaluation to best suit the needs of the child and family. Open-ended questions of a general nature can allow a parent to provide the doctor with his or her subjective experience of the child's problems and strengths. The clinician can then move to more specific, direct questioning of the parent.

The history should attempt to determine the types, severity, and possible causes of the learning problem while excluding other conditions that may imitate or be associated with the learning problem, such as attentional problems. A framework of the neurodevelopmental history is presented in Table 20-2.

The history should include a detailed exploration of prenatal and perinatal events, although these are more closely related to the development of cerebral palsy than to learning problems. There is a high prevalence of learning disorders among very low birthweight infants. The medical history should explore any chronic medical problem that could impede development. A neurologic history should be obtained to determine the presence of major neurologic events such as meningitis, seizures, or concussions. A review of early motor milestones can provide important information about the time course of the child's problems. The parents should be asked about clumsiness of fine or gross motor skills, gait problems, or difficulty with tying shoes and drawing.

Table 20-2

Framework for the Neurodevelopmental History

School
- Preschool performance. Hyperactive children have more trouble than learning disabled children.
- At which grade did the child begin to experience difficulty? Sometimes this is of gradual onset. Note that not all learning disabilities show themselves as present in first grade. Note that above average intelligence can mask or at the very least significantly delay the appearance of learning disabilities, since schools equate learning problems with failure rather than underachievement.
- Review each full report card and standardized achievement batteries at the annual physical and scan for discrepancies.

Social
- Consider the possibility that symptoms suggesting poor self-esteem, low self-image, anxiety, or depression in the younger school-age children are more likely to reflect learning problems than underlying psychopathology.

Family
- Parental educational level and employment history
- Parent, siblings, and other close relatives' early development and receipt of special education services

Preconception and prenatal
- Substance abuse
- Medication exposure
- Medical complications
- Level of prenatal care
- Genetic history: history of fetal demise

Perinatal
- Length of gestation
- Birth weight
- Complications

Medical
- Exposure to toxins (including lead)
- Sensory impairment (hearing/vision)
- Chronic illness
- Neurologic disorders (seizures)
- Puzzling somatic symptoms (headache, stomachache, leg pains) as possible markers for school problems, especially if the history associates them with school (or test) days with remission of symptoms during vacation periods

Early developmental milestones
- Developmental risk factors: early speech/language delays, toe walking, motor clumsiness, etc.
- Drawing skills, handwriting

Attention/impulsivity/hyperactivity

A through family history is very helpful in detecting the risk of possible inherited forms of learning problems and the environmental factors contributing to the problem. The family history should ascertain the level of parental educational achievement and any difficulties they may have encountered in school. The history should also explore the child's relationships with family and peers and include an assessment of social skills and self-esteem. This social history can provide insight into the possibility of psychiatric comorbidity, such as depression, anxiety, substance abuse, or sleep disorders.

It is very important to interview the middle school or high school student alone to get his or her own perception of details and possible causes for underachievement in school. Parents of elementary school children are generally better historians for detailing the child's learning-deficit profile than the child is. Some questions that may be helpful in this respect are listed in Table 20-3.

Physical Examination

A thorough physical examination should be performed as part of a neurodevelopmental evaluation of any learning disorder. Although the examination will not yield specific data leading to the diagnosis of a learning disability, certain neurologic diseases of childhood and forms of developmental disabilities with brain impairment are associated with an increased likelihood of learning disabilities (Table 20-4). Despite the perception of many educators, the traditional neurologic evaluation is rarely helpful in the evaluation of a child with suspected learning difficulties. So called soft-neurologic signs are difficult to measure, do not correlate directly with learning or behavior, and do not contribute to management.

It is important to rule out hearing loss or poor visual acuity during the examination, but

---

Table 20-3

Interview Questions Regarding Academic Performance

Mathematics

Do you understand the teacher when he or she is explaining something in mathematics class?

Do you prefer to learn mathematics by having the teacher explain it to you, or would you prefer to see how a mathematics problem is solved correctly?

Do you have trouble remembering things in math? What kinds of things do you have trouble remembering?

When you have a word problem, can you figure out what operation you should use (addition, subtraction, etc.)?

Do you make a lot of careless mistakes in math?

Reading

What is the hardest thing about reading?

Is it hard to sound out words?

Do you know words by just looking at them (sight-word vocabulary)?

Do you forget things that you read at the beginning of a paragraph when you reach the end of the paragraph?

Do you understand what you read?

Table 20-4

Organic Factors Associated with Learning Problems

Most genetic syndromes
Most neurosurgical conditions
Prenatal alcohol exposure
Pre- and perinatal insults to the central
    nervous system
Prematurity
Sensory impairment
Seizure disorder
Neurofibromatosis

the screening procedures used in the typical office settings may not be adequate when learning problems are suspected. Referral for more extensive testing by an audiologist or optometrist/ophthalmologist may be warranted.

A search for dysmorphic features may help to specify genetic syndromes. Even in the absence of a specific syndrome, the presence of an unusually high number of minor dysmorphic features can be a nonspecific marker of learning problems.[6] If, on examination, the child has a significant number of dysmorphic features or neurologic soft signs, then a central nervous system (CNS) contribution to the child's learning difficulties should be considered. However, the absence of such signs should not be considered reassuring in dealing with the learning problem.

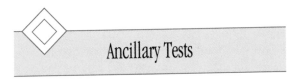

Ancillary Tests

Many children undergo evaluations within a school setting under the auspices of the Individuals with Disabilities Education Act (IDEA). Some parents fear that evaluations in schools are possibly biased toward not providing services to needy children. Available services, rigid regulations, and funding constraints can influence the outcome of these school-based evaluations. It is uncommon for these evaluations to include information from clinicians, much less have a clinician participate directly in the evaluation. As a result, there is a growing demand for independent evaluations, or second opinions outside of school. Often clinicians are asked to participate in such evaluations.

NEURODEVELOPMENTAL EXAMINATION

Neurodevelopmental examination by a clinician can be useful in generating an independent, functional descriptive profile of a child's cognitive and neurologic status. Such an examination can also serve as an adjunct to educational and psychological testing in order to confirm the diagnosis of learning disabilities. Comparing findings on neurodevelopmental examination with other tests and historical data will permit the discovery of recurring themes that can provide insight into the child's strengths and weaknesses.

A single professional cannot adequately assess the diverse sources and broad effects of learning problems. An interdisciplinary approach to evaluation provides a high level of expertise in the diagnosis and management of learning disability. Primary care clinicians should attempt to participate in or contribute to these interdisciplinary evaluations whenever possible. Expertise in learning disabilities is not a requirement. Rather, he or she can often mediate between strongly held ideologic views and advocate for the child.

An optimal evaluation team should consist of a clinician, nurse, psychologist, social worker, and psychoeducational specialist. Other professionals who may be asked to contribute to the team include a speech and language pathologist and an occupational therapist.

STANDARDIZED TESTS

Schools commonly use individually administered, standardized measures of cognitive ability and academic achievement in order to determine eligibility for special education services (Table 20-5). However these tests contain inherent inadequacies involving content, scoring, and sensitivity.[7] The most common (and minimally appropriate) evaluation for a learning problem is the combination of a Weschler Intelligence Scale for Children—3rd ed. (WISC-III) and the Woodcock-Johnson Psychoeducational Bat-

tery—Revised (WJ-R). The Wechsler Individual Achievement Test (WIAT) and Wide Range Achievement Test—3 (WRAT-3) are not the most sensitive tests for possible learning problems. A primary care clinician should become familiar with these tests and their interpretation. The key items for which one should look for are (1) discrepancy between IQ and achievement scores, (2) patterns of scores within tests, and (3) achievement standard scores equal to or less than 90 (percentile scores ≤ 25). Whether or not the state discrepancy criteria make such allowances, the impact of a given discrepancy can vary with the age and intelligence level of the child.

As stated earlier, clinicians should be familiar with the discrepancy criteria used by their state to qualify a child for services for learning problems. Significant discrepancies of scores within tests, which may not be apparent on composite scores, can also be possible indicators of learning problems. For example, on the Wechsler Intelligence Scales for Children—3rd ed. (WISC-III), there can be discrepancies between verbal and performance portions of the test that are associated with but not necessarily diagnostic of specific learning problems. Children with language-based learning problems in reading and spelling may have significantly lower scores on the Verbal IQ than on the Performance IQ. The opposite pattern may be seen in children with nonverbal learning disabilities, such as dyscalculia. There can be significant variability among subtests (scatter) and pattern analysis (e.g. the ACID profile: low arithmetic, coding, information, and digit span scores suggestive of problems in learning).

An educational diagnostician or psychoeducational specialist can expand upon standardized testing by performing an educational assessment that reflects the developmental demands of reading or mathematical tasks, assess specific skill acquisition and application, and observe and analyze specific academic parameters. The evaluation should take into account the child's age and grade level.

Table 20-5

Commonly Used School Assessments

> **Cognitive functioning (IQ)**
> Weschler Intelligence Scale for Children, 3rd ed. (WISC-III)
> Kaufman Assessment Battery for Children (K-ABC)
> **Individual achievement**
> Kaufman Individual Achievement Test (K-TEA)
> Wechsler Individual Achievement Test (WIAT)
> Wide Range Achievement Test—3 (WRAT-3)
> Woodcock-Johnson Psychoeducational Battery—Revised (WJ-R)
> **Domain-specific: reading**
> Formal Reading Inventory
> Gates-MacGinitie Reading Tests
> Gray Oral Reading Test—3
> Test of Reading Comprehension—Revised
> Test of Early Reading Ability—2
> Woodcock-Johnson Reading Mastery Tests—Revised
> **Domain-specific: mathematics**
> Key Math Diagnostic Arithmetic Test—Revised
> Sequential Assessment of Mathematics Inventories
> Stanford Diagnostic Mathematics Test—3
> Test of Early Mathematics Ability—2
> Test Mathematics Abilities—2

ERROR ANALYSIS

Error analysis is one of the tools that can be utilized in the assessment of academic difficulties. There is more than one way for a student to make a mistake, and many of these mistakes occur in recognizable patterns. By conducting error analysis, an educational diagnostician can collect sufficient information to be able to determine where the breakdowns in an individual student's performance occur, what neurodevelopmental subcomponents are involved, and how a plan for remediation can be developed.

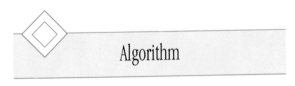

Algorithm

Figure 20-1 shows the steps in the well-child analysis.

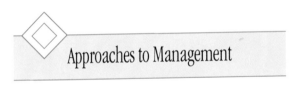

Approaches to Management

Just as assessment of learning problems requires an interdisciplinary approach, the management of children with learning problems necessitates a team approach using multimodal intervention. Public schools are required to develop an individual education plan (IEP) to provide a free, appropriate education in the least restrictive environment to children with disabling conditions. There is a specific, legislated time frame from the initial parental request for screening to the development and implementation of an IEP. Members of the evaluation team, the child's teachers, and the child's parents participate in the development of an IEP. Clinicians are often invited to these meetings but often cannot attend, since they predominantly occur during clinic hours. Nevertheless, the clinician has a role in helping parents in managing the appropriate remedial activities as well as advocating for the child.

Demystification

Because learning problems are taken so seriously by children, parents, and teachers, it is imperative that the nature of the individual child's learning problems be fully explained in terms that are developmentally appropriate. This must be accomplished in a manner that permits the child a measure of optimism. Clear explanations of individual neurodevelopmental strengths and weaknesses and their relationships to academic performance can be helpful. Children should also learn about their strengths. They need to know that they are competent individuals despite their current difficulties with school.

Controlling the Sequelae

Parents and teachers need to be aware of the effects that learning disabilities have on a child's self-esteem. A child with a learning problem is likely to be exquisitely sensitive and even embarrassed when a parent tries to help him or her with homework. Often the child seeks to conceal the learning problem from parents whom she or he wants so much to impress. This felt need to cover up or minimize the problem at the same time that parents are trying to help with homework frequently leads to major conflagrations at home. At school, a measure of privacy in academics may be in order, whereby a child is not called to answer a problem in front of the class or have other students correct his or her quizzes. Teachers and parents need to be as supportive as possible when working with a child with a learning disability. They must offer considerable praise and positive reinforcement. Whenever possible, parents and teachers need to collaborate to try to make learning fun. The use of games and rewards can sometime facilitate this effort.

Figure 20-1

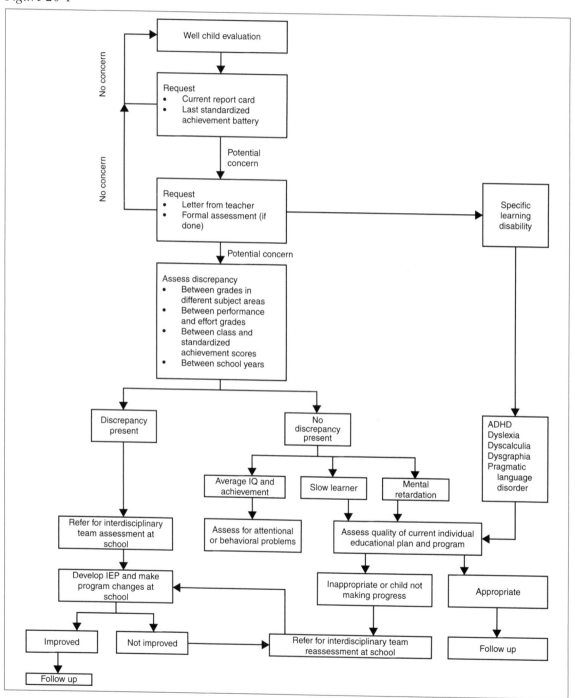

Algorithm demonstrating the steps in the well-child evaluation.

Educational Management

Effective management of learning disabilities requires the coordinated efforts of regular classroom teachers, special education teachers, students, parents, and clinicians. There is a wide range of special education services available for those children who qualify: consultation in the regular classroom, small-group or individual instruction in a resource room, placement (full or part time) in a self-contained special education classroom, specialized therapies, or a combination of the above. Educational interventions can include direct remediation of specific skill deficits, development of study skills, the use of by-pass strategies, accommodations in the classroom or a combination of the above.

Some parents will choose alternatives to public school services such as private tutoring and therapy or transfer to a private school. The availability of such services does not relieve the public school system of it's mandate to provide a free and appropriate education to all students in the least restrictive environment.

Selection of the type, location and amount of intervention depends on the availability of services, the child's eligibility status, the severity and pervasiveness of the learning problem, and the age of the child. For younger children who have not been previously served, direct remediation is usually the treatment of choice. If the child is older or has received services for awhile, the use of accommodations and by-pass strategies may be considered.

Direct Remediation of Learning Problems

Intervention should begin at the level of the individual underdeveloped subcomponents described earlier in this chapter. A regular or resource classroom teacher—or, under certain circumstances, a parent—can work specifically on an underdeveloped subcomponent. In general, remediation should include activities that make the deficient subcomponent an end in itself. That is to say, the child works not so much to obtain the correct answer but to master the subcomponent itself. For example, a student who is good at mathematical computation (a good knowledge of facts) but is having trouble identifying the operations necessary to solve word problems (poor pattern recognition) might be asked to look over a number of word problems in mathematics and identify the key words or patterns that suggest a particular operation. This might be done instead of actually solving the problem. A child with delayed automatization of math facts should be given practice drills, recalling facts under timed conditions. He or she might be given a page of simple problems and asked to see how many can be solved in 2 min. In reading, students can work on rapidly recalling the sounds attached to basic letter combinations on flash cards to improve their memory for basic sound-symbol associations.

Methods and materials that utilize a child's developmental strengths, preferred learning styles, and subject-area affinities should be exploited. Success at *something* promotes self-esteem. Children should read about topics they know a lot about. Topical magazines, television and film scripts, and technical manuals often provide a more meaningful medium for instruction. This approach also helps reduce reading avoidance. Visual learners may grasp new concepts more effectively by using models, graphics, and demonstrations. In some instances, educational software may aid learning at the level of the deficient subcomponents.

Remedial work performed outside the regular classroom must be directly relevant to what is being taught in the regular class. Skills taught in the context of regular classroom work are more likely to be used, maintained, and generalized. Good coordination between special education and regular classroom teachers is necessary so that skills and strategies are applied consistently across all subjects.

Students need to be active participants in learning. Cooperative, small-group learning activities and group problem solving will help to keep the child with learning problems involved in learning. Students will benefit from instruction in study skills such as note taking, time management, test-taking skills, mnemonic aids, and self-monitoring.

Bypass Strategies

Within regular classroom settings, it is often desirable to accommodate or bypass a deficient learning subcomponent. This enables a child to continue to learn despite the presence of a deficient subcomponent. For example, if a student is weak at recalling mathematical facts, he or she might be able to use a calculator while solving word problems. Other strategies include giving a child more time on a test, giving an open-book test to offset memory problems, using fewer reading assignments, or not grading for spelling when demonstration of knowledge is important. These techniques should be used discreetly so as not to attract public notice of the child with a learning problem. A private arrangement between the student, parent and teacher is typical. *Bypass strategies require a teacher to be flexible and sensitive to a student's struggles. This flexibility should not be confused for laxity.* Bypass strategies should not be provided freely but should carry an appropriate cost that ensures student accountability and integrity. Reduction of a reading assignment should be linked with extra time spent on drill practice in word identification. Reducing a five-page report to three pages should require the child to use a graphic or diagram to explain a point of interest.

Treatment of Other Neurodevelopmental Problems

Management of learning problems may require treatment of an underlying neurodevelopmental dysfunction. For example, if a child has an attention deficit that is compromising accuracy in mathematics performance, treatment with stimulant medication as well as other behavioral and cognitive management techniques may be indicated. Language therapy for children with language disabilities may result in some improvement in reading comprehension. Certain kinds of cognitive training may be deployed to improve concept formation, problem-solving skill, and memory.

Controversies

Grade Retention

The greatest controversy in the diagnosis and management of learning problems is the phenomenon of retention.[8] Although this may shock many teachers and parents and even some clinicians, it should be held as a universal rule that *no child should ever be retained in grade (i.e., held back) without the benefit of a diagnostic assessment.* Whenever parents casually inform the clinician that the school is considering retention, they should be strongly advised to refuse that option. Retention (repeating a grade, being left back) is a specific treatment intervention. The vast majority of children who are held back are never even considered for a diagnostic assessment, much less receive it. *School failure is a symptom and not a diagnosis; there are many diagnostic possibilities that must be considered and eliminated before inaugurating an intervention that carries such a heavy emotional impact for children. School retention will reduce the child's motivation to continue his or her academic efforts. Research has consistently demonstrated that retention and its converse, social promotion, both ultimately fail to meet children's needs. They merely delay an accurate diagnosis and appropriate treatment. Whenever a child is provided with a comprehen-*

sive diagnostic assessment, a better alternative than school retention will almost always be found.

Alternative Therapies

Because learning and attentional difficulties are difficult to diagnose and require lengthy therapy with varying prospects of improvement, several alternative therapies have emerged offering families a "quick cure." Clinicians should be aware of these "therapies" and be ready to provide parents with clear, understandable, and accurate advice concerning them.[9]

SPECIAL DIETS, VITAMINS, AND SUPPLEMENTS

The plethora of foods, food allergies, and food additives have been blamed for various developmental and behavioral problems underlying school failure also exemplify the persistent controversies in the field.[10] Over time, these three explanations have been combined, resulting in recommendations to restrict sugar, additives, and preservatives in children's diets in order to improve or prevent learning or attentional problems. Considerable efforts have been made to refute these myths, but they persist. Reviews of the objective evidence about dietary therapies can be presented to parents who seek such therapies.[11]

Megavitamin therapy is another controversial approach to the treatment of learning and attentional problems. There is considerable evidence that megavitamin therapy is both ineffective and potentially dangerous. Specific warnings about the dangers of this approach and its lack of validity were published over 20 years ago. Despite these warnings, some individuals continue to propose and use it. Continued objective studies of this approach have not only failed to demonstrate efficacy but more disruptive behavior and potential hepatotoxicity were documented during vitamin therapy.[12] Treatment with trace elements and/or antioxidants is also unproven.

NEUROPHYSIOLOGIC THERAPIES

Several neurophysiologic therapies purport to improve functioning of the CNS by stimulating specific sensory inputs or exercising specific motor patterns. These methods include patterning (the Doman-Delacato method), sensory integration, various visual techniques (including the use of colored lenses), and auditory integration. All of these techniques are unproven and have been refuted by position statements from medical organizations including American Academy of Cerebral Palsy, American Academy of Neurology, American Academy of Pediatrics, American Academy of Physical Medicine and Rehabilitation, American Congress of Rehabilitation Medicine, American Academy of Orthopedics, Canadian Association for Children with Learning Disabilities, Canadian Rehabilitation Council for the Disabled, American Association for Pediatric Ophthalmology and Strabismus, American Academy of Ophthalmology, and National Association for Retarded Children (U.S.A.).[9]

References

1. Levine MD, Lindsay RL, Reed MS: The wrath of math: deficiencies of mathematical mastery in the school child. *Pediatr Clin North Am* 39:525–536, 1992

2. Kosc L: Developmental dyscalculia. *J Learning Disabil* 7:164–177, 1974.

3. Badian NA: Dyscalculia and nonverbal disorders of learning, in Myklebust HR (ed): *Progress in Learning Disabilities.* Vol 15. New York; Stratton, 1983, p 235–264.

4. Gross-Tsur V, Manor O, Shalev RS: Developmental dyscalculia: prevalence and demographic features. *Dev Med Child Neurol* 38:25–33, 1996.

5. Shaywitz SE, Fletcher JM, Shaywitz BA: Issues on the definition and classification of attention deficit disorder. *Topics Lang Disord* 14:1–25, 1994.

6. Accardo PJ, Tomazic T, Morrow J, et al: Minor malformations, hyperactivity, and learning disabilities. *Am J Dis Child* 145:1184–1187, 1991.

7. Reed M: Educational Testing, in Levine MD, Crocker A, Carey W (eds.): *Developmental*

Behavioral Pediatrics, 3rd ed. Philadelphia, Saunders, 1999, pp 713–724.

8. Accardo PJ, Lindsay RL: Learning disabilities don't add up. *J Pediatr* 133:320–321, 1998.

9. Lindsay RL: Alternative therapies, in Levine MD, Carey WB, Crocker AC (eds.): *Developmental-Behavioral Pediatrics*, 3rd ed. Philadelphia, Saunders, 1999, pp 836–842.

10. Accardo PJ, Lindsay RL: Nutrition and behavior: the legend continues. *Pediatrics* 93:127, 1994.

11. Wolraich ML: Diet and behavior: what the research shows. *Contemp Pediatr* 13:29, 1996.

12. Haslam RH: Is there a role for megavitamin therapy in the treatment of attention deficit hyperactivity disorder? *Adv Neurol* 58:303–310, 1992.

Index

Page numbers in *italics* denote figures; those followed by "t" denote tables.